Workbook for

Timby's Fundamental
Nursing Skills and Concepts

Twelfth Edition

Loretta A. Donnelly-Moreno, DNP, RN, MSN

LVN/LPN Program Director
Nurse Faculty
Schreiner University
Kerrville, Texas

Brigitte Moseley, RNC-OB, MSN

Nursing Faculty, Vocational Nursing Program
Schreiner University
Kerrville, Texas

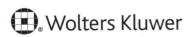 Wolters Kluwer

Philadelphia • Baltimore • New York • London
Buenos Aires • Hong Kong • Sydney • Tokyo

Vice President and Publisher: Julie K. Stegman
Acquisitions Editor: Jonathan Joyce
Director of Product Development: Jennifer K. Forestieri
Associate Development Editor: Rebecca J. Rist
Editorial Coordinator: Michael Jeffrey Cohen
Marketing Manager: Brittany Clements
Editorial Assistant: Molly Kennedy
Design Coordinator: Teresa Mallon
Art Director, Illustration: Jennifer Clements
Production Project Manager: Justin Wright
Manufacturing Coordinator: Karin Duffield
Prepress Vendor: S4Carlisle Publishing Services

Twelfth edition

9 8 7 6 5 4 3 2 1

Printed in China

Library of Congress Cataloging-in-Publication Data
ISBN-13: 978-1-975159-65-8
ISBN-10: 1-975159-65-9

Library of Congress Control Number: 2020940711

Preface

This workbook was developed to accompany the twelfth edition of *Timby's Fundamental Nursing Skills and Concepts* by Loretta A. Donnelly-Moreno. There is a diversity of exercises in each chapter of the workbook that are designed to help you practice and retain knowledge gained from the accompanying textbook. The workbook is structured to help you integrate that foundational knowledge and apply it to your nursing practice.

ASSESSING YOUR UNDERSTANDING

The beginning of each workbook chapter concentrates on the basic information in the textbook chapter. These exercises help you remember key concepts, vocabulary, and principles.

- **Fill in the blanks**
  Fill-in-the-blank exercises help you recall important chapter information. They also test key chapter information and encourage you to recall key points.
- **Labeling**
  Labeling exercises ask you to remember certain visual representations of the concepts presented in the textbook.
- **Match the following**
  Matching questions test your knowledge of key term definitions.
- **Sequencing**
  Sequencing exercises ask you to remember the order of particular steps in testing processes and/or prioritizing nursing actions, for example.
- **Short answers**
  Short answer questions cover facts, concepts, procedures, and principles of the chapter. These questions ask you to recall information and demonstrate comprehension of that information.

REVIEWING WHAT YOU HAVE LEARNED

The section of each workbook chapter consists of challenging activities that are designed to help master critical material and prepare for the NCLEX-PN.

- Fill in the blanks
- True or false
- Identifying terms and procedures
- Problem-solving exercises

APPLYING YOUR KNOWLEDGE

The section of each workbook chapter consists of case study–based exercises. These exercises seek for you to apply knowledge gained from the textbook as well as knowledge reinforced as you progress through workbook exercises. A case study scenario derived from the textbook's chapter content is presented, and you are asked to write the answers to some questions related to the case study. The questions cover the following areas:

- Assessment
- Planning nursing care
- Communication
- Reflection

PRACTICING FOR NCLEX

The final section of the workbook chapters help you practice NCLEX-style questions. The questions presented are multiple-choice and scenario-based to remain aligned with the NCLEX. They ask you to reflect, consider, apply what you know, and choose the best answer. These exercises will help you to apply the knowledge that you have gained from the textbook as well as reinforce this information as you progress through the workbook exercises.

ANSWER KEY

The answers for all of the exercises and questions in the workbook are found at the back of the book so that you can assess your own learning as you complete each chapter.

Acknowledgments

Teaching Vocational Nursing is a pleasure and an experience. The information learned during nursing skills and their related concepts courses will follow a nurse throughout their life and nursing career. Foundational nursing skills are truly the backbone of nursing, and this workbook can help you achieve your nursing goals by supporting your learning.

Brigitte Moseley, RNC-OB, MSN

Contents

SECTION I

Fundamental Nursing Concepts

UNIT 1

Exploring Contemporary Nursing

CHAPTER 1
Nursing Foundations   1

CHAPTER 2
Nursing Process   7

UNIT 2

Integrating Basic Concepts

CHAPTER 3
Laws and Ethics   14

CHAPTER 4
Health and Illness   22

CHAPTER 5
Homeostasis, Adaptation, and Stress   29

CHAPTER 6
Culture and Ethnicity   36

UNIT 3

Fostering Communication

CHAPTER 7
The Nurse–Client Relationship   41

CHAPTER 8
Client Teaching   47

CHAPTER 9
Recording and Reporting   53

SECTION II

Fundamental Nursing Skills

UNIT 4

Performing Basic Client Care

CHAPTER 10
Asepsis   59

CHAPTER 11
Admission, Discharge, Transfer, and Referrals   65

CHAPTER 12
Vital Signs   70

CHAPTER 13
Physical Assessment   76

CHAPTER 14
Special Examinations and Tests   82

UNIT 5

Assisting with Basic Needs

CHAPTER 15
Nutrition   89

v

CHAPTER **16**
Fluid and Chemical Balance   95

CHAPTER **17**
Hygiene   101

CHAPTER **18**
Comfort, Rest, and Sleep   108

CHAPTER **19**
Safety   114

CHAPTER **20**
Pain Management   120

CHAPTER **21**
Oxygenation   126

CHAPTER **22**
Infection Control   132

UNIT **6**
Assisting the Inactive Client

CHAPTER **23**
Body Mechanics, Positioning, and Moving   138

CHAPTER **24**
Therapeutic Exercise   144

CHAPTER **25**
Mechanical Immobilization   149

CHAPTER **26**
Ambulatory Aids   156

UNIT **7**
The Surgical Client

CHAPTER **27**
Perioperative Care   161

CHAPTER **28**
Wound Care   167

CHAPTER **29**
Gastrointestinal Intubation   173

UNIT **8**
Promoting Elimination

CHAPTER **30**
Urinary Elimination   180

CHAPTER **31**
Bowel Elimination   187

UNIT **9**
Medication Administration

CHAPTER **32**
Oral Medications   193

CHAPTER **33**
Topical and Inhalant Medications   199

CHAPTER **34**
Parenteral Medications   205

CHAPTER **35**
Intravenous Medications   211

UNIT **10**
Intervening in Emergency Situations

CHAPTER **36**
Airway Management   217

CHAPTER **37**
Resuscitation   224

UNIT **11**
Caring for the Terminally ILL

CHAPTER **38**
End-of-Life Care   230

ANSWERS   237

Nursing Foundations

Learning Objectives

- Identify the historical event that led to the demise of nursing in England before the time of Florence Nightingale.
- Identify the reforms for which Florence Nightingale is responsible.
- Name the ways that nurses used their skills in the early history of U.S. nursing.
- Describe the ways in which early U.S. training schools deviated from those established under the direction of Florence Nightingale.
- Explain how art, science, and nursing theory have been incorporated into contemporary nursing practice.
- Discuss the evolution of definitions of nursing.
- Identify the factors that influence choice of educational nursing programs.
- List the types of educational programs that prepare students for beginning levels of nursing practice.
- Explain the importance of continuing education in nursing.
- List examples of current trends affecting nursing and health care.
- Discuss the shortage of nurses and methods to reduce the crisis.
- Describe four skills that all nurses use in clinical practice.

SECTION I: ASSESSING YOUR UNDERSTANDING

Activity A   FILL IN THE BLANKS

1. Florence Nightingale started the first training school for nurses at _____ hospital in England.

2. In 1890, one of the first courses for training "attendants for the sick" was begun in New York by the Brooklyn Young Women's Christian Association. These attendants became what is known as today's _____ nurses.

3. The development of a unique scientific body of knowledge predicting the best nursing interventions to produce desired outcome is referred to as _____.

4. The ability to perform an act skillfully or the _____of nursing was the focus of the first nurse training by mentors.

5. The word _____ comes from a Greek word that means "vision" and refers to an opinion, belief, or view that explains a process.

6. One tenet of the self-care theory developed by _____ is that nurses assist clients with self-care to improve or maintain health.

7. _____ are a vital link between the registered nurse and unlicensed assistive personnel (UAP).

8. _____ programs are considered a stepping stone to associate and baccalaureate nursing degrees.

9. Nurses with a _____ degree usually are preferred in areas requiring substantial independent decision-making, such as hospital administrative positions, out-client care centers, and public health and home health nursing.

10. A(n) _____ is one who listens to a client's needs, responds with information based on their area of expertise, and facilitates the outcome that a client desires.

Activity B *Consider the following figure.*

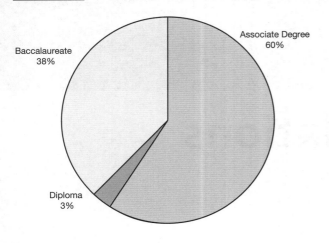

1. What are the educational options available in a nursing career?

_____

_____

_____

2. What are the factors that affect the choice of a nursing program?

_____

_____

_____

Activity C *Match the types of nursing skills in Column A with the examples in Column B.*

Column A

____ **1.** Assessment skills

____ **2.** Comforting skills

____ **3.** Counseling skills

____ **4.** Caring skills

Column B

a. A nurse assists a senior client with grooming

b. A nurse takes the vital signs of clients in an acute care facility

c. A nurse listens to the concerns of a new mother whose baby was born with a cleft palate

d. A nurse helps a client diagnosed with anorexia to devise a nutritious meal plan

Activity D *Write the correct sequence of the line of authority and delegation of work in a nursing unit in the boxes provided.*

1. Registered nurse

2. Unlicensed assistive personnel

3. Licensed practical nurse (LPN)

4. Physician

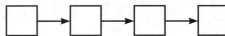

The following are accomplishments of Florence Nightingale. Arrange the events in chronologic order in the boxes provided.

1. Florence Nightingale establishes a training school for nurses in England.

2. Florence Nightingale works with the Institution for the Care of Sick Gentlewomen in Distressed Circumstances.

3. Florence Nightingale works with nursing deaconesses, a Protestant order of women.

4. Florence Nightingale provides nursing care to soldiers during the Crimean War.

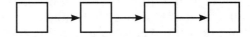

Activity E *Briefly answer the following questions.*

1. What selection criteria were established by Dorothea Lynde Dix for recruitment of nurses?

_____

_____

_____

2. What is the definition of nursing according to Virginia Henderson?

_____

_____

_____

3. According to the ANA, what are the six essential features that characterize nursing?

_____

_____

_____

4. What are the factors that influence the choice of a nursing program?

_____

_____

_____

5. What are the guidelines to be kept in mind while delegating nursing tasks to staff members?

_____

_____

_____

SECTION II: APPLYING YOUR KNOWLEDGE

Activity F   *Nursing skills are activities that are unique to the practice of nursing. One of these skills is the counseling skill that the nurse implements during exchanges of information, offering pertinent health teaching and providing emotional support to the clients. Answer the following questions, which involve implementation of nursing skills.*

An 8-year-old with a tapeworm infection visits their primary care doctor along with their mother. The mother is worried that her child seems to be weak and is not gaining weight.

1. What nursing skills should the nurse use to provide effective nursing care to this client?

_____

_____

_____

2. What are the advantages of active listening in communicating with a client?

_____

_____

_____

SECTION III: PRACTICING FOR NCLEX

Activity G   *Answer the following questions.*

1. Florence Nightingale was instrumental in changing the negative image of nursing to a positive

one. What was the most important nursing contribution of Florence Nightingale and her team of nurses during the Crimean War?
  a. The death rate of soldiers decreased from 60% to 1%
  b. Sanitary conditions for the sick and injured were improved
  c. The soldiers were given hygienic food to eat
  d. Infection and gangrene in the soldiers were controlled

2. A client reports to the primary health care center for their regular checkup. Which nursing action demonstrates the use of assessment skills?
  a. Telling the client to exercise daily
  b. Palpating the abdomen for liver enlargement
  c. Educating the client about the hepatitis B vaccination program
  d. Ensuring that the client is taking their medication regularly

3. A mother is informed by the oncologist that her son has been diagnosed with terminal cancer. What nursing skills should the nurse use to help the mother cope with this news?
  a. Assessment skills
  b. Caring skills
  c. Comforting skills
  d. Counseling skills

4. As a result of diabetic complications, a client has had a leg amputated. The nurse uses empathy to perceive the client's emotional state and need for support. How would empathy help the nurse in dealing with this client?
  a. It helps to avoid hurting the client's emotions and feelings unknowingly
  b. It helps to provide effective care while remaining compassionately detached
  c. It helps to provide emotional support to the emotionally unstable client
  d. It helps to counsel the client effectively by suggesting available rehabilitation options

5. A 50-year-old client is admitted to nursing care in an unconscious state. What nursing

skills does the nurse demonstrate by interviewing the client's spouse?
a. Counseling skill
b. Comforting skill
c. Caring skill
d. Assessment skill

6. The nurse, after assessing the client's needs, delegates nursing tasks to the nursing staff. Which factor should the nurse keep in mind while delegating the work?
a. Knowing the unique competencies of the caregiver
b. Ensuring that care is given to the right client
c. Confirming that the caregiver is sincere in their work
d. Ensuring that the client deserves the care

7. A nurse delegates the task of changing the colostomy bag of a client to the LPN. The LPN informs the nurse that they have never done the procedure on a client. What is the appropriate action of the nurse delegator?
a. Perform the procedure with the LPN and teach them
b. Request that the LPN refer to the procedure manual
c. Request that the LPN take the manual along and do the procedure
d. Request that the LPN observe another LPN who knows the procedure

8. A nurse assigns an LPN to change the position of a comatose client. Which statement demonstrates the correct direction guideline while delegating the nursing task?
a. "Change the position of the comatose client and report back to me"
b. "Change the position of the client in cubicle number 3 and give them a back rub"
c. "Change the position of the client, give them a back rub, and report back to me"
d. "Change the position of the comatose client in cubicle no. 3 and give them a back rub"

9. The nurse is caring for a client who is experiencing pain at the surgical incision site during the postoperative period. Which statement would indicate assessment?

a. "Please take this analgesic medication; it will reduce the pain"
b. "Can you rate the pain on the pain scale, from 1 to 10?"
c. "Don't worry; it is the result of surgery; it will subside after some time"
d. "Guard the incision site with your palm during movements"

10. A client is scheduled to undergo arthroplasty of the knee. On the day of surgery, the client expresses anxiety, because they are undergoing surgery for the first time. What statement should the nurse use to comfort the client and alleviate anxiety?
a. "The operating team is very competent and the surgery has had good outcomes"
b. "You should not worry; there is always a first time for everything"
c. "Don't worry; even I underwent the same surgery a few months back"
d. "There are many people who undergo this surgery without any problem"

11. Several types of programs prepare graduates in registered nursing. Each educational track provides the knowledge and skills for a particular entry level of practice. Which factors affect a student's choice of a nursing program? Select all that apply.
a. Career goals
b. Type of training
c. Length of program
d. Job availability
e. Cost involved

12. Nurses use active listening to facilitate therapeutic interactions. By active listening, the nurses demonstrate full attention to what is being said, hearing both the content being communicated and the unspoken message. Which actions are examples of active listening? Select all that apply.
a. The nurse nods their head when the client speaks
b. The nurse repeats what the client has said
c. The nurse expresses their own emotions
d. The nurse observes the client's body language
e. The nurse relates what they are hearing to an incident that happened to them

13. A client reports to the emergency department with pain in the leg as a result of a fall in the garden. The nurse tells the client to describe the incident. What nursing skill is the nurse using?
    a. Assessment skills
    b. Comforting skills
    c. Counseling skills
    d. Caring skills

14. Shortage of nurses is a major issue today. Which factors have contributed to the nursing shortage? Select all that apply.
    a. Increased aging population requiring health care
    b. Limited scope for educational growth
    c. Policies regarding mandatory overtime
    d. Heavier workloads and sicker clients
    e. Rigorous training and difficult life

15. A student wishes to pursue a career in nursing. Which nursing program offers the shortest course in registered nursing?
    a. Graduate nursing programs
    b. Baccalaureate programs
    c. Associate degree programs
    d. Hospital-based diploma programs

SECTION IV: REVIEWING WHAT YOU HAVE LEARNED

Activity H *Fill in the blanks by choosing the correct word from the options given in parentheses.*

1. A _____ develops from observing and studying the relationship of one phenomenon to another. (science, skill, theory)

2. _____ defined nursing as "putting individuals in the best possible condition for nature to restore and preserve health." (Henderson, Herbert, Nightingale)

Activity I *Mark the statement as either T (True) or F (False). Correct any false statements.*

1. **T F** Advanced practice nurses fill roles as clinical specialists, nurse practitioners, certified nurse anesthetists, certified midwives, administrators, and collegiate educators.

Activity J *Match the nursing skills in Column A with their descriptions in Column B.*

Column A

____ 1. Assessment skills
____ 2. Caring skills
____ 3. Counseling skills
____ 4. Comforting skills

Column B

a. Assisting with activities of daily living
b. Offering pertinent health teaching
c. Providing interventions that allow for stability and security during a health-related crisis
d. Interviewing, observing, and examining the client

Activity K *Answer the following questions.*

1. How did Florence Nightingale improve the image of nursing?

   _____
   _____
   _____

2. How did Virginia Henderson define nursing?

   _____
   _____
   _____

Activity L *Give a rationale for the following question.*
Why is the use of empathy so important when nurses care for clients?

   _____
   _____
   _____

Activity M *Answer the following questions focusing on nursing roles and responsibilities.*
A family member brings a senior client with severe back pain following a fall to the health care facility.

1. What should the nurse do before determining the nursing care that the client requires?

   _____
   _____
   _____

2. What skills must the nurse possess to perform the previous intervention?

_____

_____

_____

Activity N *Consider the following questions. Discuss them with your instructor or peers.*
Question 1. A client with lung cancer is undergoing chemotherapy. Recently, they have been losing their hair, looks pale and tired, and has significantly reduced activities. Family members are worried about the drastic changes in appearance and health. In the beginning, the client was eager to comply with the treatment, but now they tell the nurse that they would rather suffer the consequences of the disease than the side effects of the treatment. How might the nurse approach this situation using assessment, caring, counseling, and comforting skills?

_____

_____

_____

SECTION V: GETTING READY FOR NCLEX

Activity O *Answer the following questions.*

1. Several factors contributed to the demise of nursing in England prior to the contributions of Florence Nightingale. Which factor had the greatest negative impact on nursing?

  a. Use of untrained workers, some of whom lacked good character, as nurses
  b. Recruitment of lay people by monasteries to assist in physical care
  c. Engagement of religious groups in many of the roles of nursing
  d. Lack of resources during periods of plague and pestilence

2. A nursing student wishes to take the National Council Licensure Examination-Registered Nurse (NCLEX-RN) upon graduation. Which programs would qualify the nurse for this type of licensing? Select all that apply.

  a. A practical nurse program
  b. A hospital-based diploma program
  c. A licensed practical nursing (LPN) program
  d. An associate degree in nursing
  e. A baccalaureate nursing program

CHAPTER 2

Nursing Process

Learning Objectives

- Define the term "nursing process."
- Describe characteristics of the nursing process.
- List the steps in the nursing process.
- Identify sources of assessment data.
- Differentiate among database, focus, and functional assessment.
- List the parts of a nursing diagnostic statement.
- Distinguish between a nursing diagnosis and a collaborative problem.
- Describe the rationale for setting priorities.
- Discuss appropriate circumstances for short- and long-term goals.
- Identify ways to document a plan of care.
- Describe the information that is documented in a plan of care.
- Discuss the outcomes that result from evaluation.
- Identify learning strategies educators use to help students implement the nursing process.

SECTION I: ASSESSING YOUR UNDERSTANDING

Activity A FILL IN THE BLANKS

1. The _____ is an organized sequence of problem-solving steps used by nurses to identify and manage the health problems of clients.

2. The first step in the nursing process, known as _____, is the systematic collection of facts or data.

3. The assessment of pitting edema in a client's leg is an example of _____ data.

4. When performing an assessment, the _____ is the primary source for information.

5. A nurse who administers medications according to the plan of care is carrying out the _____ step of the nursing process.

6. A(n) _____ assessment contains information that provides more details about specific problems and expands the original database.

7. A(n) _____ results from analyzing the collected data and determining whether they suggest normal or abnormal findings.

8. A client complaint of stomach pain is considered _____ data.

9. Problems interfering with the _____ needs of a client have priority over those affecting other levels of needs.

10. _____ problems are physiologic complications that require both nurse- and physician-prescribed interventions.

Activity B *Consider the following figure.*

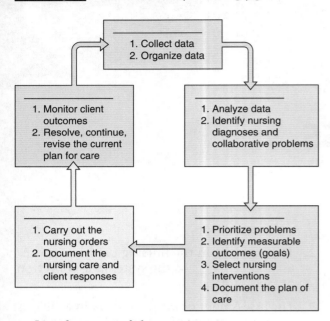

1. Collect data
2. Organize data

1. Analyze data
2. Identify nursing diagnoses and collaborative problems

1. Prioritize problems
2. Identify measurable outcomes (goals)
3. Select nursing interventions
4. Document the plan of care

1. Carry out the nursing orders
2. Document the nursing care and client responses

1. Monitor client outcomes
2. Resolve, continue, revise the current plan for care

1. List the steps of the nursing process.

_____

_____

_____

2. What are the types of data collected during assessment?

_____

_____

_____

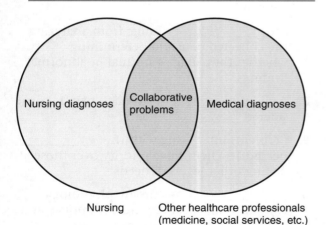

Nursing diagnoses

Collaborative problems

Medical diagnoses

Nursing

Other healthcare professionals (medicine, social services, etc.)

3. What are collaborative problems?

_____

_____

_____

4. What is the role of nurses in managing collaborative problems?

_____

_____

_____

Activity C *Match the steps of the nursing process in Column A with their descriptions in Column B.*

Column A

_____ **1.** Assessment

_____ **2.** Diagnosis

_____ **3.** Planning

_____ **4.** Implementation

Column B

a. Process of carrying out the plan of care

b. Process of prioritizing nursing diagnoses and collaborative problems

c. Systematic collection of facts or data

d. Identification of health-related problems

Activity D *Presented here, in random order, are the steps of the nursing process. Write the correct sequence in the boxes provided below.*

1. Implementation
2. Planning
3. Evaluation
4. Assessment
5. Diagnosis

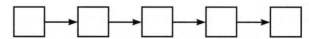

Activity E *Briefly answer the following questions.*

1. What is meant by the nursing process?

_____

_____

_____

2. What are the characteristics of the nursing process?

_____

_____

_____

3. What are the three types of assessments?

_____

_____

_____

4. What is concept mapping?

_____

_____

_____

5. What are the characteristics of short-term goals?

_____

_____

_____

SECTION II: APPLYING YOUR KNOWLEDGE

Activity F *During assessment, the nurse collects information to determine areas of abnormal function, risk factors that contribute to health problems, and client strengths. Read the scenario and answer the questions that follow.*

A client reports to the emergency room with chest pain. The medical file shows that the client has a history of hospitalization for chest pain. The family members inform the nurse that the client is a chain smoker. The nurse performs an initial assessment to plan the care.

1. What are the sources of data in this case?

_____

_____

_____

2. What types of assessment data should be obtained in this case? Group them into subjective and objective data.

_____

_____

_____

SECTION III: PRACTICING FOR NCLEX

Activity G *Answer the following questions.*

1. A client is admitted to a health care facility with cramping pain in the abdomen.

The nurse interviews the client, performs the initial assessment, and records the vital signs. Which data collected by the nurse can be classified as objective data?

a. Pain in the abdomen
b. High blood pressure
c. Tingling sensation
d. Itching in the nose

2. A client with Cushing's disease is admitted to the emergency department after falling on the road. They have an open leg wound. Which nursing diagnosis should be given the highest priority?

a. Risk for infection
b. Impaired physical mobility
c. Disturbed body image
d. Risk for delayed recovery

3. When caring for a client who has had a stroke, which action should the nurse perform first?

a. Implement nursing care
b. Plan nursing action
c. Perform physical assessment
d. Ascertain nursing goals

4. Of the following nursing diagnoses entered in a client's plan of care, which one would be of least priority?

a. Altered breathing pattern
b. Ineffective coping
c. Altered elimination needs
d. Risk for body image disturbance

5. A nurse is caring for a client who receives anticoagulant therapy after mitral valve replacement. The nurse understands that the nursing diagnosis of highest priority would be:

a. Risk for physical injury
b. Risk for infection
c. Risk for imbalanced fluid volume
d. Ineffective health maintenance

6. A nurse is giving postoperative care to a client after total hip replacement. What is a short-term goal for this client?

a. To ambulate the client to a bedside chair
b. To help the client return to activities of daily life
c. To maintain a healthy and active lifestyle
d. To prevent repeat surgery in the client

7. A client is admitted to the health care center with profuse, watery stools. The client informs the nurse that they have eaten out the previous evening with family and friends and had rich food because they wanted to fit in with their peers. The client has a history of ulcerative colitis and is restricted from having fat-rich food. Which nursing diagnosis is most appropriate for this client?

   a. Risk for body image disturbance
   b. Risk for situational self-esteem
   c. Ineffective health maintenance
   d. Risk for impaired nutritional intake

8. A client complains of pain in the right flank. Which data gathered from the client are objective data?

   a. Pricking pain in the flank
   b. Grade 2 pain on the pain scale
   c. Dull, throbbing pain
   d. Cramping pain in the flank

9. A client is brought to the postoperative room after surgery for disc prolapse. What is a long-term goal for the client?

   a. To prevent infection at the surgical site
   b. To avoid putting strain on the back during the immediate postoperative period
   c. To prevent recurrence by practicing body mechanics
   d. To ambulate and perform activities of daily life

10. A nurse is assessing a client with renal calculus. The client received one shot of analgesic 2 hours earlier. The client is scared that the pain will come back, noting that it was the worst pain they have ever experienced. Taking into account the client's concerns, what nursing diagnosis would be appropriate?

    a. Impaired coping mechanism related to severe pain
    b. Anxiety related to anticipation of recurrent severe pain
    c. Pain related to presence of calculus in the kidney
    d. Impaired elimination resulting from obstruction of urinary tract

11. Which risk nursing diagnosis is appropriate for a comatose client?

    a. Risk for disuse syndrome
    b. Ineffective breathing pattern
    c. Impaired physical mobility
    d. Total self-care deficit

12. A pregnant woman in her third trimester is admitted with spotting. She is tense and continuously inquires about the safety of her baby. Which nursing diagnosis is most appropriate for the client?

    a. Risk for deficient fluid volume
    b. Fear related to unpredictable outcome
    c. Activity intolerance as a result of pregnancy
    d. Risk for impaired urinary elimination

13. A nurse is caring for a diabetic client who has a wound. Which component of the nursing care plan should be performed first?

    a. To change the dressing of the wound
    b. To arrange articles for dressing
    c. To assess the condition of the wound
    d. To record the findings of the wound

14. A nurse is planning care for a client who is receiving nasogastric feeds. Which nursing diagnosis should the nurse identify as the highest priority?

    a. Altered bowel elimination
    b. Risk for imbalanced fluid volume
    c. Risk for imbalanced nutrition
    d. Risk for lung aspiration

15. A client is brought to the emergency room with a head injury. After an initial assessment, the client is taken to the operating room for removal of a blood clot. Which actions would be part of the focus assessments for the client? Select all that apply.

    a. Conducting postoperative surgical assessments
    b. Conducting urine analysis on admission
    c. Monitoring pain before and after administering medications
    d. Checking the neurologic status of a client with a head injury
    e. Inquiring about the dietary habits of the client

16. A client with a spinal cord injury is paralyzed from their neck down. The client frequently picks a fight with fellow patients on petty issues and often complains about the nursing staff. The nurse interprets that the client is inappropriately using the defense mechanism of displacement. What would be an appropriate nursing diagnosis for the client?

    a. Risk for disuse syndrome
    b. Deficient diversional activity

    c. Ineffective coping
    d. Disturbed self-esteem

17. A nurse is caring for a patient on hormone therapy. The client has a nursing diagnosis of disturbed body image related to alopecia. Which plan should be implemented, based on the nursing diagnosis?

    a. Teach the client about use of wigs
    b. Teach the client about use of cosmetics
    c. Teach the client to use mild shampoo
    d. Teach the client the method to wash the hair and scalp

18. A client reports to the health care center with complaints of diarrhea and vomiting after having pizza at a party. The nurse conducts an interview and collects the following assessment data. Which data are considered subjective data? Select all that apply.

    a. High temperature
    b. Pain in abdomen
    c. Tenesmus
    d. Nausea
    e. High blood pressure

SECTION IV: REVIEWING WHAT YOU HAVE LEARNED

Activity H *Fill in the blanks by choosing the correct word from the options given in parentheses.*

1. A nursing _____ is a health issue that can be prevented, reduced, resolved, or enhanced through independent nursing measures. (assessment, diagnosis, evaluation)
2. _____ data are observable and measurable facts and are referred to as signs of a disorder. (Historical, Objective, Subjective)

Activity I *Mark the statement as either T (True) or F (False). Correct any false statements.*

1. T F Concept mapping is a method of organizing information in a graphic or pictorial form.
2. T F The primary health care provider refers to the plan of care, reviews it for appropriateness, and revises it according to changes in the client's condition.
3. T F Nurses frequently use Maslow's Hierarchy of Human Needs to determine priorities when caring for clients.

Activity J *Write the correct term for each description that follows.*

1. An expected or desired outcome that helps the nursing team know whether nursing care has been appropriate for managing the client's nursing diagnoses and collaborative problems _____

2. The standard for clinical nursing practice _____

Activity K *Differentiate between a database assessment and a focus assessment based on the criteria given.*

1. Definition
2. Purpose
3. Example

Activity L *The nursing process is an organized sequence of problem-solving steps used to identify and manage the health concerns of clients. When nursing practice follows the nursing process, clients receive quality care in minimal time with maximum efficiency. Write in the boxes provided the correct sequence in which the actions of the nursing process are performed.*

1. Implementation
2. Diagnosis
3. Assessment
4. Evaluation
5. Planning

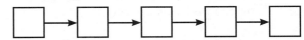

Activity M *Answer the following questions.*

1. What are the different types of nursing diagnoses?

_____

_____

_____

2. What is a collaborative problem?

_____

_____

_____

SECTION V: APPLYING YOUR KNOWLEDGE

Activity N *Give rationales for the following questions.*

1. Why are short-term goals most appropriate for clients receiving care in acute care settings?

   _____

   _____

   _____

2. Why should the nurse document and sign a nursing order?

   _____

   _____

   _____

Activity O *Answer the following questions focusing on nursing roles and responsibilities.*

1. A family member brings a senior client with severe back pain, following a fall, to the health care facility.

   a. What should the nurse do before determining the nursing care that the client requires?

   _____

   _____

   _____

   b. What skills must the nurse possess to perform the previous intervention?

   _____

   _____

   _____

2. A nurse is providing care to a client with respiratory distress.

   a. What are the requirements for preparing a nursing diagnosis?

   _____

   _____

   _____

b. What are the different parts of a problem-focused nursing diagnosis?

   _____

   _____

   _____

3. A nurse is identifying short-term and long-term goals for a client who has been admitted to the health care facility with a fractured right leg.

   a. What should the nurse keep in mind when setting short-term goals?

   _____

   _____

   _____

   b. What are long-term goals?

   _____

   _____

   _____

   c. Identify one possible short-term goal and one possible long-term goal for this client.

   _____

   _____

   _____

Activity P *Consider the following questions. Discuss them with your instructor or peers.*

A 50-year-old client is in a long-term care facility following a stroke. Their left arm is paralyzed. The client is having problems with urinary incontinence; recently, they also developed constipation and are not eating well. Full or partial return of the left limb's function is one of the long-term goals for this client, who eventually will undergo occupational therapy.

1. How should the nurse prioritize care given to this client?

   _____

   _____

   _____

2. What client needs require immediate attention?

_____

_____

_____

3. Identify some other short- and long-term goals for this client.

_____

_____

_____

SECTION VI: GETTING READY FOR NCLEX

Activity Q   *Answer the following questions.*

1. A nurse is assessing a client who is recovering from a stroke. Which data should the nurse record as subjective data?

   a. Temperature
   b. Abdominal pain
   c. Pulse rate
   d. Blood pressure

2. Nursing diagnoses for a client with a fractured hip include "Impaired Skin Integrity related to inactivity." To which category does this nursing diagnosis belong?

   a. Problem-focused
   b. Risk
   c. Syndrome
   d. Health promotion

CHAPTER 3

Laws and Ethics

Learning Objectives

- Identify different types of laws.
- Discuss the purpose of nurse practice acts and the role of the state board of nursing.
- Explain the difference between intentional and unintentional torts.
- Describe the difference between negligence and malpractice.
- Identify reasons why a nurse should obtain professional liability insurance.
- List the ways that a nurse's professional liability can be mitigated in the case of a lawsuit.
- Define the term "ethics."
- Explain the purpose of a code of ethics.
- Describe two types of ethical theories.
- Name and explain the ethical principles that apply to health care.
- List ethical issues common in nursing practice.

SECTION I: ASSESSING YOUR UNDERSTANDING

Activity A   FILL IN THE BLANKS

1. A nurse practice act (statute that legally defines the unique role of the nurse and differentiates it from that of other health care practitioners) is one example of a _____ law.

2. The ethical principle _____ means the duty to be honest and to avoid deceiving or misleading a client.

3. _____ is the ethical study based on duty or moral obligations, which proposes that the outcome is not the primary issue; rather, decisions must be based on the morality of the act itself.

4. _____ insurance is a contract between a person or corporation and a company willing to provide legal services and financial assistance when the policyholder is involved in a malpractice lawsuit; it is a necessity for all practicing nurses.

5. _____ is an unlawful act in which untrue information harms a person's reputation.

6. _____ is a litigation in which one person asserts that a physical, emotional, or financial injury was a consequence of another person's actions or failure to act.

7. _____, also known as utilitarianism, is an ethical theory based on final outcomes resulting in decisions that are best for the most people involved.

8. A(n) _____ is a serious criminal offense, such as murder, falsifying medical records, insurance fraud, and stealing narcotics.

9. _____ law, also known as judicial law, interprets legal issues based on previous court decisions in similar cases (legal precedents).

10. _____ laws are legal provisions through which federal, state, and local agencies maintain self-regulation.

Activity B   *Consider the following figure.*

```
THREE RIVERS AREA HOSPITAL INCIDENT REPORT                         Addressograph
Confidential - DO NOT DUPLICATE
Forward to Risk Management within 48 hours
Identification  Sex  Age  Incident Date  Time   Shift   Department
__Inpatient      _M  ___  __/__/__        __:    __1st
__Outpatient     _F                              __2nd   _____
__Visitor                                        __3rd
=================================================================================
Reason for hospitalization/presence on premises: _____

I.   Location of Incident          II.  Type of Incident
     __Patient Room #_____             __Fall              __Treatment/Procedure
     __Patient Bathroom                 __Medication         __Equipment
     __Corridor                         __Infusion           __Needle/Sponge Count
     __Other _____         __Lost/Found         __Other_____
                                        __Burn
III. Description of Incident   _____
     _____
     _____

IV.  Nature of Incident
     A.  Falls:
     Activity Order:       Pt. Condition Prior to:   Fall Involved:      Patient/Visitor was:
     __Restraints          __Weak, unsteady          __Chair, W/C        __Lying
     __Bedrest only        __Alert, oriented         __Stretcher         __Standing
     __BRP                 __Disoriented/confused     __Tub/Shower        __Getting on/off
     __Up w/asst.          __Senile                   __Toilet            __Sitting
     __Up AD LIB           __Unconscious              __Floor Condition(below) __Ambulating
                           __Medicated/Sedated        __Bed               __Other
                           Med. Name _____         __Side Rails Up     _____
                           Last Dose _____         __Side Rails Down   _____

     B.  Medications:
     Incident Involved:                              Factors:
     __Wrong Med, Tx, Procedure   __Adverse Reaction  __Patient I.D. Not Checked
     __Wrong Patient              __Infiltration      __Transcription
     __Wrong Time                 __Other_____    __Labeling
     __Omission                   _____          __Physician orders not clear
     __Incorrect Dose             _____          __Physician orders not checked
     __Incorrect Method of        _____          __Misread label/dose
        Administration                                __Charting
                                                      __Wrong Med from Pharmacy
                                                      __Defective equipment
                                                      __Communications
                                                      __Other_____

     C.  Other:
     __Loss of Property          __Equipment malfunction   __Patient ID
     __Struck by object, equipment  __Anesthesia           __Other_____
V.   Nature of Injury (Injury sustained as a result of incident):
     __Asphyxia, Strangulation,   __Fracture or dislocation  __Burn or Scald
        Inhalation                __Viscera Injury           __Chemical Burn
     __Head Injury                __Sprain or strain         __No injury
     __Contagious or infectious   __Contusion, Cut,          __No apparent injury
        Disease Exposure             Laceration              __Other_____
VI.  Action Taken:
     Physician   __Yes    PT/Visitor seen by MD/T&EC    MD Name
     Notified    __No     __Yes        __No             _____  Time  :___
     Physician's Findings: _____
     _____
     Other follow up:  __No   __Yes - Specify_____
     _____

     _____  __/__/__    _____  __/__/__
     Name of Person Reporting  Date      Department Director      Date

     _____  __/__/__    _____  __/__/__   8311-109
     Supervisor               Date       Risk Management         Date
```

1. Identify the figure.

_____

_____

_____

2. What is the role of the nurse in filling out an incident report?

_____

_____

_____

3. What are the important factors the nurse should keep in mind while completing an incident report?

_____

_____

_____

LIVING WILL

TO: My family, physicians and all those concerned with my care

I, _____, the undersigned "principal", presently residing at _____, _____, and being an adult of sound mind, make this declaration as a directive to be followed if for any reason I become unable to make or communicate decisions regarding my medical care.

I do not want medical treatment that will keep me alive if I am unconscious and there is no reasonable prospect that I will ever be conscious again (even if I am not going to die soon in my medical condition) or if I am near death from an illness or injury with no reasonable prospect of recovery. The procedures and treatment to be withheld and withdrawn include, without limitation, surgery, antibiotics, cardiac and pulmonary resuscitation, respiratory support, and artificially administered feeding and fluids. I direct that treatment be limited to measures to keep me comfortable and to relieve pain, even if such measures shorten my life.

[OPTIONAL] I wish to live out my last days at home rather than in a hospital, if it does not jeopardize the chance of my recovery to a meaningful and conscious life and does not impose an undue burden on my family.

[OPTIONAL] If, upon my death, any of my tissue or organs would be of value for transplantation, therapy, advancement of medical or dental science, research, or other medical, educational or scientific purpose, I freely give my permission to the donation of such tissue or organs.

These directions are the exercise of my legal right to refuse treatment. Therefore, I expect my family, physicians, health care facilities and all concerned with my care to regard themselves as legally and morally bound to act in accordance with my wishes, and in so doing to be free from any liability for having followed my directions.

IN WITNESS WHEREOF, I have executed this declaration, as my free and voluntary act and deed, this _____ day of _____, 2003.

_____   _____

Principal's name: WITNESS:

---

4. Identify the figure.

_____

_____

_____

5. What is meant by advance directives?

_____

_____

_____

6. Can the nurse sign as a witness in a living will?

_____

_____

_____

Activity C *Match the legal terms in Column A with their descriptions in Column B.*

Column A

_____ **1.** Assault

_____ **2.** Battery

_____ **3.** Slander

_____ **4.** Libel

Column B

a. Damaging statements written and read by others

b. An act in which bodily harm is threatened or attempted

c. Unauthorized physical contact that includes touching a person's body, clothing, chair, or bed

d. Character attack uttered orally in the presence of others

Activity D *Briefly answer the following questions.*

1. What is meant by allocation of scarce resources?

_____

_____

_____

2. What is meant by code status?

_____

_____

_____

3. What is a living will?

_____

_____

_____

4. What are some common ethical issues that recur in nursing practices?

_____

_____

_____

5. What is the meaning of autonomy in client care?

_____

_____

_____

SECTION II: APPLYING YOUR KNOWLEDGE

Activity E *Battery is unauthorized physical contact that can include touching a person's body, clothing, chair, or bed. A plaintiff can claim battery even if the contact causes no actual physical harm. The criterion is that contact happened without the plaintiff's consent. Nurses have great responsibility to avoid lawsuits regarding client care. Please answer the following questions in this regard:*

A client is brought to the emergency department with blunt injury on the abdomen resulting from a motor vehicle accident. The client is unconscious and not accompanied by their family, but has identification in their pocket. The surgeon decides that the client has to be taken up for surgery because they are bleeding in their abdomen.*

1. What should the health care team do in case there is nobody to provide consent for surgery?

_____

_____

_____

2. Should the act be considered battery?

_____

_____

_____

SECTION III: PRACTICING FOR NCLEX

Activity F *Answer the following questions.*

1. A client is experiencing chest pain and asks to see the physician. The nurse calls upon the physician, who is busy. When the physician visits the client, the nurse overhears them telling the client that the nurse is very inefficient. For which illegal act could the physician be charged?

   a. Battery
   b. Assault
   c. Slander
   d. Libel

2. A physician asks the nurse to remove the nasogastric tube from a client who has been in a coma for the past few months. The physician informs the nurse that the family members had requested them to do so. What should be the first action of the nurse with regard to the legal implication of removing the feeding tube?

   a. The nurse should carry out the order as told by the physician
   b. The nurse should check the records for the physician's written order
   c. The nurse should check the records for the family's authorization
   d. The nurse should check the records for the court order

3. A nurse on duty finds that their colleague is accepting money from a client for the care provided. What appropriate action should the nurse take?

   a. Inform the supervisor about the incident
   b. Ignore the incident and keep silent
   c. Call the local police to the nursing unit
   d. Confront the colleague and ask for an explanation

4. A client is brought to the emergency department with a head injury sustained from a motor vehicle accident. The surgeon determines that the client needs to undergo immediate surgery for the removal of a clot to save their life. The client is not accompanied by any family member. Which action should be a priority?

   a. Contact the client's family and wait for them to give consent for surgery
   b. Arrange for the operation, assuming that the consent is implied
   c. Sign the consent form yourself and later explain to the family
   d. Inform the supervisor and request that they sign the consent form

5. A well-known television personality has been admitted to the health care facility with chest pain. A person approaches the nurse posing as the client's family member and asks about the client's health details. The nurse reveals the medical details about the client. Later, it is discovered that this person was a press reporter and not a family member. Which legal provision has the nurse violated?

   a. Right to information
   b. Breach of nursing duty
   c. Client's right to privacy
   d. Defamation of the client

6. A physician on a client visit tells the nurse to increase the insulin dose to 10 units. They request that the nurse write down the orders on their behalf, because they have to rush to the intensive care unit (ICU). What should be the nurse's response in this case?

   a. Tell the physician to come back and write the orders
   b. Carry out the instruction without a written order
   c. Write the order on behalf of the physician
   d. Inform the client about the change in drug dosage

7. While administering regular insulin shots to a client, the nurse notices that the client is sweating profusely. Assuming that the sweating is a result of the warm weather, the nurse ignores the client's condition. Later, the client is found unconscious due to hypoglycemia. Which legal term appropriately describes the nurse's action?

   a. Defamation
   b. Negligence
   c. Battery
   d. Assault

8. A nurse is caring for a client who has terminal cancer. The client states that their lawyer would be coming to prepare their living will and requests the nurse to sign as a witness. What is the appropriate nursing response?

   a. Willingly signing as a witness to the living will
   b. Calling the physician to sign as a witness
   c. Politely informing the client that the nurse providing care is not authorized to sign
   d. Calling the nurse supervisor to sign as a witness

9. A nurse enters the client's room and finds that the plug point for the cardiac monitor has a short circuit. The nurse turns off the main switch and calls for the electrician. The nurse assesses whether the client has sustained any injury, makes them comfortable, and proceeds to fill in the incident report. What should be the nurse's next action?

   a. Informing the physician and nurse supervisor about the incident
   b. Making a copy of the incident report to give to the physician
   c. Making a copy of the incident report and putting it in the client's record
   d. Making a note in the client's record about the incident report

10. A client who has undergone arthroscopy is advised to ambulate only with assistance. The nurse finds that the client is trying to walk without any support and warns that they may fall and hurt themselves. Later, the client loses their balance and falls down, sustaining an injury to the forehead. Which legal defense should provide the nurse immunity from a possible lawsuit?

    a. Good Samaritan Law
    b. Assumption of risk
    c. Statute of limitation
    d. Judicial law

11. Which situation is an example of assault that a nurse may experience when performing their nursing duties?

   a. A nurse telling the client they cannot leave the health care facility
   b. A nurse restraining a client from being discharged without physician consent
   c. A nurse threatening to turn off the signal system of communication
   d. A nurse discussing confidential client information with a friend

12. A client who is scheduled for barium ingestion tests receives a food tray at mealtime. The client refuses to eat the food because the physician had instructed them not to take anything orally. The nurse insists that it is not necessary to be fasting before a barium investigation. The client takes dinner and, as a result, cannot undergo the barium ingestion test. The determination of negligence in this situation is based on which factor?

   a. The dietary department sent a meal for the client
   b. Harm resulted because the nurse did not act reasonably
   c. The nurse did not confirm the order with the physician
   d. The nurse insisted that the patient have the meal

13. A client feels that they are not getting appropriate treatment and wants to leave the hospital. They inform their caregiver of this. On realizing that the client is leaving without proper discharge, the nurse tries to stop the client by physically restraining them. What legal charges could occur based on the nurse's action? Select all that apply.

   a. Assault
   b. Battery
   c. Slander
   d. False imprisonment
   e. Libel

14. A nurse has published a research report on human immunodeficiency virus (HIV). A client finds that their name is mentioned in the report, along with the fact that the client had contracted the infection from a prostitute. Which legal provisions apply to the nurse? Select all that apply.

   a. Felony
   b. Invasion of privacy
   c. Libel
   d. Slander
   e. Misdemeanor

15. A client is experiencing psychotic symptoms and is becoming violent. The nurse determines that the client needs to be restrained because they can be potentially harmful. Which nursing actions are appropriate? Select all that apply.

   a. The nurse should sedate the client and then restrain them
   b. The nurse should take orders from the physician for restraining
   c. The nurse should document the type and duration of restraint
   d. The nurse should make their own decision and restrain the client
   e. The nurse should explain to the family the reason for restraining

SECTION IV: REVIEWING WHAT YOU HAVE LEARNED

Activity G *Fill in the blanks by choosing the correct word from the options given in parentheses.*

1. _____ means damaging statements written and read by others. (Libel, Misdemeanors, Slander)

2. _____ is the ethical principle that emphasizes the duty to be honest and to avoid deceiving or misleading clients. (Autonomy, Justice, Veracity)

Activity H *Mark each statement as either T (True) or F (False). Correct any false statements.*

1. T F An anecdotal note cannot be used as evidence in court.

2. T F Malpractice is harm that results from acting carelessly in a given circumstance.

Activity I   *Question 1. Differentiate between teleologic theory and deontologic theory.*

1. Definition
2. Ideology
3. Example

Activity J   *Answer the following questions.*

1. What are laws? What are the different types of laws?

   _____

   _____

   _____

2. What is the purpose of a nurse practice act?

   _____

   _____

   _____

Activity K   *Answer the following questions.*

1. Why is it important for nurses to obtain their own personal liability insurance?

   _____

   _____

   _____

2. Why can a nurse be charged with a criminal offense in the case of gross negligence?

   _____

   _____

   _____

3. Why should the nurse refuse the assistance of untrained interpreters, volunteers, or family when caring for a client with whom the nurse does not share a common language?

   _____

   _____

   _____

4. Why must the nurse avoid making or writing negative comments about clients, physicians, or other coworkers?

   _____

   _____

   _____

Activity L   *Answer the following questions focusing on nursing roles and responsibilities.*

An unconscious client has been admitted to the health care facility after a motor vehicle crash. When the client regains consciousness, they want to leave the facility without being medically discharged.

1. Can the nurse prevent the client from leaving?

   _____

   _____

   _____

2. What procedure should the nurse follow if the client refuses to stay at the facility?

   _____

   _____

   _____

Activity M   *Consider the following questions. Discuss them with your instructor or peers.*

A client with a fractured left leg is learning how to use crutches. The nurse has asked the client not to leave the room without assistance. The client ignores this suggestion and falls. How should the nurse handle this situation?

   _____

   _____

   _____

SECTION V: GETTING READY FOR NCLEX

Activity N *Answer the following questions.*

1. A nurse at a health care facility has been stealing narcotics for personal use and has been attempting to conceal the theft by altering records of narcotic drug administration. What offense would the nurse most likely be charged with in the case of legal proceedings?

   a. Misdemeanor
   b. Felony
   c. Malpractice
   d. Negligence

2. The nurse has asked a client who is likely to experience orthostatic hypotension to use the nurse's call light if they need to use the bathroom. The client refuses to comply with this request. Which nursing action would be appropriate to ensure the client's safety?

   a. Raise the side rails of the bed
   b. Obtain a medical order to use a restraint
   c. Threaten to use a restraint
   d. Use a wanderer alarm

CHAPTER 4

Health and Illness

Learning Objectives

- Describe how the World Health Organization (WHO) defines health.
- Discuss the difference between values and beliefs, and list health beliefs common among Americans.
- Explain the concept of holism.
- Identify the five levels of human needs.
- Define illness and terms used to describe illness.
- Differentiate primary, secondary, tertiary, and extended care.
- Name programs that help finance health care for the aged, disabled, and low-income population.
- List methods for control escalating health care costs.
- Identify national health goals targeted for the year 2030.
- Discuss methods that nurses use to administer client care.

SECTION I: ASSESSING YOUR UNDERSTANDING

Activity A   FILL IN THE BLANKS

1. Abraham Maslow is a psychologist who identified five levels of human needs and grouped them into a(n) _____.

2. The sum of physical, emotional, social, and spiritual health is called _____.

3. The term _____ denotes the number of people who died from a particular disease or condition.

4. A disorder acquired from the genetic codes of one or both parents is called a(n) _____ condition.

5. Health services provided by the first health care professional or agency a person contacts is called _____ care.

6. WHO defines health as a state of complete physical, mental, and social well-being, not merely the absence of disease or _____

7. _____ refers to incidence of a specific disease, disorder, or injury and the rate or numbers of people affected.

8. A foot ulcer that develops in a patient who has uncontrolled diabetes is an example of a(n) _____ illness.

9. _____ is a federal program that finances health care costs of persons 65 years and older, permanently disabled workers of any age and their dependents, and those with end-stage renal disease.

10. The nursing care pattern in which nursing personnel divide clients into groups and complete their care together is called _____ nursing.

Activity B *Consider the following figure.*

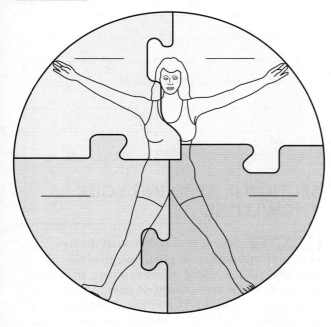

1. Identify and label the figure.

   _____

   _____

   _____

2. List the components of holism that determine how "whole" or well a person feels.

   _____

   _____

   _____

3. How are the components of holism related to each other?

   _____

   _____

   _____

4. Label the figure to indicate members of the nursing team.

   _____

   _____

   _____

5. What is the main purpose of the nursing team?

   _____

   _____

   _____

Activity C *Match the types of illness in Column A with their descriptions in Column B.*

Column A

_____ 1. Primary illness

_____ 2. Acute illness

_____ 3. Terminal illness

_____ 4. Chronic illness

Column B

a. Illness that comes on slowly and lasts a long time

b. Illness that develops independently of any other disease

c. Illness that comes on suddenly and lasts a short time

d. Illness for which there is no potential for cure

Activity D   *The following are the five levels of human needs in random order as identified by Maslow in his hierarchy of human needs. Write the correct sequence in the boxes provided.*

1. Physiologic needs

2. Esteem and self-esteem

3. Safety and security

4. Love and belonging

5. Self-actualization

☐ → ☐ → ☐ → ☐ → ☐

The following are some of the agencies and institutions, in random order, where people seek treatment for health problems or assistance with maintaining or promoting their health. Write the correct sequence in which health care is obtained, in the boxes provided.

1. Physiotherapy center

2. Family physician

3. Multispecialty hospital

4. Diagnostic center

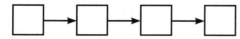

Activity E   *Briefly answer the following.*

1. Why is the first level of Maslow's hierarchy of human needs very important?

   _____

   _____

   _____

2. What are the types of illness based on duration?

   _____

   _____

   _____

3. What are managed care organizations?

   _____

   _____

   _____

4. What is capitation?

   _____

   _____

   _____

5. What is nurse-managed care?

   _____

   _____

   _____

SECTION II: APPLYING YOUR KNOWLEDGE

Activity F   *Nursing care is based on five common management patterns: functional nursing, case method, team nursing, primary nursing, and nurse-managed care. Nurse-managed care involves a clinical pathway and is typically used in a managed care approach. Answer the following questions, which involve the nurse's role as a nurse manager.*

A client is admitted to the nursing unit for a hernioplasty. The nursing unit follows the nurse-managed care pattern of nursing care.

1. What are the responsibilities of a nurse manager?

   _____

   _____

   _____

2. What are the advantages of the nurse-managed care pattern?

   _____

   _____

   _____

SECTION III: PRACTICING FOR NCLEX

Activity G   *Answer the following questions.*

1. A client has undergone amputation of the left leg. The wound has healed well with no complications. The client will need a prosthesis to

enable them to walk. The nurse understands that the client at this stage of recovery would require:
a. Primary care of a general physician
b. Secondary care of a reconstructive surgeon
c. Tertiary care of a sophisticated hospital
d. Extended care of a rehabilitation center

2. A client is depressed after the death of their spouse. They do not want to meet their friends or other family members. The client has low self-esteem because they were dependent on their spouse. Which aspect of this client's health requires immediate attention?
a. Inability to cope
b. Depression
c. Low self-esteem
d. Dependency

3. An LPN is caring for a senior client recently diagnosed with osteoarthritis. The client informs the nurse that they have been experiencing pain in the knees for the past 4 months. The nurse understands that osteoarthritis has a:
a. Gradual onset
b. Genetic predisposition
c. Short disease course
d. Short treatment regimen

4. The nurse understands that secondary illness is a disorder that develops from a preexisting condition. Which example is a secondary disorder?
a. Lung disease resulting from smoking
b. Smoking because of social causes
c. Heart disease resulting from a damaged lung
d. Heart disease resulting from fetal abnormalities

5. An LPN understands that remission is the disappearance of signs and symptoms associated with a particular disease. They are aware that although remission resembles a cured state, the relief may be only temporary. Which disease condition has a remission state?
a. Gout
b. Heart attack
c. Common cold
d. Varicose veins

6. A student nurse is posted to a new nursing unit in their rotation. They observe that the nursing staff follows the functional nursing approach of nursing. The nurse understands that functional nursing is a nursing model wherein:
a. The nursing staff is headed by a team leader
b. The nurse manager plans the nursing care of clients
c. One nurse plans and provides individualized nursing care
d. A head nurse assigns specific tasks to other members

7. A nurse manager plans the nursing care of clients based on their type of case or medical diagnosis. The nurse evaluates whether predictable outcomes are met on a daily basis. The nurse manager is an important person in:
a. Team nursing
b. Functional nursing
c. Nurse-managed care
d. Case method

8. The LPN understands that managed care organizations are private insurers and agencies that provide health care services. Federal policies like Medicare and Medicaid also exist for people who cannot afford services of managed care organizations. Which statement describes an important component of Medicare?
a. They bargain with providers for quality care at reasonable costs
b. They reimburse hospital charges based on the diagnostic-related group
c. They provide client education to decrease the risk of disease
d. They monitor and manage fiscal and client outcomes

9. An LPN is caring for a client with hemophilia, a hereditary disorder. What is another example of a hereditary disorder?
a. Atrial septal defect
b. Myositis
c. Cystic fibrosis
d. Macular edema

10. A baby is born with multiple fingers (polydactyly). The nurse explains to the mother that it is a congenital disorder. Which statement from the mother indicates the need for further education on the subject?
a. It is the result of an abnormality in genes
b. It is the result of faulty embryonic development
c. It is the result of maternal exposure to infections
d. It is the result of maternal exposure to certain drugs

11. Mortality and morbidity are measures of disease burden relating to specific diseases or conditions. Which statement indicates neonatal mortality rate?
    a. Number of neonatal deaths per 1,000 deliveries
    b. Number of neonatal deaths before 1 year of age
    c. Number of neonatal deaths per 1,000 live births
    d. Number of neonatal deaths per year

12. A 50-year-old client who underwent surgery for prolapsed disk is to undergo physiotherapy after discharge. The nurse understands that a physiotherapy center is an example of:
    a. Continuity of care
    b. Extended care
    c. Secondary care
    d. Tertiary care

13. In a nursing unit, the nurse leader delegates specific tasks to the team members and tells them to report on the completion of the task. The nurse assigns the task, supervises, and obtains feedback. Which type of nursing care is being implemented?
    a. Team nursing
    b. Functional nursing
    c. Primary nursing
    d. Nurse-managed care

14. A client admitted for arthroscopy is discharged 2 days earlier than the estimated time because they had a fast recovery and are doing well. The client is insured through a capitation scheme. In the event of early discharge of the client, who receives the monetary profit?
    a. The client
    b. The hospital
    c. The provider
    d. The government

15. A client presents to a family physician with symptoms of chest pain. After initial examination, the physician refers the client to a medical specialist. This is an example of:
    a. Extended care
    b. Continuity of care
    c. Secondary care
    d. Primary care

16. Which statement indicates a measure of mortality?
    a. Lung cancer accounts for 1% of all cigarette smoking–attributable illnesses
    b. Each year, 440,000 people die of a cigarette smoking–attributable illness
    c. Cigarette smoking results in 5.6 million potential lives lost each year
    d. Seventy-five billion dollars is lost in the direct medical costs of smoking-attributable illnesses

17. Assessment of a client with minor burns on the face and hands reveals the following main findings. Place the needs in order of priority of nursing care.
    a. Inability to perform daily activities
    b. Pain in the open wound
    c. Anxiety and apprehension about the treatment
    d. Inability to interact with friends and family

18. A nurse is caring for several clients in a health care facility. What are examples of acute disorders? Select all that apply.
    a. Diabetes mellitus
    b. Influenza
    c. Measles
    d. Hypertension
    e. Conjunctivitis

19. Team nursing is a pattern in which nursing personnel divide the clients into groups and complete their care together. What is the responsibility of the team leader?
    a. To care for clients who are confined to bed
    b. To administer medicines and injections
    c. To assign, supervise, and evaluate care
    d. To act as a liaison with other departments for client care

20. The nurse understands that there are five common management patterns. Each has advantages and disadvantages. Which pattern of nursing has a conference as its most important component?
    a. Functional nursing
    b. Case method
    c. Team nursing
    d. Nurse-managed care

SECTION IV: REVIEWING WHAT YOU HAVE LEARNED

Activity H *Fill in the blanks by choosing the correct word from the options given in parentheses.*

1. A(n) _____ disorder is acquired from the genetic codes of one or both parents. (congenital, hereditary, idiopathic)

2. Health services to which health care providers refer clients for consultation and additional testing, such as cardiac catheterization, are an example of _____ care. (primary, secondary, tertiary)

Activity I *Mark each statement as either T (True) or F (False). Correct any false statements.*

1. T F Capitation is a payment system that provides incentives to control the number of tests and services rendered as a means of making a profit.

2. T F In the case method of nursing, one nurse manages all the care needs of a client or group of clients for a designated period.

Activity J *Write the correct term for each description below.*

1. Sum of physical, emotional, social, and spiritual health, which determines how "whole" or well a person feels _____.

2. Ill effect that results from permanent or progressive organ damage caused by a disease or its treatment _____.

3. Period during which signs and symptoms of a particular disease temporarily disappear _____.

Activity K *Match the terms in Column A with their definitions in Column B.*

Column A

____ 1. Morbidity

____ 2. Mortality

____ 3. Acute illness

____ 4. Chronic illness

Column B

a. An illness that comes on slowly and lasts a long time

b. Incidence of a specific disease, disorder, or injury, referring to the rate or numbers of people affected

c. Incidence of death from a particular disease or condition

d. An illness that comes on suddenly and lasts a short time

Activity L *Answer the following questions.*

1. How does the World Health Organization (WHO) define health?

_____
_____
_____

2. What are the five common management patterns that nurses use to administer client care?

_____
_____
_____

SECTION V: APPLYING YOUR KNOWLEDGE

Activity M   *Answer the following questions focusing on nursing roles and responsibilities.*

Personnel at a health care facility follow a team nursing pattern of care, with one member as the team leader.

1. What is team nursing?

   _____

   _____

   _____

2. What are the roles and responsibilities of the team leader?

   _____

   _____

   _____

SECTION VI: GETTING READY FOR NCLEX

Activity N   *Answer the following questions.*

1. A nurse admits a client to a health care facility and plans and evaluates care for the client during the stay. The same nurse prepares discharge planning for the client. What type of nursing care is this nurse practicing?

   a. Primary nursing
   b. Functional nursing
   c. Nurse-managed care
   d. Case method

2. A nurse manager plans nursing care for clients on a burn unit using a clinical pathway based on their medical diagnosis. In the majority of cases, the clients are ready for discharge by the time designated by prospective payment systems, if not before. This type of nursing is termed:

   a. Primary nursing
   b. Functional nursing
   c. Nurse-managed care
   d. Case method

Homeostasis, Adaptation, and Stress

- Explain homeostasis, and list categories of stressors that affect homeostasis.
- Identify beliefs about the body and mind based on the concept of holism.
- Identify the purpose of adaptation and possible outcomes of unsuccessful adaptation.
- Trace the structures through which adaptive responses take place.
- Differentiate between sympathetic and parasympathetic adaptive responses.
- Define stress, and list factors that affect the stress response.
- Discuss the stages and consequences of the general adaptation syndrome.
- Explain psychological adaptation and possible outcomes.
- Name three levels of prevention that apply to reducing or managing stress-related disorders.
- Describe the nursing activities helpful to the care of clients prone to stress and approaches for preventing, reducing, or eliminating a stress response.

SECTION I: ASSESSING YOUR UNDERSTANDING

Activity A FILL IN THE BLANKS

1. _____ are chemical messengers synthesized in the neurons, which allow for communication across the synaptic cleft between neurons.

2. Neurotransmitters, when released, temporarily bind to receptor sites on the _____ neuron and transmit their information.

3. Another chemical messenger, called a(n) _____, is a type of neuromodulator that helps neurons communicate with each other.

4. _____ stabilizes mood, induces sleep, and regulates temperature.

5. The neurotransmitter _____ heightens arousal and increases energy.

6. The central nervous system is composed of the brain and _____.

7. The _____ enables people to think abstractly, use and understand language, accumulate and store memories, and make decisions about information received.

8. The _____ is responsible for regulating and maintaining blood pressure.

9. The pituitary gland is connected to the _____ through both vascular connections and nerve endings.

10. The _____ gland in the brain is known as the master gland, and it produces hormones that influence other endocrine glands.

Activity B   *Consider the following figure.*

1. Identify and label the figure.

   _____

   _____

   _____

2. What is the function of each component?

   _____

   _____

   _____

Activity C   *Match the physiologic stress response in Column A with its corresponding characteristics in Column B.*

Column A

____ 1. Alarm stage

____ 2. Stage of resistance

____ 3. Stage of exhaustion

Column B

a. Adaptation/resistance can no longer protect the person experiencing the stressor

b. Prepares the person for a "fight-or-flight" response

c. Returns the person experiencing the stressor to the stage of normalcy

Activity D   *Presented here, in random order, are stress-related responses. Write the correct sequence in the boxes provided below.*

1. Adrenal glands secrete additional norepinephrine and epinephrine.
2. Storage vesicles release norepinephrine.
3. The body might return to the homeostasis stage.
4. The adrenal cortex releases cortisol, a stress hormone.
5. The person is at a risk of severe infections or cancer.
6. The person is prepared for a fight-or-flight response.

☐→☐→☐→☐→☐→☐

Presented here, in random order, are steps for nurses to follow while treating a stressed client. Write the correct sequence in the boxes provided below.

1. Eliminate or reduce the stressors.

2. Identify the stressors.

3. Prevent additional stressors.

4. Assess the client's response to stress.

5. Implement stress reduction and stress management techniques.

6. Promote the client's physiologic adaptive responses.

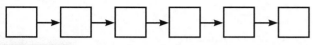

Activity E   *Briefly answer the following questions.*

1. What is the difference between the sympathetic and the parasympathetic nervous systems?

_____

_____

_____

2. Define feedback loop.

_____

_____

_____

3. What is the scientific definition of stress?

_____

_____

_____

4. Briefly describe the three stages of stress.

_____

_____

_____

5. What are coping strategies? List the types of coping strategies people use to deal with stress-provoking events or situations.

_____

_____

_____

6. How can you help prevent or minimize stress-related illnesses?

_____

_____

_____

SECTION II: APPLYING YOUR KNOWLEDGE

Activity F   *Stress is a physiologic and behavioral response to disequilibrium. It has physical, emotional, and cognitive effects. Although all humans have the capacity to adapt to stress, not everyone responds to similar stressors exactly the same. Read the scenario and answer the questions that follow, which involve the nurse's role in caring for the client with stress.*

A 50-year-old client with a high glucose level is undergoing stress-related treatment. The client seems to be getting aggressive. The nurse stands in front of the client and says, "Tell me about the incident that is disturbing you." The client, who is seated, seems disturbed and is sweating profusely. The nurse repeats the instructions, but the client becomes agitated and does not respond to the nurse.

1. What measures could the nurse take to ensure an accurate assessment of the client's condition?

_____

_____

_____

2. What actions should the nurse take during further discussions and care of the client?

_____

_____

_____

SECTION III: PRACTICING FOR NCLEX

Activity G   *Answer the following questions.*

1. A client with a family history of hypertension and high blood pressure visits the health care facility for a physical examination. As a primary level of stress prevention, what should the nurse do?

  a. Regularly monitor the client's blood pressure

  b. Teach principles to maintaining blood pressure

  c. Prescribe medicines for hypertension

  d. Prescribe a strict diet and exercise routine

2. A client who had been involved in a minor car accident is stressed about the cost of recovery. Under the nurse's guidance, the client starts focusing on the positive aspect of being physically unharmed. What technique is the nurse implementing?

   a. Alternative thinking
   b. Alternative behavior
   c. Alternative lifestyle
   d. Adaptive activities

3. The nurse is caring for a client with a family history of hypertension. As a secondary level of stress prevention, what should the nurse do?

   a. Regularly monitor the client's blood pressure
   b. Teach principles to maintain the blood pressure
   c. Prescribe medicines for hypertension
   d. Prescribe a strict diet and exercise routine

4. A client visits the medical center with complaints of stress. They had lost their left arm in an accident and have been complaining that their family has not been treating them properly since the accident. They feel they have become a burden. What should be the nurse's observation in this case?

   a. The client is resorting to nontherapeutic coping strategies.
   b. The client is adopting therapeutic coping strategies.
   c. The client is using coping mechanisms to deal with their situation.
   d. The client is suffering from stress-related disorders.

5. A client diagnosed with stress and depression is advised by the nurse to share their frustrations with other supportive people and also to adopt an assertive approach to the situation. Which stress management technique is the nurse implementing?

   a. Alternative thinking
   b. Alternative behaviors
   c. Alternative lifestyles
   d. Adaptive activities

6. A nurse is caring for a client with insomnia. Which neurotransmitter would help induce sleep in the client?

   a. Norepinephrine
   b. Serotonin
   c. Dopamine
   d. Endorphins

7. A client complains of pain in the arm muscles. The nurse suggests a body massage for pain relief. Identify the chemical that will be released by the massage, which will help stop the pain.

   a. Endorphins
   b. γ-Aminobutyric acid
   c. Substance P
   d. Acetylcholine

8. A client is admitted to the clinic with high blood pressure. Upon interviewing the client, the nurse finds that they are suffering from stress at the workplace. The client is very timid in nature and is unable to refuse any work that comes from their colleagues or boss. What should the nurse advise the client?

   a. The nurse should advise that the client change their job
   b. The nurse should advise that the client accept their duties and situation
   c. The nurse should advise the client to adopt alternative behavior
   d. The nurse should advise the client to undergo therapy to reduce stress

9. A 10-year-old child, who has gone into depression after the death of their mother, is accompanied by their father to the health care facility. The nurse performs routine tests and finds that the child has very high blood pressure. Their heartbeat is irregularly high. What should the nurse conclude in this case?

   a. The child is in the exhaustion stage of stress
   b. The child is in the alarm stage of stress
   c. The child is in the resistance stage of stress
   d. The child is in a state of homeostasis

10. Many factors affect the ability of humans to respond to stress. Which situation represents the greatest stressor for a client?

    a. The spouse of the client has died recently
    b. The client has lost a lot of money from gambling
    c. The client has recently lost their job
    d. The client has moved to a low-income neighborhood

11. A 55-year-old client is suffering from depression after their spouse died. The children of the client are married and settled in other states. The nurse advises them to get a pet dog to stay with them for company and to listen to soothing music to uplift their mood. Which technique is the nurse implementing?

    a. Alternative thinking
    b. Alternative behaviors
    c. Alternative lifestyles
    d. Adaptive activities

12. A client has been admitted to the medical center with severe depression and stress. What initial action should the nurse take to treat the client?

    a. Teach the client the importance of being happy and unstressed
    b. Administer therapies that alter mood and feelings
    c. Administer antidepressants to counter stress
    d. Find the factors that have caused stress and depression

13. A client who has been facing financial distress for a long time manifests bowel infections and allergies. The client has also developed rheumatoid arthritis. The nurse feels that the immune system of the client is compromised. What might the nurse conclude?

    a. The client is in the exhaustion stage of stress
    b. The client is in the resistance stage of stress
    c. The client is in the alarm stage of stress
    d. The client is in a state of homeostasis or balance

14. The nurse is caring for a client who is admitted to the medical center with high levels of stress and anxiety. Upon questioning, the client states that their mother also suffered from stress. How should the nurse help the client? Select all that apply.

    a. Advise the client to undergo stress management therapy
    b. Advise the client to accept their duties and situation
    c. Advise the client to adopt assertive behavior at the workplace
    d. Advise the client to make changes to their home environment
    e. Advise the client to take medication to counter stress

15. A client is admitted to the medical center with a high level of stress. Order the following tasks in the most likely sequence in which the nurse should perform them while caring for this client.

    a. Prevent other factors from causing stress
    b. Analyze how the client responds to stress
    c. Identify the reasons for stress
    d. Implement stress reduction and stress management techniques
    e. Eliminate or reduce the factors causing stress

16. The nurse is caring for a client with high levels of stress. The client was involved in an accident, during which their car was severely damaged. Order the stress-related responses that occur in the client's brain in the most likely sequence in which they would have occurred.

    a. The hypothalamus releases corticotropin-releasing factor
    b. The storage vesicles within the sympathetic nervous system neurons rapidly release norepinephrine
    c. The adrenal glands secrete additional norepinephrine and epinephrine
    d. The adrenal cortex releases cortisol, a stress hormone
    e. The pituitary gland secretes adrenocorticotropic hormone

SECTION IV: REVIEWING WHAT YOU HAVE LEARNED

Activity H *Fill in the blanks by choosing the correct word from the options given in parentheses.*

1. The term _____ means physiologic and behavioral responses to disequilibrium. (adaptation, holism, stress)

2. _____ stabilizes mood, induces sleep, and regulates temperature. (dopamine, norepinephrine, serotonin)

Activity I *Mark each statement as either T (True) or F (False). Correct any false statements.*

1. T F   Coping mechanisms are stress-reduction activities people select consciously to help them deal with challenging events or situations.

2. T F   Receptors for neurotransmitters are found throughout the central nervous, endocrine, and immune systems.

Activity J *Write the correct term for each description below.*

1. A relatively stable state of physiologic equilibrium _____

2. Natural body chemicals that produce effects similar to those of opiate drugs _____

Activity K *Differentiate between the sympathetic and parasympathetic nervous systems.*

1. Function
2. Effect on physiologic functions
3. Example

Activity L *Consider the following figure.*

Label the structures in the figure.

Activity M *Answer the following questions.*

1. What is homeostasis? What are the four categories of stressors that affect homeostasis?

   _____

   _____

   _____

2. What factors affect the stress response?

   _____

   _____

   _____

Activity N *Answer the following questions focusing on nursing roles and responsibilities.*

A nurse is caring for a client scheduled for minor surgery who is unusually quiet. The nurse believes that the client is under stress.

1. What can the nurse do if the client is experiencing stress?

   _____

   _____

   _____

2. What stress-reduction techniques can the nurse employ for this client?

_____

_____

_____

Activity O *Consider the following questions. Discuss them with your instructor or peers.*

1. A client is unhappy with the lunch served at the health care facility. When the nurse arrives to check if the client has eaten, the client pushes away the tray, spilling its contents on the floor. What should the nurse do in this case?

2. A client who is to undergo chemotherapy expresses concern about the side effects of the drug treatment and the effects that the cancer is causing on their family roles. The client mentions to the nurse that they try to combat stress by sleeping most of the time. What interventions can the nurse suggest to help reduce the client's stress?

SECTION V: GETTING READY FOR NCLEX

Activity P *Answer the following questions.*

1. The nurse is caring for a client who has been diagnosed with cancer. The client refuses to believe the diagnosis and wants all the diagnostic tests repeated. The nurse is aware that the client is using the coping method known as:

a. Displacement
b. Projection
c. Sublimation
d. Denial

2. A nurse is caring for a client whose right hand had to be amputated following an accident. The client, whose employment involves using a computer keyboard to enter data, may have to look for another job. Which factor is the highest contributor to stress in this client's situation?

a. Moving to a different job
b. Adjusting to a change in financial status
c. Dealing with a personal injury
d. Changing living conditions

Culture and Ethnicity

Learning Objectives

- Differentiate culture, race, and ethnicity.
- Discuss factors that interfere with perceiving others as individuals.
- Explain why U.S. culture is described as anglicized.
- List characteristics of Anglo-American culture.
- List the predominant cultures present in the United States.
- List the diversities in people according to their cultures.
- Describe characteristics of culturally sensitive care.
- List ways to demonstrate cultural sensitivity.

SECTION I: ASSESSING YOUR UNDERSTANDING

Activity A   FILL IN THE BLANKS

1. _____ is a term used when referring to a collective group of people who differ from the dominant group in terms of cultural characteristics, such as language, and physical characteristics, such as skin color, or both.

2. African Americans and people from _____ countries lack the glucose 6-phosphate dehydrogenase (G-6-PD) enzyme.

3. _____ are unique cultural groups that coexist within the dominant culture.

4. _____ is a supposition that a person shares cultural characteristics with others of a similar background.

5. _____ is the belief that one's own ethnicity is superior to all others.

6. _____ is a digestive enzyme that converts lactose, the sugar in milk, into the simpler sugars glucose and galactose.

7. _____ medicine refers to the health practices unique to a particular group of people and has come to mean the methods of disease prevention or treatment outside mainstream conventional practice.

8. A(n) _____ is a holy man with curative powers in folk medicine.

9. Mongolian spots, an example of _____, are dark-blue areas on the lower back and sometimes on the abdomen, thighs, shoulders, or arms of darkly pigmented infants and children.

10. _____ is the ability to speak a second language.

Activity B   *Consider the following figure.*

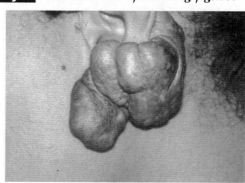

1. Identify the skin condition shown in the figure.

   _____

   _____

   _____

2. Which skin types commonly show this condition and why?

   _____

   _____

   _____

Activity C *Match the names of beliefs concerning illness in Column A with its description in Column B.*

Column A

_____ **1.** Yin/yang

_____ **2.** Hot/cold

_____ **3.** Naturalistic

_____ **4.** Magico-religious

Column B

a. Supernatural forces contribute to disease or health

b. Humans and nature must be in balance or harmony to remain healthy

c. Balanced forces promote health

d. Illness is an imbalance between components described as having hot or cold attributes

Activity D *Briefly answer the following questions.*

1. What is meant by culture?

   _____

   _____

   _____

2. What are the characteristics of minority groups?

   _____

   _____

   _____

3. What is the difference between stereotyping and generalizing?

   _____

   _____

   _____

4. What is the current impact of ethnocentrism on different parts of the world?

   _____

   _____

   _____

5. What are the various subcultures in the United States?

   _____

   _____

   _____

SECTION II: APPLYING YOUR KNOWLEDGE

Activity E *To provide culturally sensitive care, nurses must become skilled at managing language differences, understanding biologic and physiologic variations, promoting health teaching that will reduce prevalent diseases, and respecting alternative health beliefs or practices.*

A client who is Native American is admitted to the nursing unit for abdominoplasty. The nurse understands that behavioral patterns of Native Americans differ from one culture to another. Answer the following questions, which involve the nurse's understanding of cultural differences and their application.

1. What should the nurse keep in mind while interviewing the client?

   _____

   _____

   _____

2. How should the nurse demonstrate culturally sensitive nursing care?

   _____

   _____

   _____

SECTION III: PRACTICING FOR NCLEX

Activity F *Answer the following questions.*

1. The nurse is interviewing a Latino/a client who is scheduled for a routine physical examination after chemotherapy. What action by the nurse demonstrates cultural sensitivity?

   a. Sit far away from the client
   b. Provide information and ask questions slowly
   c. Use medical terminology during the interview
   d. Ask the client to express themselves emotionally

2. The nurse is assisting with eating for an Asian American client who has minor burns on their hands. The nurse is aware that people of Asian descent may feel threatened with physical closeness. What would be the nurse's most appropriate action?

   a. Do not assist the client if they feel uneasy
   b. Assist the client and leave the client's room
   c. Explain to the client the purpose of the assistance
   d. Give instructions to the client regarding how to eat

3. A nurse is caring for a client with lactase deficiency. Which action should the nurse perform either to reduce or eliminate lactose?

   a. Avoid giving lactose-free milk to the client
   b. Ask the client to eat breads and cereals
   c. Avoid using foods with pareve on the label
   d. Ask the client to use nondairy creamers

4. After bathing a dark-skinned client, the nurse notices that the washcloth has brown discoloration on it. What should be the reaction of the nurse in this case?

   a. Assume it is dirt and bathe the client again
   b. Consider it to be normal for the client
   c. Educate the client about personal hygiene
   d. Consider it a symptom of the disease

5. On a home visit to an African American family, the nurse finds that the 3-month-old baby has dark-blue spots on the lower back. What would be the appropriate nursing action?

   a. Inform the police of child abuse
   b. Ask the family about the spot
   c. Advise the mother to consult a doctor
   d. Consider it normal for the ethnic group

6. A client is admitted to the nursing unit with cramps, intestinal gas, and diarrhea, approximately 30 minutes after ingesting milk. Which condition should the nurse suspect?

   a. Lactase deficiency
   b. G-6-PD deficiency
   c. Antidiuretic hormone (ADH) deficiency
   d. Thyroid deficiency

7. On examining a dark-skinned client, the nurse detects the presence of keloids. What should be the nurse's reaction?

   a. Consider it pathologic
   b. Inform the physician
   c. Consider it normal
   d. Perform biochemical tests

8. A male nurse is assigned to change the dressing of a female Southeast Asian client who has an accidental wound on the knee. Keeping in mind that the people of this culture consider the female body as private from knee to waist, what actions should the nurse take while dressing the wound? Select all that apply.

   a. Relieve the client's anxiety by offering an explanation
   b. Request permission from the client's husband
   c. Include a female attendant during the procedure
   d. Instruct the husband to do the procedure
   e. Allow the client's husband to stay in the room

9. A nurse is caring for an African American client who is noncooperative with the health care team. What can the nurse do to make the client comfortable? Select all that apply.

   a. Address the client by their last name
   b. Follow up thoroughly with requests
   c. Respect the client's privacy
   d. Maintain eye contact during communication
   e. Ask direct questions to the client

10. A registered nurse delegates the task of combing a client's hair to the LPN. The client is an African American woman with curly hair. What nursing actions are appropriate? Select all that apply.

    a. Ask the client to help you comb her hair
    b. Apply a moisturizing cream or gel
    c. Use a wide-toothed comb or pick
    d. Wet the hair with water before combing
    e. Let the client's hair remain as it is currently

SECTION IV: REVIEWING WHAT YOU HAVE LEARNED

Activity G *Fill in the blanks by choosing the correct word from the options given in parentheses.*

1. _____ is a bond or kinship that a person feels their country of birth or place of ancestral origin. (culture, ethnicity, race)

2. A fixed attitude about all people who share a common characteristic related to age, sex, race, sexual orientation, or ethnicity is called a _____. (belief, generalization, stereotype)

Activity H *Mark each statement as either T (True) or F (False). Correct any false statements.*

1. T F Ethnocentrism refers to the belief that one's own ethnicity is superior to all others.

2. T F A G-6-PD deficiency makes red blood cells vulnerable during stress, which increases metabolic needs.

Activity I *Write the correct term for each description below.*

1. Digestive enzyme that converts lactose into glucose and galactose _____.

2. When a person consumes alcohol, a process of chemical reactions involving enzymes, one of which is _____, eventually breaks down the alcohol into acetic acid and carbon dioxide.

Activity J *Match the skin disorders in Column A with their descriptions in Column B.*

Column A

_____ 1. Keloids

_____ 2. Hypopigmentation

_____ 3. Vitiligo

_____ 4. Mongolian spots

Column B

a. Dark-blue areas on the lower backs of darkly pigmented infants and children

b. Irregular, elevated thick scars

c. Damaged skin with temporary redness that fades to a lighter hue

d. Irregular white patches on the skin from a lack of melanin

Activity K *Answer the following question.*

What is transcultural nursing care?

_____

_____

_____

SECTION V: APPLYING YOUR KNOWLEDGE

Activity L *Answer the following question.*

1. Why should the nurse refuse the assistance of untrained interpreters, volunteers, or family when caring for a client with whom the nurse does not share a common language?

_____

_____

_____

2. Why is it important for the nurse to inspect the skin of the palm, foot, and abdomen during a skin assessment of a dark-skinned person?

_____

_____

_____

Activity M *Answer the following questions focusing on nursing roles and responsibilities.*

A nurse is assessing a client who immigrated to the United States years ago and understands English well but does not speak the language fluently. The client does not want an interpreter.

1. How should the nurse communicate with the client during the assessment?

_____

_____

_____

2. Why is it important for the nurse to be patient when communicating with this client?

_____

_____

_____

Activity N *Consider the following questions. Discuss them with your instructor or peers.*

A nurse who works in a large urban clinic assesses clients from various subcultures.

1. What data should the nurse obtain during an assessment to provide culturally sensitive care?

   _____

   _____

   _____

2. What variations is a nurse likely to observe when assessing these clients?

   _____

   _____

   _____

3. A nurse is working at a health care facility where most clients do not speak English. How should the nurse prepare to meet the challenges of this job?

   _____

   _____

   _____

SECTION VI: GETTING READY FOR NCLEX

Activity O *Answer the following questions.*

1. The nurse is assigned to care for an Asian American woman. Which nursing action would be culturally appropriate when providing care for this client?

   a. Touch the client's head gently
   b. Avoid touching the client's hand
   c. Provide personal care in the presence of family members
   d. Avoid lingering eye contact with the client

2. When assessing a client who does not speak the same language as the nurse, the nurse seeks the assistance of an interpreter. What action would a skilled interpreter perform in this role?

   a. Explain the interpreter role to the client
   b. Express personal views on the client's statement
   c. Inform the client's family about the client's condition
   d. Translate the client's statements without conveying the client's emotions

CHAPTER 7

The Nurse–Client Relationship

Learning Objectives

- Name the roles that nurses perform in nurse–client relationships.
- Describe the current role expectations for clients.
- List the principles that form the basis of the nurse–client relationship.
- Identify the phases of the nurse–client relationship.
- Differentiate between social communication and therapeutic verbal communication.
- Provide examples of therapeutic and nontherapeutic communication techniques.
- List factors that affect oral communication.
- Describe the forms of nonverbal communication.
- Differentiate task-related touch from affective touch.
- List situations in which affective touch may be appropriate.

SECTION I: ASSESSING YOUR UNDERSTANDING

Activity A FILL IN THE BLANKS

1. A nurse–client _____ is established between the nurse and the client when nursing services are provided.

2. Nurses use _____ (an intuitive awareness of what a client is experiencing) to perceive the client's emotional state and need for support.

3. _____ occurs when the nurse and the physician share information and exchange findings with other health care workers as well as when the nurse responsible for managing care delegates care.

4. A _____ is one who assigns a task to someone; they must know what tasks are legal and appropriate for particular health care workers to perform.

5. The nurse–client relationship can be called a _____ relationship because the desired outcome of the association is almost always improving health.

6. The relationship between a client and the nurse begins with the _____ phase, the period of getting acquainted.

7. _____ communication or body language is the exchange of information without using words.

8. _____ refers to vocal sounds that are not actually words but communicate a message.

9. _____ is an activity that includes attending to and becoming fully involved in what the client says.

10. The _____ phase of the nurse–client relationship is a period when the relationship comes to an end and the nurse and client agree that the client's immediate health problems have improved.

Activity B   *Consider the following figure.*

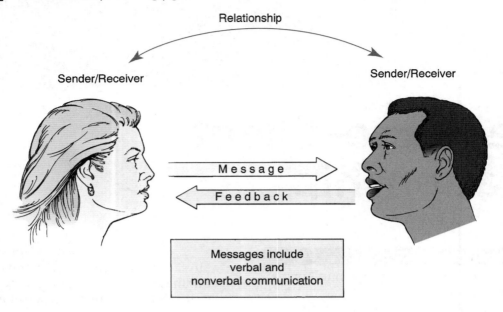

1. What is meant by therapeutic verbal communication?
2. What is the role of active listening in therapeutic communication?

Activity C   *Match the techniques of communication in Column A with their description in Column B.*

Column A	Column B
____ **1.** Kinesics	**a.** Vocal sounds that are not actually words but communicate a message
____ **2.** Silence	
____ **3.** Proxemics	**b.** Body language that includes nonverbal techniques such as facial expressions, posture, gestures, and body movements
____ **4.** Touch	
____ **5.** Paralanguage	
	c. Tactile stimulus produced by making personal contact with another person or object
	d. Use and relationship of space to communication
	e. Intentional withholding of verbal commentary

Activity D   *Presented here, in random order, are steps that occur during a client's stay in the hospital. Write the correct sequence in the boxes provided.*

1. Admission to the nursing unit
2. Discharge from the unit
3. Treatment and recovery
4. Diagnosis of the disease condition

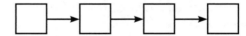

Activity E   *Briefly answer the following questions.*

1. What are the various roles of a nurse?

  _____

  _____

  _____

2. What is meant by a therapeutic relationship?

  _____

  _____

  _____

  _____

3. What are the phases of a nurse–client relationship?

_____

_____

_____

4. What are the factors that affect the ability to communicate by speech or in writing?

_____

_____

_____

5. What is nonverbal communication?

_____

_____

_____

SECTION II: APPLYING YOUR KNOWLEDGE

Activity F *Therapeutic verbal communication refers to using words and gestures to accomplish a particular objective. It is extremely important, especially when the nurse is exploring problems with the client or encouraging expression of feelings. Answer the following questions, which involve the nurse's role when communicating with the client.*

A client is informed by the physician that their leg needs to be amputated because of a diabetic ulcer. The client is distraught and begins to cry. They are angry and blame the nursing staff for the amputation.

1. How should the nurse handle the client at this stage?

_____

_____

_____

2. What should be the nurse's action to help the client deal with their loss?

_____

_____

_____

SECTION III: PRACTICING FOR NCLEX

Activity G *Answer the following questions.*

1. A nurse is caring for a client who is recovering from a cerebrovascular accident. The nurse discovers that the client has become irritable and angry because their activities are limited. What is the best nursing approach to keep the client motivated?

   a. Ignore the behavior, knowing that the client is grieving
   b. Use supportive statements to correct the client's behavior
   c. Allow frequent and longer visits by family members
   d. Tell the client that they know how the client feels

2. A postoperative client has been vomiting. The physician diagnoses them as having paralytic ileus and advises the insertion of a nasogastric tube. The nurse explains the purpose and the procedure to the client. The client expresses that they are fed up with the treatment and cannot take it any longer. What would be the most appropriate nursing response?

   a. "If you don't have this tube inserted, you will keep on vomiting."
   b. "You have every right to refuse the treatment. Shall I call the physician?"
   c. "Get this nasogastric tube inserted and you will feel a lot better."
   d. "Are you feeling tired and frustrated with your recovery from surgery?"

3. A client is admitted to a health care facility with bowel obstruction secondary to Crohn disease and is scheduled for surgery. They are concerned if surgery will cure their condition permanently. What is the most appropriate therapeutic statement?

   a. "Let us give this surgery a chance. You may improve."
   b. "You have every right to refuse surgery. Shall I call the physician?"
   c. "Are you wondering if this surgery will work for you?"
   d. "I have seen a similar case that was cured by surgery."

4. A new parent is trying to decide whether to circumcise their baby boy. What is the most appropriate statement from the nurse to help the parents decide about the circumcision?

    a. "Read this pamphlet and then we can talk if you have any doubts."
    b. "The physician is the best person to give advice about circumcision."
    c. "I got my son circumcised without any problem and he is healthy now."
    d. "I would certainly recommend it, because it prevents cancer and sexually transmitted diseases."

5. A nurse in a neonatal intensive care unit is caring for a newborn diagnosed with neonatal jaundice. Which statement by the nurse is most appropriate for the situation?

    a. "The baby is very sick and the next 24 hours are crucial for the baby."
    b. "The baby care unit has all the necessary equipment to take care of the baby."
    c. "Ask me any questions that you have regarding baby care."
    d. "This is common in neonates, so you should not worry."

6. A school nurse is conducting a health education program for high school children about sexually transmitted diseases. What should be the nurse's opening statement to encourage student participation?

    a. The objective of the session is to learn about sexually transmitted diseases.
    b. Feel free to share your personal experience with the class to learn more.
    c. At the end of the class, everyone should fill out a questionnaire survey form.
    d. The topic is very personal, so whatever we discuss here will be kept confidential.

7. A client confides to the nurse that they know they are going to die and really wish their family would stop hoping for a cure. They feel angry and frustrated when they see their family trying to be helpful. Which statement is the best therapeutic response?

    a. "We should talk more about your anger toward your family."
    b. "You feel angry that your family hopes for your cure?"
    c. "It sounds as if you are being very pessimistic."
    d. "Have you shared your feelings with your family?"

8. A nurse is caring for a senior client. The client tells the nurse that they would rather speak to the physician than talk to a mere nurse. What should be the nurse's immediate response?

    a. "I am your nurse, not your servant."
    b. "Would you prefer to speak to your physician?"
    c. "I will leave you now and call your physician."
    d. "Your physician has placed you in my hands."

9. A teenage client tells the nurse that they are unhappy with themselves because they are unable to do anything right. What should be the nurse's appropriate response?

    a. "You don't do anything right?"
    b. "You always do things right."
    c. "Everything will get better."
    d. "You must be holding up well."

10. A client with suicidal thoughts admits to the nurse that they do not find any reason to live and would like to end it all. Which response would help the nurse to assess the client further?

    a. "Did you sleep well last night?"
    b. "Tell me what you mean by that."
    c. "I am sure your family cares for you."
    d. "I know you had a stressful night."

11. A nurse is caring for a toddler who has recovered from a seizure. The mother is worried that the seizure may recur. What is the most therapeutic statement?

    a. "Most children will never experience a second seizure."
    b. "Medicines can prevent the occurrence of seizures."
    c. "Why worry about something that you cannot control?"
    d. "Tell me more about what frightens you about seizures."

12. A client expresses to the nurse that the physician purposely provided wrong information about their physical condition. Which statement by the nurse would *prevent* effective communication?

    a. "I am not sure what information you are referring to."
    b. "I am certain that the physician would not lie to you."
    c. "Do you want to talk to the physician again to clarify issues?"
    d. "Describe the information to which you are referring."

13. The nurse is caring for a client who is in depression and expresses that they wish to die because they feel like a failure. What would be the best therapeutic response?

    a. "Have you been feeling like a failure for some time now?"
    b. "I see a lot of positive things in you."
    c. "It is the result of your illness that you feel this way."
    d. "You have so many purposes in life to live for."

14. A client who has been diagnosed with renal failure asks the nurse if the diagnosis means that they will die soon. What should be the nurse's immediate response?

    a. "You will do just fine."
    b. "What are you thinking about?"
    c. "You sound discouraged today."
    d. "Death is a beautiful experience."

15. A nurse is caring for a client with urticaria and pruritus. The client expresses their concern because they are getting married within a week. They are worried about having rashes and itching. What would be the nurse's most appropriate response?

    a. "The medications will help a lot to reduce the rashes."
    b. "You are worried that this will extend into your marriage?"
    c. "It is probably just the result of pre-wedding tension."
    d. "I hope that your fiancé is aware of it."

SECTION IV: REVIEWING WHAT YOU HAVE LEARNED

Activity H *Fill in the blanks by choosing the correct word from the options given in parentheses.*

1. _____ includes nonverbal components such as facial expressions, posture, gestures, and body movements. (Kinesics, Paralanguage, Proxemics)

2. _____ is the technique of restating what the client has said to demonstrate listening. (Paraphrasing, Reflecting, Structuring)

Activity I *Mark each statement as either T (True) or F (False). Correct any false statements.*

1. T F Health teaching promotes the client's ability to meet their health needs independently.

2. T F Therapeutic verbal communication involves the use of words alone to accomplish a particular objective.

3. T F Silence is a form of therapeutic communication that encourages the client to participate in verbal discussions.

Activity J *Write the correct term for each description below.*

1. Nursing role that involves assigning a task, checking on completion of that task, and evaluating the outcome _____

2. Person who performs health-related activities that a sick person cannot perform independently _____

Activity K *Match the phases of the nurse–client relationship in Column A with the descriptions of what happens during those phases in Column B.*

Column A

____ 1. Introductory phase

____ 2. Working phase

____ 3. Terminating phase

Column B

a. The nurse and client plan and implement the client's care.

b. The nurse and client mutually agree that the client's immediate health problems have improved.

c. The client identifies one or more health problems for which they are seeking help.

Activity L *Answer the following questions.*

1. How does task-oriented touch differ from affective touch?

    _____

    _____

    _____

2. What factors affect the ability to communicate by speech or in writing?

_____

_____

_____

SECTION V: APPLYING YOUR KNOWLEDGE

Activity M *Give a rationale for the following question.*

Why is the nurse–client relationship called a therapeutic relationship?

_____

_____

_____

Activity N *Answer the following questions focusing on nursing roles and responsibilities.*

A nurse at an extended-care facility is caring for a client with impaired hearing who has undergone knee surgery.

1. How might the nurse approach teaching for this client?

_____

_____

_____

A young male client is bedridden with limited use of his arms following a motorcycle accident. A female nurse needs to assist this client with activities of daily living, such as bathing and shaving.

2. What actions can the nurse take to prevent the client from misinterpreting physical nearness and hands-on nursing procedures as sexual advances?

_____

_____

_____

3. Why should nurses use affective touch cautiously?

_____

_____

_____

Activity O *Think over the following questions. Discuss them with your instructor or peers.*

A nurse is caring for a middle-aged client who has been diagnosed with cancer. The client is worried about the expenses involved in treatment, their future, and their dependent family members.

1. How can the nurse begin to build a therapeutic relationship with this client?

_____

_____

_____

2. What communication techniques should the nurse use with this client?

_____

_____

_____

SECTION VI: GETTING READY FOR NCLEX

Activity P *Answer the following questions.*

1. A nurse is caring for a senior client who lives alone and is recovering from a fall. The client is in severe pain and angry that the fall could have been avoided if someone else had been at home. Which response by the nurse is most appropriate?

a. Ask why the client is living alone

b. Allow the client to express emotions

c. Ask the client to stop complaining

d. Tell the client to stay calm and take pain medication

2. A nurse is teaching an American-born client about a medication regimen. What is the appropriate distance that the nurse should maintain from the client during teaching?

a. 12 or more feet

b. 4 to 12 feet

c. 6 inches to 4 feet

d. 6 inches or less

Client Teaching

Learning Objectives

- Identify the authoritative bases that mandate client teaching.
- List examples of client teaching provided by nurses.
- List five benefits of client teaching.
- Identify factors that nurses assess before teaching clients.
- Describe the three domains of learning.
- Discuss age-related categories of learners.
- Discuss characteristics unique to older adult learners.

SECTION I: ASSESSING YOUR UNDERSTANDING

Activity A   FILL IN THE BLANKS

1. To implement effective teaching, the nurse must determine the client's _____, or purpose for acquiring new information.

2. Client teaching generally focuses on a combination of subjects such as _____ instructions and rehabilitation programs.

3. Twenty percent of Americans are considered _____ illiterate (possess minimal literacy skills), which means they can sign their name and perform simple mathematical tasks but read at or below fifth-grade level.

4. The best teaching and learning takes place when both are _____ to meet the client's needs.

5. _____ care refers to visiting clients electronically in their home for the purpose of seeing and communicating in real time.

6. _____ is optimal when a person has a purpose for acquiring new information.

7. _____ teaching is unplanned and occurs spontaneously at the bedside.

8. Learning depends on a person's _____ and developmental level.

9. "_____ generation" or "Generation Z" refers to those born at the beginning of the 21st century.

10. For the person to receive, remember, analyze, and apply new information, they must have a _____ to learn, that is, a certain amount of intellectual ability.

Activity B   *Consider the following figure.*

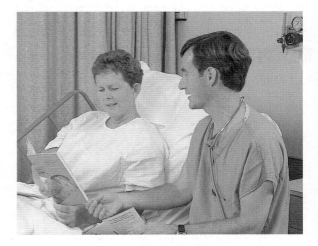

1. Identify the style of learning from the figure.

   _____

   _____

   _____

2. What are the other styles of learning?

_____

_____

_____

Activity C *Match the learning styles in column A with their description in column B.*

Column A

____ **1.** Cognitive

____ **2.** Affective

____ **3.** Psychomotor

Column B

a. It means learning using feelings, beliefs, or values.

b. It means learning by doing.

c. It means learning by listening or reading facts and descriptions.

Activity D *A client visits a health care facility for a session on blood sugar testing. Presented here, in random order, are steps that the nurse should perform before and during the session. Write the correct sequence of the steps in the boxes provided.*

1. Show how to take the test to evaluate the blood sugar level.

2. Demonstrate the blood sugar test on a client.

3. Create charts and diagrams.

4. Explain why the blood sugar level increases.

5. Plan how to make the session effective.

☐ → ☐ → ☐ → ☐ → ☐

Activity E *Briefly answer the following questions.*

1. Explain briefly the stages of learning.

_____

_____

_____

2. What should the nurse keep in mind while implementing effective teaching to a client?

_____

_____

_____

3. What is meant by learning styles? Describe briefly the three styles of learning.

_____

_____

_____

4. Describe briefly the science involved in teaching learners of different age groups.

_____

_____

_____

5. Describe briefly the three types of age groups. What are the common learning characteristics for people born in the computer age?

_____

_____

_____

6. How do you define functionally illiterate? Give an example.

_____

_____

_____

SECTION II: APPLYING YOUR KNOWLEDGE

Activity F *Teaching is one of the most important uses of communication for nurses. Health teaching promotes the client's ability to independently meet their health needs. Answer the following questions, which involve the nurse's role in the health teaching of the client.*

A client brought to a health care facility with symptoms of food poisoning has been asked by the physician to get admitted for observation and treatment. The nurse who is caring for the client has been asked to teach them ways to achieve a healthy lifestyle.

1. What question should the nurse ask to assess the learning of the client?

_____

_____

_____

2. What points should the nurse include to ensure complete health teaching before the discharge of the client?

_____

_____

_____

SECTION III: PRACTICING FOR NCLEX

Activity G _Answer the following questions._

1. A nurse is caring for a client with influenza and is imparting health teaching to the client. Which action will help the client retain the key points of the teaching?

  a. The nurse helps the client in self-administration of medications

  b. The nurse gives the client a pamphlet on how to clear nasal debris

  c. The nurse shows the client how to measure body temperature

  d. The nurse explains how to use a nebulizer mask

2. A nurse, caring for a 45-year-old client, observes that the client has very low motivation and feels that they cannot be cured. Which learning style is best suited for the client?

  a. Cognitive domain

  b. Affective domain

  c. Psychomotor domain

  d. Interpersonal domain

3. A nurse is caring for a client who has to undergo hip surgery in a week. The nurse observes that the client likes to watch videos and demonstrations, and is an avid reader. Which learning style is best suited for the client?

  a. Cognitive domain

  b. Affective domain

  c. Psychomotor domain

  d. Interpersonal domain

4. A nurse is teaching a diabetic client the self-administration of insulin. The nurse shows the client how to hold the syringe and read the calibration. What is this learning style a part of?

  a. Cognitive domain

  b. Affective domain

  c. Psychomotor domain

  d. Interpersonal domain

5. A nurse is caring for an 8-year-old client who has been admitted to a health care facility with tonsillitis. Which teaching method should the nurse use for this client?

  a. Show enthusiasm

  b. Use colorful materials

  c. Vary tone and pitch

  d. Use the client's name frequently

6. A 25-year-old client has been admitted to a health care facility for hernioplasty. Which teaching method is best suited for the client?

  a. Limit the teaching session to 15 to 20 minutes

  b. Offer praise and encouragement for accomplishments

  c. Provide the client total attention

  d. Assess previous learning and literacy abilities of the client

7. A 73-year-old client has been admitted to a health care facility with abdominal pain. Which teaching method is best suited for the client?

  a. Involve the client during the teaching session to impart learning

  b. Implement the teaching session when the client is most alert and comfortable

  c. Use diagrams to aid teaching during the teaching session

  d. Motivate the client to understand the importance and benefits of the session

8. A nurse is caring for a 65-year-old client with symptoms of an eye infection. Which teaching strategy will best promote health teaching for this client?

  a. Obtain pamphlets in large print

  b. Speak in a louder tone

  c. Use flash cards

  d. Select red print on white paper

9. While teaching an adult client how to self-administer insulin, which strategy is the best choice to implement health teaching?

  a. Collaborate with the client on content

  b. Determine the client's learning style

  c. Begin with basic concepts

  d. Divide information into manageable amounts

10. A nurse involves an adult client actively in health teaching by encouraging feedback and handling of equipment. In which phase should this activity take place?

    a. Assessment
    b. Planning
    c. Implementation
    d. Evaluation

11. A nurse observes that a client's behavior consists of the following features: supporting, accepting, refusing, and defending. In which learning domain does the client's learning style fall?

    a. Cognitive domain
    b. Affective domain
    c. Psychomotor domain
    d. Interpersonal domain

12. A nurse motivates a client and promises a reward when the client can name the number of recommended servings in each category within the food pyramid. To which age category does the client likely belong?

    a. Child
    b. Adult
    c. Older adult
    d. Net Generation

13. A nurse is caring for a client from Generation Y. Which learning characteristic do clients from Generation Y share with Generation X and the Net Generation?

    a. Craving for stimulation and quick response
    b. Enthusiastic about performing repetitive tasks
    c. Preference for verbal or practical methods of participatory learning
    d. Avoidance of choosing a variety of instructional methods

14. When teaching a client the benefits of following proper toilet hygiene, the nurse observes that the client is fatigued, has low energy levels, and is not able to pay proper attention to the health teaching. Which age category does the client likely belong to?

    a. Child
    b. Adult
    c. Older adult
    d. Net Generation

15. When a nurse asks a client what they want to accomplish at the end of the health training, what aspect of learning is being assessed by the nurse?

    a. Preferred learning style
    b. Capacity to learn
    c. Learning readiness
    d. Learning needs

16. A nurse is caring for a 7-year-old client. What are the characteristics of a pedagogic learner? Select all that apply.

    a. Lack of experience
    b. Physically mature
    c. Rote learning
    d. Responds to competition
    e. Crisis learner

17. A nurse is caring for a 73-year-old client who has been admitted to a health care facility with a slipped disk. What are the characteristics of a gerogogic learner? Select all that apply.

    a. Vast experience
    b. Learning is self-centered
    c. Needs direction and supervision
    d. Responds to family encouragement
    e. Long-term retention

18. A nurse is caring for a 40-year-old client who has been diagnosed with asthma. What are the characteristics of an androgogic learner? Select all that apply.

    a. Vast experience
    b. Prefers simulation
    c. Needs direction and supervision
    d. Responds to family encouragement
    e. Long-term retention
    f. Physically mature

19. A nurse is caring for a 5-year-old client with diarrhea. Which teaching styles are best suited for this client? Select all that apply.

    a. Show enthusiasm
    b. Use colorful materials
    c. Vary tone and pitch
    d. Use the client's name frequently
    e. Limit the teaching session to 15 to 20 minutes
    f. Offer praise and encouragement for accomplishments
    g. Assess previous learning and literacy abilities

SECTION IV: REVIEWING WHAT YOU HAVE LEARNED

Activity H *Fill in the blanks by choosing the correct word from the options given in parentheses.*

1. The _____ domain is a learning style through which information is presented in such a way as to appeal to a person's feelings, beliefs, or values. (affective, cognitive, psychomotor)
2. Learning _____ refers to the client's current physical and psychological well-being. (readiness, style, ability)

Activity I *Mark each statement as either T (True) or F (False). Correct any false statements.*

1. **T F** Health teaching promotes the client's ability to meet their health needs independently.

2. **T F** People belonging to Generation X are technologically literate, having grown up with computers.

Activity J *Write the correct term for each description below.*

1. Learning style in which a person processes information by listening or reading facts and descriptions _____
2. Science of teaching children or those with cognitive ability comparable to that of children _____

Activity K *Match the terms in column A with their descriptions in column B.*

Column A	Column B
____ **1.** Psychomotor domain	**a.** The principle of teaching adult learners
____ **2.** Androgogy	**b.** A style of processing information that focuses on learning by doing
____ **3.** Gerogogy	**c.** A term given to a person who possesses minimal literacy skills
____ **4.** Functionally illiterate	**d.** A technique that enhances learning in older adults

Activity L *Differentiate between informal and formal teaching based on the components listed below.*

1. Definition
2. Requirements
3. Disadvantages

Activity M *Consider the following figure.*

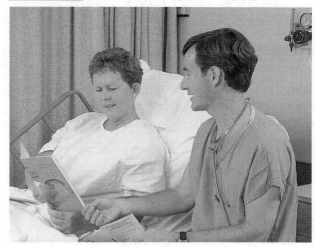

1. Identify what is happening in the figure shown above.
2. What learning style might this client prefer?

Activity N *Limited hospitalization time demands that nurses begin teaching as soon as possible after admission rather than waiting until discharge. Early attention to the client's educational needs is essential because learning takes place in four progressive stages. Write down the correct sequence of the progressive stages of learning in the boxes below:*

1. Using new learning independently
2. Recalling or describing information to others
3. Recognizing what has been taught
4. Explaining or applying information

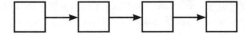

Activity O *Answer the following questions.*

1. What subject areas should the nurse focus on when teaching a client?

_____

_____

_____

2. How can the nurse implement effective teaching?

_____

_____

_____

SECTION V: APPLYING YOUR KNOWLEDGE

Activity P   *Give a rationale for the following question.*

Why should a nurse select black print on white paper when providing instructions to a visually impaired client?

_____

_____

Activity Q   *A nurse at a dermatology clinic is caring for a 12-year-old child who has just had a cyst removed from the soft tissue on their forearm.*

1. What important first step should the nurse follow after the surgical procedure?

_____

_____

_____

2. Describe skin care techniques that the nurse should explain to this client.

_____

_____

_____

Activity R   *Think over the following questions. Discuss them with your instructor or peers.*

A nurse is caring for three clients in a health care facility:

- A functionally illiterate senior man who has undergone cataract surgery
- A 58-year-old woman with diabetes who has undergone hand amputation
- An 18-year-old Asian American girl who cannot speak English and has to learn how to use a hearing aid

1. How can the nurse determine each client's preferred learning style and developmental level?

_____

_____

_____

2. How should the nurse provide teaching to these clients?

_____

_____

_____

3. What kind of processes or techniques should the nurse follow?

_____

_____

_____

SECTION VI: GETTING READY FOR NCLEX

Activity S   *Answer the following questions.*

1. A nurse is caring for a client who uses prescription eyeglasses for reading. Which action facilitates the reading process for this client?

- **a.** Provide pamphlets in 12- to 16-point type and serif lettering
- **b.** Provide teaching material printed on glossy paper
- **c.** Ensure that the room is well lit by a ceiling light
- **d.** Stand in front of a window letting in bright sunlight

2. A nurse tailors teaching for a 10-year-old client who is learning to walk with crutches. Which characteristics of pedagogic learners would the nurse keep in mind? Select all that apply.

- **a.** Need direction and supervision
- **b.** Need immediate feedback
- **c.** Think abstractly
- **d.** Learn analytically
- **e.** Respond to competition

CHAPTER 9

Recording and Reporting

Learning Objectives

- Identify uses for medical records.
- List components generally found in any client's medical record.
- List legally defensible characteristics of written charting.
- Differentiate between source-oriented records and problem-oriented records.
- Identify methods of charting.
- List advantages and disadvantages of an electronic medical record.
- Explain the purpose and applications associated with the Health Insurance Portability and Accountability Act (HIPAA).
- List aspects of documentation required in the medical records of all clients cared for in acute settings.
- Discuss why it is important to use only approved abbreviations when charting.
- Explain how to convert traditional time to military time.
- Identify written forms used to communicate information about clients.
- List ways that health care workers exchange client information other than by reading the medical record.

SECTION I: ASSESSING YOUR UNDERSTANDING

Activity A FILL IN THE BLANKS

1. When writing source-oriented records, a _____ style of charting is generally used.

2. _____ electronic charting is most useful for nurses when a terminal is available at the point of care or at the bedside.

3. _____ time is based on a 24-hour clock.

4. Charting by exception is a method in which nurses chart only _____ assessment findings or care that deviates from a standard norm.

5. The _____ legislation was introduced to ensure the privacy of health records and to protect the rights of US citizens to retain their health insurance when changing employment.

6. Auditors examine client medical records to determine whether the care provided meets established criteria for _____.

7. _____ charting is a modified form of SOAP charting.

8. Nurses use _____ to avoid document-ing types of care that are regularly repeated.

9. When agencies can release private health information without the client's prior autho-rization, it is called _____ disclosures.

10. According to HIPAA rules, client information is _____ when transmitting via the Internet.

Activity B   *Consider the following figure.*

1. Identify the figure.

   _____

   _____

   _____

2. Explain the need for this procedure.

   _____

   _____

   _____

Activity C   *Match the methods of charting in Column A with their features in Column B.*

Column A

_____ **1.** Narrative

_____ **2.** SOAP

_____ **3.** Compu-terized

_____ **4.** PIE

_____ **5.** Charting by exception

Column B

a. Recording the client's progress under the head-ings of problem, interven-tion, and evaluation

b. Writing information about the client and client care in chronologic order

c. Documenting style more likely to be used in prob-lem-oriented records

d. Documenting abnormal assessment findings

e. Documenting the client information electronically

Activity D   *Presented here, in random order, are steps taken by a nurse when exchanging information using the telephone. Write the correct sequence in the boxes provided.*

1. Identifies themselves by name, title, and nursing unit
2. Obtains or states the reason for the call
3. Repeats information to ensure it has been heard accurately
4. Answers as promptly as possible

☐ → ☐ → ☐ → ☐

Activity E   *Briefly answer the following questions.*

1. What are the reasons for maintaining a medi-cal record?

   _____

   _____

   _____

2. What evidence does the Joint Commission need in order to provide a health care facility with accreditation?

   _____

   _____

   _____

3. How is a medical record maintained and who is responsible for maintaining the records?

   _____

   _____

   _____

4. What measures should a nurse take when documenting a medical record?

   _____

   _____

   _____

5. What are the different methods of communi-cating a client's health-related details to other personnel of the agency?

   _____

   _____

   _____

SECTION II: APPLYING YOUR KNOWLEDGE

Activity F   *Many health care facilities maintain computerized health records for their clients. Answer the following question, which involves a nurse's role in keeping client health records confidential.*

A nurse at a health care facility uses the computer to store the health records for all the clients. All nurses caring for a particular client and using the system are required to ensure that the records are confidential.

1. What care should the nurse take to ensure that these data are not available to unauthorized personnel and are not misused?

   _____

   _____

   _____

SECTION III: PRACTICING FOR NCLEX

Activity G   *Answer the following questions.*

1. A nurse documents information about a client and client care in chronologic order in the format resembling a log. What method of documentation is the nurse using in this case?

   a. SOAP charting
   b. Narrative charting
   c. PIE charting
   d. Focus charting

2. A nurse needs to access a client's data stored on a computer by a colleague. What would the nurse enter into the computer to begin the process?

   a. Password
   b. User name
   c. Employee identification (ID)
   d. Name

3. A nurse caring for a client documents information regarding health care in the medical record. For what reason can the medical record be used without the client's permission?

   a. Sharing information among the client's health care personnel
   b. Sharing information with personnel involved in research

   c. Sharing the client's health condition with the client's relatives
   d. Sharing the client's health condition with insurance agencies

4. A nurse involved in a malpractice lawsuit obtains information on a particular client to provide evidence of the health care provided. What method should the nurse use to obtain this patient data?

   a. Calling the client's nurse for verification
   b. Checking with other staff members
   c. Checking the nursing Kardex
   d. Calling the client's physician for verification

5. A nurse who has just taken charge in a shift is caring for a client who complains of severe pain in the abdomen. What measure should the nurse take prior to administering any medication to the client?

   a. Ask the client when they last took pain medication
   b. Check the medical record for details of medication
   c. Provide medication as requested by the client
   d. Check for the severity of pain experienced by the client

6. An officer from the Joint Commission is visiting a community health clinic. What is a possible reason for the officer's visit?

   a. To discuss career plans with clinic staff
   b. To discuss an employee-related medical problem
   c. To inspect the health care agency for the level of facilities provided
   d. To inspect the health care agency for evidence of quality care

7. A nurse in a health care facility is caring for a client diagnosed with hypertension. The client's family observes the nurse diligently maintaining the health record and asks why a health record is used. What is an appropriate response by the nurse?

   a. It verifies care through quality assurance programs
   b. It helps in employment and disability applications
   c. It helps in providing safe and effective care
   d. It helps in meeting standards of care set by the government

8. A nurse caring for clients in an acute-care facility accurately documents patient data on the medical records to ensure reimbursement from insurance companies. For what reason might the insurance company deny this reimbursement?

    a. Absence of health care personnel signatures
    b. Documents shared with family
    c. Documents shared with researchers
    d. Presence of abbreviated instructions

9. A nurse documenting patient data uses a format that contains separate forms on which each member of the health care team documents their own patient care activities. Which method of data organization is the clinic following?

    a. Problem-oriented records
    b. Source-oriented records
    c. PIE charting records
    d. Focus charting records

10. Nurses at a health agency compile and arrange all the client information according to the client's health problems. They also emphasize goal-directed care to promote recording of pertinent information and to facilitate communication among health care professionals. Which method of data organization is this?

    a. Problem-oriented records
    b. Source-oriented records
    c. Narrative charting
    d. Computerized charting

11. A nurse records client data under four different components—the data base, the problem list, the plan of care, and progress notes—and stores all these records in one location. Which style of data recording is this?

    a. Focus charting
    b. SOAP charting
    c. Narrative charting
    d. PIE charting

12. A nurse uses the PIE charting method for recording the information about a client. What nursing action would be included in this format?

    a. The nurse gives the client's listed problems corresponding numbers
    b. The nurse documents assessments on one form

    c. The nurse makes entries in the same location in the chart
    d. The nurse organizes data according to the client's health problems

13. A health agency has been providing health care to multiple clients for more than 6 months and applies to the Joint Commission for accreditation. What measures should be taken to ensure accreditation? Select all that apply.

    a. The medical records should show the nursing diagnoses or client needs
    b. The number of people working in the health agency should be more than 50
    c. The nursing standards of care for meeting client nursing care needs should be planned
    d. The latest equipment should be available to treat all kinds of health issues
    e. Client response to interventions and outcomes of care for pain management should be recorded

14. A health agency is following the computerized charting method to store data electronically. What are the advantages of this charting method? Select all that apply.

    a. It automatically records the date and time of the documentation
    b. It reduces overtime costs for uncompleted end-of-shift charting
    c. The expense of purchasing a computer system is minimal
    d. The abbreviations and terms are consistent with agency-approved lists
    e. Electronic data require less storage space and are quickly retrievable

15. The nurse notes that a medication order for a client states "a.c." When or how would the nurse administer this medication based on this abbreviation?

    a. Before meals
    b. After meals
    c. By mouth
    d. At bedtime

16. A medical record states that the client has had their last medication at 2:00 PM. The nurse needs to enter this detail in the computer. How should the nurse document this information in military time?

    a. 1400 hours
    b. 1600 hours
    c. 1800 hours
    d. 2000 hours

SECTION IV: REVIEWING WHAT YOU HAVE LEARNED

Activity H *Fill in the blanks by choosing the correct word from the options given in parentheses.*

1. Charting by exception is a documentation method in which nurses chart only _____ assessment findings. (abnormal, physical, psychological)

2. The nursing _____ is a quick reference for current information about the client and their care. (checklist, Kardex, care plan)

3. _____ charting follows a data, action, response (DAR) model to reflect the steps in the nursing process. (Exception, Flow, Focus)

Activity I *Mark each statement as either T (True) or F (False). Correct any false statements.*

1. T F PIE charting is a method of recording the client's progress under the headings of patient, implementation, and education.

2. T F A change-of-shift report is a discussion between a nurse from a shift that is ending and the personnel coming on duty.

Activity J *Write the correct term for each description below.*

1. Written collections of information about a person's health, the care provided by health practitioners, and the client's progress _____

2. Method of documentation that involves writing information about the client and their care in chronologic order _____

Activity K *Differentiate between source-oriented records and problem-oriented records based on the items listed below.*

1. Definition
2. Components

Activity L

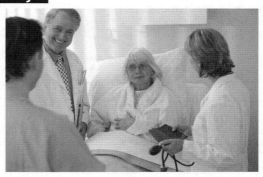

1. Identify what is happening in the figure shown above.

   _____

   _____

   _____

2. What are the benefits of this activity?

   _____

   _____

   _____

Activity M *Answer the following questions.*

1. What are the seven uses of medical records?

   _____

   _____

   _____

2. What are the steps for converting traditional time into military time?

   _____

   _____

   _____

SECTION V: APPLYING YOUR KNOWLEDGE

Activity N *Give rationales for the following questions.*

1. Why should the nurse document information they have taught and evidence demonstrating the client's understanding?

   _____

   _____

   _____

2. Why is it important for nurses to follow their agency's documentation policy?

_____

_____

_____

3. Why do some health care agencies use military time instead of traditional time?

_____

_____

_____

Activity O *Answer the following questions focusing on nursing roles and responsibilities.*

A nurse caring for multiple clients in a health care facility has completed shift duties and is preparing to leave for the day.

1. How should the nurse proceed when completing a shift and preparing to leave the facility?

_____

_____

_____

2. What actions should the nurse receiving the shift report take to ensure maximum efficiency during this process?

_____

_____

_____

A physician returns a nurse's call about a change in a client's health condition.

3. What actions should the nurse take when answering the telephone and reporting the client's condition?

_____

_____

_____

4. What information should the nurse document following communication with the physician?

_____

_____

_____

Activity P *Think over the following questions. Discuss them with your instructor or peers.*

A nurse is working at a health care facility that has a computer terminal at every client's bedside. The nurse is required to use computerized charting for each client.

1. What actions should the nurse take when completing computerized charting?

_____

_____

_____

2. What are the advantages and disadvantages of this documentation system?

_____

_____

_____

SECTION VI: GETTING READY FOR NCLEX

Activity Q

1. A nurse is caring for a client undergoing treatment following a stroke. The nurse needs to document routine care, such as bathing and oral hygiene. Which form should the nurse use to document this care?

   a. Kardex
   b. Flow sheet
   c. Care plan
   d. Checklist

2. A nurse is caring for a client who cannot have any food or oral fluids for 4 hours before the scheduled surgery. Which abbreviation should the nurse note on the client's chart?

   a. AMA
   b. NKA
   c. NPO
   d. NSS

CHAPTER 10

Asepsis

Learning Objectives

- Describe microorganisms.
- Name and describe specific types of microorganisms.
- Differentiate between nonpathogens and pathogens and between aerobic and anaerobic microorganisms.
- Give examples of the ways some microorganisms have adapted for their survival.
- Name the components of the chain of infection.
- Cite examples of biologic defense mechanisms.
- Define health care–associated infection.
- Discuss the concept of asepsis.
- Differentiate between medical and surgical asepsis.
- Identify principles of medical asepsis.
- List examples of medical aseptic practices.
- Name techniques for sterilizing equipment.
- Identify principles of surgical asepsis.
- List nursing activities that require application of the principles of surgical asepsis.

SECTION I: ASSESSING YOUR UNDERSTANDING

Activity A   FILL IN THE BLANKS

1. The most effective method for preventing infections is _____, an essential nursing activity that must be performed repeatedly when caring for clients.

2. _____, commonly called germs, are living animals or plants that are visible only with a microscope.

3. _____, or normal flora, live abundantly and perpetually on and in the human body, which is their host.

4. Pathogens have _____, which are tiny hairs that prevent pathogens from being eliminated during urination.

5. Pathogens may cause _____ when the host is immunosuppressed from acquired immune deficiency syndrome (AIDS), chemotherapy, or steroid drug therapy.

6. The three types of fungal (mycotic) infections are superficial, intermediate, and _____.

7. Helminths are classified into three major groups: nematodes, trematodes, and _____.

8. A _____, the last link in the chain of infection, is one whose biologic defense mechanisms are weakened in some way.

9. Before each use of a sterile solution, a nurse pours and discards a small amount from the mouth of the container to wash away airborne contaminants in a process called _____ the container.

Activity B   *Consider the following figure.*

A   B   C
_____   _____   _____

1. Identify and label the figure. Give the scientific names for each.

_____

_____

_____

2. What are the two types of bacteria?

_____

_____

_____

3. Which type of drug is used most often to combat bacterial infections?

_____

_____

_____

Activity C   *Match the garments health care personnel don in Column A with their functions and features in Column B.*

Column A

____ 1. Gloves

____ 2. Hair and shoe covers

____ 3. Protective eyewear

____ 4. Clean laboratory coat

____ 5. Scrub suits or gowns

Column B

a. Helps when working in the nursery, operating room, and delivery room; worn during other sterile procedures as well

b. Helps reduce the spread of microorganisms onto or from the surface of clothing worn from home

c. Helps reduce transmission of pathogens present on the hair or shoes; usually worn during surgical or obstetric procedures

d. Helps when there is a potential transfer of microorganisms from one client or object to another client during subsequent nursing care

e. Helps when there is a possibility that body fluids will splash into the eyes

Activity D   *Presented here, in random order, are the six essential components of the chain of infection. In the boxes provided below, write the correct sequence that enables the spread of disease-producing microorganisms from one location or person to another.*

1. A port of entry
2. An infectious agent
3. A mode of transmission
4. A reservoir for growth and reproduction
5. An exit route from the reservoir
6. A susceptible host

□→□→□→□→□→□

Activity E   *Briefly answer the following questions.*

1. What are the factors that influence the development of an infection or an infectious disease in the human body?

_____

_____

_____

2. What are the various types of viruses?

_____

_____

_____

3. What are rickettsiae?

_____

_____

_____

4. What are the classifications of protozoans?

_____

_____

_____

5. Why are mycoplasmas termed "pleomorphic"?

_____

_____

_____

6. Define and list examples of the types of biologic defense mechanisms that exist.

_____

_____

_____

SECTION II: APPLYING YOUR KNOWLEDGE

Activity F *Asepsis means practices to decrease or eliminate infectious agents, their reservoirs, and vehicles for transmission. It is the major method for controlling infection. Answer the following questions that involve the various aspects of asepsis that a nurse should follow while caring for clients.*

A nurse practices medical and surgical asepsis to accomplish care for a client suffering from an infection. There are other clients around who should be protected from the spread of infection.

1. What are the principles or measures the nurse should follow to break the chain of infection?

   _____

   _____

   _____

2. What are antimicrobial agents?

   _____

   _____

   _____

3. Which antimicrobial agents should the nurse use and why? Define the role of each type of agent.

   _____

   _____

   _____

SECTION III: PRACTICING FOR NCLEX

Activity G *Answer the following questions.*

1. A nurse visits a client at their home. At a nearby wash basin, the nurse notices a bar of soap and towel that are shared by the entire family. To prevent the spread of germs and infection, the nurse performs hand antisepsis with an alcohol-based hand rub instead of a hand wash. How would the nurse explain their actions to the family involved in the client's health care?

   a. The hand rub destroys active microorganisms but not spores
   b. The hand rub provides the fastest and greatest reduction in microbial counts on the skin
   c. The hand rub is as effective as using soap and water on visibly soiled hands
   d. The hand rub controls viral replication or release from any infected cells

2. A nurse is preparing to attend an emergency case at a health clinic. Because of lack of time, the nurse follows a faster process of hand antisepsis with an alcohol-based hand rub. What interventions should the nurse follow when decontaminating?

   a. Dip hands in the product for a minimum of 15 seconds
   b. Apply a nickel- to a quarter-size volume of the product
   c. Apply anti-infective drugs to the product
   d. Remove the product from the clean utility room

3. A nurse visits a client with a skin infection at the client's home. What is the most important teaching point for this client?

   a. Apply antiseptics
   b. Apply an antiviral lotion
   c. Stop sharing soaps, towels, and washcloths
   d. Use only sterilized instruments

4. A client is being taken to the labor room with severe contractions. The nurse is preparing to attend the client who may require a cesarean birth. What kind of medical asepsis or cleaning technique should the nurse follow?

   a. Hand washing
   b. Hand antisepsis
   c. Surgical scrub
   d. Sterile technique

5. A nurse manager is checking whether the technique of concurrent disinfection is being carried out appropriately by the housekeeping staff. What is one of the principles of concurrent disinfection that the staff should follow?

   a. Scrub the mattress and the insides of the drawers
   b. Clean the grossly soiled areas before the less dirty ones
   c. Wet-mop the floors and damp-dust the furniture
   d. Boil contaminated equipment for 15 minutes at 212°F (100°C)

6. A nurse puts on examination gloves to attend to a client admitted to a hospital with a severe injury. Latex causes the nurse to suffer from skin rash, flushing, and itching. Which of the

following set of gloves should the nurse wear when handling the client's wounds?

a. A pair of latex gloves
b. A pair of vinyl gloves
c. A double pair of latex gloves
d. A double pair of vinyl gloves

7. A nurse is handling a saline water bottle to sterilize used equipment and syringes. Which intervention should the nurse follow while using the sterile solution?

a. Hold the container below waist level while pouring
b. Keep the cap upside down on a flat surface or hold it during pouring
c. Pour a small amount of solution at a time to avoid contamination
d. Touch only sterile areas within the field

8. A nurse needs to use a new scalpel for an operation. It is important that the nurse checks all the new equipment packages that have arrived in the health agency. Which agency-sterilized surgical instrument should a nurse consider safe from contamination?

a. A partially unwrapped sterile package
b. An item sterilized that is past its expiration date
c. A dry sterile wrapper
d. A wet sterile wrapper

9. A nurse is attending a long-term resident client with an invasive indwelling catheter attached. Which practice should the nurse follow to prevent urinary tract infections?

a. The tubing should always be placed higher than the bladder
b. The tubing should never be placed higher than the bladder
c. The tubing should never be placed at the same level as the bladder
d. The tubing should never be placed lower than the bladder

10. A nurse is attending a 65-year-old client at the client's home. Which practice should the nurse suggest that the client's family follow to prevent the outbreak of any infection?

a. Those 65 years and older should receive an initial dose of the pneumococcal vaccine
b. All family members should wear masks

c. Personal contact with the client should be limited
d. The client and family should take multi-vitamin capsules between meals

11. A nurse is teaching an older female client about the ways to prevent urinary tract infections. Which of the following is the most relevant teaching?

a. Wash and clean from the urinary area back toward the rectal area
b. Use dry tissue to clean the urinary area
c. Maintain dry vaginal skin
d. Wear gloves while cleaning the urinary area

12. There is a sudden outbreak of infections at a health care facility. The nurse in charge is moving clients who are more susceptible to infections immediately to a safer environment. Who should be moved first?

a. Clients admitted for pathologic tests
b. Clients with burn injuries
c. Clients waiting for a surgery
d. Clients who have just given birth

13. A nurse follows a set order when sterilizing all used equipment and syringes. Which techniques should the nurse use to sterilize equipment? Select all that apply.

a. Physical sterilization
b. Chemical-dipped cloth
c. Radiation
d. Boiling water
e. Dry heat

14. A nurse is unwrapping a sterile package that has been delivered to a health care facility. Place the steps that the nurse should follow to unwrap the sterilized items in the sequence in which they should occur.

a. The nurse unwraps the cloth by supporting the wrapped item in one hand
b. The nurse drops the sterile contents onto the sterile field
c. The nurse then holds each of the four corners
d. The nurse separates the flaps
e. The nurse discards the cloth cover
f. The nurse places the unwrapped item on the sterile field

SECTION IV: REVIEWING WHAT YOU HAVE LEARNED

Activity H *Fill in the blanks by choosing the correct word from the options given in parentheses.*

1. _____ bacteria exist without oxygen. (Aerobic, Anaerobic, Mycoplasmic)

2. Tinea corporis is a/an _____ type of fungal infection. (intermediate, superficial, systemic)

Activity I *Mark each statement as either T (True) or F (False). Correct any false statements.*

1. **T F**   A spore is a temporarily inactive microbe that can resist heat and destructive chemicals and survive without moisture.

2. **T F**   Some pathogens have tiny hairs called flagella that enable them to attach to the host's tissue and avoid expulsion.

Activity J *Write the correct term for each description below.*

1. Practices that decrease or eliminate infectious agents, their reservoirs, and their vehicles for transmission _____

2. A haven in which microbes survive, grow, and reproduce _____

Activity K *Match the type of microorganism in Column A with its characteristics in Column B.*

Column A

____ 1. Bacterium

____ 2. Virus

____ 3. Protozoan

____ 4. Prion

Column B

a. Smallest microorganism known to cause infectious disease, visible only with an electron microscope

b. Protein that does not contain nucleic acid

c. Single-celled microorganism; may be round, rod shaped, or spiral

d. Single-celled animal classified according to its ability to move

Activity L *Differentiate between medical asepsis and surgical asepsis based on the components listed below.*

1. Definition
2. Technique
3. Methods of obtaining asepsis

Activity M *Surgical hand antisepsis extensively removes transient microorganisms from the nails, hands, and forearms before an operative procedure. Write in the boxes provided below the correct sequence in which a nurse should perform the actions of a surgical scrub.*

1. Use friction to scrub all surfaces of the hands.
2. Use friction to lather the liquid cleanser.
3. Hold the hands and arms up and away from the body.
4. Put on a mask, hair, and shoe covers.
5. Rinse the lather while keeping the hands above the elbows.
6. Dry hands with a sterile towel.
7. Wet hands to the forearms.
8. Clean under each fingernail.

□→□→□→□→□→□→□→□

Activity N *Answer the following questions.*

1. What is a health health care-associated infections infections?

_____

_____

_____

2. What are the six components of the chain of infection?

_____

_____

_____

SECTION V: APPLYING YOUR KNOWLEDGE

Activity O *Give rationales for the following questions.*

1. Why does the nurse pour out and discard a small amount of sterile solution before each use?

_____

_____

_____

2. Why is it good practice for the nurse to remove chipped or peeling nail polish before working at a health care facility?

_____

_____

_____

Activity P   *Answer the following questions focusing on nursing roles and responsibilities.*

1. A nurse at an extended care facility is caring for a senior client with a hip fracture who has developed pulmonary congestion and respiratory distress during their stay.

    a. What could have caused the pulmonary congestion and respiratory distress?

_____

_____

_____

    b. What care should the nurse take to prevent nosocomial infections at the facility?

_____

_____

_____

2. A client at a health care facility is ready to give birth. A nurse is preparing to assist the obstetrician.

    a. What steps should the nurse follow before the procedure?

_____

_____

_____

    b. What is the purpose of the previous steps?

_____

_____

_____

Activity Q   *Think over the following questions. Discuss them with your instructor or peers.*

A nurse is caring for three different clients in a health care facility. The first is an immunosuppressed 68-year-old client undergoing chemotherapy. The second is a 40-year-old client with tuberculosis. The third is a teenager with a wound infection.

1. What considerations are involved when caring for the older client undergoing chemotherapy?

_____

_____

_____

2. What techniques of asepsis should the nurse follow when caring for clients with infectious disorders?

_____

_____

_____

SECTION VI: GETTING READY FOR NCLEX

Activity R   *Answer the following questions.*

1. A nurse is caring for a client with an infection at a health care facility. What precautions should the nurse take after leaving the client's room? Select all that apply.

    a. Scrub the hands thoroughly, giving special attention to the nails

    b. Use a wet towel to turn off faucets

    c. Avoid touching any part of the sink or the faucets

    d. Discard paper towels appropriately after drying the hands

    e. Apply hand sanitizer to keep the hands free from odor

2. A nurse uses an alcohol rub after the physical assessment of each client. Which of the following is true about alcohol rubs?

    a. They remove dirt with organic material

    b. They remove 80% of microorganisms

    c. They can substitute for hand washing if the hands are visibly clean

    d. They have a prolonged antiseptic effect after initial use

CHAPTER 11

Admission, Discharge, Transfer, and Referrals

Learning Objectives

- List the major steps involved in the admission process.
- Identify common psychosocial responses when clients are admitted to a health agency.
- List the steps involved in the discharge process.
- Give examples of the use of transfers in client care.
- Describe the levels of care that nursing homes provide.
- Discuss the purpose of a minimum data set (MDS).
- Explain the difference between transferring clients and referring clients.
- Identify contributing factors to the increased demand for home health care.

SECTION I: ASSESSING YOUR UNDERSTANDING

Activity A   FILL IN THE BLANKS

1. The process of entering a health care agency for nursing care and medical or surgical treatment is called _____.

2. The envelope containing the secured valuables of the client should have the signature of the nurse, the security personnel, or the _____.

3. Termination of care from a health care agency is called _____.

4. Activities involved in discharge planning ideally begin at the time of _____.

5. Discharging a client from one unit or agency and admitting them to another without going home in the interim is called _____.

6. To qualify for Medicare benefits in a nursing home, a person must have been hospitalized for _____ days or more within 30 days without needing skilled nursing care.

7. An _____ care facility is a type of agency that provides health-related care and services to people who do not require 24-hour nursing.

8. A _____ is the process of sending someone to another person or agency for special services.

9. A person on Medicare who needs skilled nursing care intermittently may vary from getting the nursing treatment every day to once every _____ days.

Activity B *Consider the following figure.*

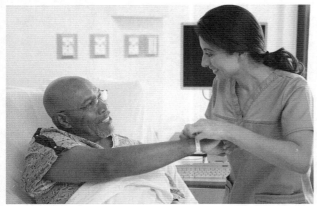

1. Identify what is occurring in the figure.

   _____

   _____

   _____

2. What information can be found on the object identified?

   _____

   _____

   _____

3. What is this object used for?

   _____

   _____

   _____

Activity C *Match the terms in Column A with their descriptions listed in Column B.*

Column A

____ **1.** Anxiety

____ **2.** Against medical advice

____ **3.** Transfer summary

____ **4.** Extended care facility

____ **5.** Basic care facility

Column B

a. Providing long-term health care

b. Leaving before the physician authorizes the discharge

c. Feeling caused by insecurity that makes the client uncomfortable

d. Providing extended custodial care

e. Briefly writing the client's current condition at the time of relocation

Activity D *Presented here, in random order, are steps of the admission process. Write the correct sequence in the boxes provided.*

1. Completion of the agency's admission database
2. Documentation of the client's medical history
3. Authorization from a physician
4. Developing the initial nursing care plan
5. Collection of billing information

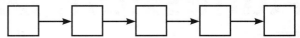

Presented here, in random order, are steps to be followed by a nurse when helping a client undress. Write the correct sequence in the boxes provided below.

1. Remove the client's shoes.
2. Cover the client with a bath blanket.
3. Lift the client's head to guide garments over it.
4. Release fasteners such as zippers and buttons.
5. Provide privacy.

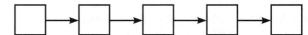

Activity E *Briefly answer the following questions.*

1. What is an initial nursing plan?

   _____

   _____

   _____

2. What nursing actions generally occur during the medical history and physical examination?

   _____

   _____

   _____

3. What actions occur during the discharge process?

   _____

   _____

   _____

4. When and why does a transfer process take place?

   _____

   _____

   _____

5. What is an extended care facility?

_____

_____

_____

SECTION II: APPLYING YOUR KNOWLEDGE

Activity F *Clients in a health care facility may be required to be transferred from one nursing unit to another within the health care facility. Answer the following questions, which involve a nurse's role in the transfer of clients.*

A nurse is caring for a client who is to be shifted from the cardiac care unit to the general nursing care unit within the facility.

1. What are the nurse's responsibilities with regard to transfer of this client?

_____

_____

_____

2. What information is provided in a transfer summary?

_____

_____

_____

SECTION III: PRACTICING FOR NCLEX

Activity G *Answer the following questions.*

1. A client who had been undergoing treatment for breast cancer at a skilled nursing facility is being discharged. At what point in the stay would the nurse begin discharge planning?

   a. During the admission process
   b. After implementing the nursing care plan
   c. When the client requests information about follow-up appointments
   d. After receiving discharge papers from the primary care provider

2. A nurse's role includes admission and discharge procedures for clients. When preparing the discharge plan for clients, which clients will have special considerations and many details on their care?

   a. Clients who are 25 to 30 years of age
   b. Clients with a terminal health condition
   c. Clients living with their families
   d. Clients living with relatives

3. A client wants to leave the health care facility before obtaining a discharge by the physician. The client is asked to sign a form and complete all the discharge formalities before leaving. What is the purpose of this form?

   a. To ensure that the client takes all medications on time
   b. To ensure that the client pays all bills before leaving
   c. To verify all the contact information of the client
   d. To release the physician and facility from future complications

4. A client who is unhappy with the treatment they received in a health care facility decides to leave. The nurse requests for them to sign a form stating that the doctor or the facility will not be responsible for any complications arising after the client is discharged. The client refuses to sign the form. What should be the nurse's appropriate action in this situation?

   a. The nurse notes in the client's medical record that the client refused to sign the form
   b. The nurse gets the form signed by the head of the agency
   c. The nurse signs the form themselves and notes that the client refused to sign it
   d. The nurse gets the form signed by the client's relative

5. A nurse has instructed the client on the medication and self-care practices to be followed after discharge from the facility. What is the next step the nurse will take to complete the discharge process?

   a. Notify the physician
   b. Notify the head of the facility
   c. Notify the business office
   d. Notify the housekeeping staff

6. A senior client being discharged from a hospital tells the nurse that they have no transportation home and is unable to drive

themselves. What action should the nurse take to assist this client? Select all that apply.

a. Call for a transportation van from the Commission on Aging 2 hours in advance
b. Call a taxicab to pick up the client
c. Arrange for an ambulance to transport the client home
d. Arrange for a staff member to drive the client home
e. Arrange for the client to stay another day until transportation is available

7. A nurse has received orders for the transfer of a client. For what reasons would a client be shifted to another agency? Select all that apply.

a. To facilitate specialized care in life-threatening conditions
b. To provide care for the change in the client's condition
c. To reduce the health care costs involved
d. To provide room for another client at the facility
e. To provide long-term care to a client after discharge

8. A client is asked to complete a Minimum Data Set for Nursing Home Resident Assessment and Care Screening form before admission to a health care agency. The form will determine the level of care the client will receive while in the agency. Which criteria are part of this assessment? Select all that apply.

a. Vision patterns
b. Oral and nutritional status
c. Financial status
d. Mood and behavior patterns
e. Continence patterns in the past month

9. A nurse is required to arrange for transfer of a client to another unit at the health care agency. Arrange the sequence of actions required for a transfer within the agency.

a. Speak with a nurse on the transfer unit to coordinate the transfer
b. Transport the client and their belongings, medications, nursing supplies, and chart to the other unit
c. Inform the client and family about the transfer
d. Complete a transfer summary that briefly describes the client's current condition and reason for transfer

10. A 5-year-old child with a high fever is admitted to a health care facility. The child is scared of being in a new place with strangers and is throwing tantrums, making it difficult to care for them. What interventions can the nurse take to help this child?

a. Ask a colleague to help in feeding the child
b. Prevent the parents from fussing over the child
c. Provide the child with toys and books
d. Ask a colleague to help in dressing the child

11. A client has been admitted to a health care facility for treatment of a fractured leg. They have a few personal items such as eyeglasses. Which of the following should the nurse do for the client regarding personal belongings?

a. Place them on the bedside table or drawer and inform the client of this action
b. Hand them over to the client's family for safekeeping
c. Keep them in the facility's safe along with other valuables
d. Tell the client that the facility is not liable for possessions

12. Nurses assist clients to transfer from one unit to another unit of health care facilities frequently. Which client requires a transfer to another unit?

a. A client who has just delivered a baby
b. A client who is capable of going home to self-care
c. A client who returns after leaving the facility without information
d. A client who might leave the facility against medical advice

SECTION IV: REVIEWING WHAT YOU HAVE LEARNED

Activity H   *Fill in the blank by choosing the correct word from the options given in parentheses.*

1. A _____ is the process of sending someone to another person or agency for special services. (discharge, referral, transfer)

Activity I   *Write the correct term for each description below.*

1. The termination of care from a health care agency _____

2. Discharging a client from one unit or agency and admitting them to another without going home in the interim _____

Activity J   *Answer the following questions.*

1. What is the purpose of a minimum data set?

_____

_____

_____

2. What are a nurse's duties when a client must be transferred within the same health care agency?

_____

_____

_____

3. Why is a physical assessment of the client upon admission to the health care facility important?

_____

_____

_____

Activity K   *Give rationales for the following questions.*

1. Why should the nurse have the signature of a second nurse, supervisor, or security person on the envelope containing a client's secured valuables?

_____

_____

_____

2. Why should the nurse drape the client during physical examinations?

_____

_____

_____

Activity L   *Answer the following questions focusing on nursing roles and responsibilities.*

A nurse at a health care facility is asked to complete admission procedures for a client scheduled for surgery.

1. What is the nurse's responsibility during the admission of the client to the facility?

_____

_____

_____

2. What should the nurse include in the initial nursing care plan?

_____

_____

_____

CHAPTER 12

Vital Signs

Learning Objectives

- List the physiologic components measured during the assessment of vital signs.
- Differentiate between shell and core body temperature.
- Identify the scales used to measure temperature.
- List temperature assessment sites and indicate the site considered the closest to core temperature.
- Name the types of clinical thermometers.
- Discuss the difference between fever and hyperthermia.
- Name the phases of a fever.
- List signs or symptoms that accompany a fever.
- Give reasons for using an infrared tympanic thermometer when body temperature is subnormal.
- List signs and symptoms that accompany subnormal body temperature.
- Identify the characteristics noted when assessing a client's pulse.
- Name the most commonly used site for pulse assessment and other assessment techniques that may be used.
- Name and explain the terms used to describe abnormal breathing characteristics.
- Discuss the physiologic data that can be inferred from a blood pressure assessment.
- Explain the difference between systolic and diastolic blood pressure.
- Name the pieces of equipment used to assess blood pressure.
- Describe the phases of Korotkoff sounds.
- Identify alternative techniques for assessing blood pressure.

SECTION I: ASSESSING YOUR UNDERSTANDING

Activity A FILL IN THE BLANKS

1. _____ is a term used to describe a warmer-than-normal set point.

2. A(n) _____ scale is commonly used in the United States to measure and report body temperature.

3. _____ is a structure within the brain that helps control various metabolic activities and acts as the center for temperature regulation.

4. _____ stiffens body hairs and gives the appearance of what commonly is described as "goose flesh."

5. _____ rhythms are physiologic changes, such as fluctuations in body temperature, and other vital signs that happen during 24-hour cycles.

6. _____ affect metabolic rate by triggering hormonal changes through the sympathetic and parasympathetic pathways of the autonomic nervous system.

7. The _____, or the underarm, is an alternative site for assessing body temperature.

8. A(n) _____ thermometer uses a temperature-sensitive probe covered with a disposable sheath and attached by a coiled wire to a display unit.

9. A(n) _____ ultrasound device is an electronic instrument that detects the movement of blood through peripheral blood vessels and converts the movement to a sound.

10. _____ sounds result from the vibrations of blood within the arterial wall or changes in blood flow.

Activity B *Consider the following figures.*

1. Identify the equipment.

_____

_____

_____

2. Explain the use of this equipment.

_____

_____

_____

3. Identify the equipment.

_____

_____

4. Describe the use of this equipment.

_____

_____

_____

Activity C *Match the terms related to measuring vital signs in Column A with their descriptions in Column B.*

Column A

____ **1.** Tachypnea

____ **2.** Bradycardia

____ **3.** Drawdown effect

____ **4.** Metabolic rate

____ **5.** Hypotension

Column B

a. Cooling of the ear when it comes in contact with the probe of the thermometer

b. Use of calories for sustaining body functions

c. Rapid respiratory rate

d. Blood pressure measurements are below the normal systolic values for the person's age

e. Pulse rate is less than 60 bpm

Activity D *Presented here, in random order, are four distinct phases through which fever progresses. Write the correct sequence of these events in the boxes provided.*

1. Invasion phase

2. Defervescence phase

3. Prodromal phase

4. Stationary phase

☐ → ☐ → ☐ → ☐

Activity E *Briefly answer the following questions.*

1. What is systolic pressure?

_____

_____

_____

2. What should the nurse do if the client's temperature is not normal?

_____

_____

_____

3. What are objective assessment data?

_____

_____

_____

4. What causes an increase in body temperature during ovulation?

_____

_____

_____

5. How does emotion affect body temperature?

_____

_____

_____

6. When is a paper chemical thermometer used?

_____

_____

_____

SECTION II: APPLYING YOUR KNOWLEDGE

Activity F   *Shell temperature in normal, healthy adults generally ranges from 96.6 to 99.3°F (35.8 to 37.4°C). On the other hand, the core body temperature ranges from 97.5 to 100.4°F (36.4 to 37.3°C). The nurse measures the temperature of the client routinely. Answer the following questions, which involve the nurse's role in the physical assessment of clients.*

A nurse is caring for a client with a high fever. The nurse notices that the client is shivering and their body is hot. The nurse has been instructed by the physician to record the client's body temperature regularly.

1. How should the nurse ensure that the temperature measured reflects the core body temperature?

_____

_____

_____

2. How should the nurse document the different assessment sites in the client's medical record?

_____

_____

_____

SECTION III: PRACTICING FOR NCLEX

Activity G   *Answer the following questions.*

1. A nurse is regularly assessing the temperature of a client with hyperthermia. At what temperature would the chances for survival of a client be diminished?
   a. Body temperatures exceeding 120°F or falling below 95°F
   b. Body temperatures exceeding 105°F or falling below 84°F
   c. Body temperatures exceeding 110°F or falling below 84°F
   d. Body temperatures exceeding 115°F or falling below 95°F

2. When assessing the temperature of a client after the afternoon meal, the nurse notes an increase in the temperature of the client from the last assessment. What condition could have led to the increase in the client's temperature in this case?
   a. The client was sleeping during the day
   b. The amount and type of food eaten
   c. The client has a rapid respiratory rate
   d. The medication used by the client

3. A nurse is caring for an asthmatic client at the health agency. The nurse notes an increase in the client's temperature after the client has taken their medication. What medication could have possibly led to an increase in the client's body temperature?
   a. Aspirin
   b. Ibuprofen
   c. Ephedrine
   d. Acetaminophen

4. A nurse needs to measure the body temperature of an infant client. Which site is the best choice?
   a. Oral
   b. Rectal
   c. Ear
   d. Axillary

5. The nurse is caring for a 26-year-old client. When measuring their temperature, the nurse notes an increase in the body temperature of the client, even though they show no symptoms of fever. Which condition could have led to this increase?
   a. Lack of perspiration
   b. Depression
   c. Ovulation
   d. Use of aspirin

6. When assessing the client, the nurse notes that the slightest bit of pressure obliterates the client's pulse. How should the nurse record the client's pulse?
   a. Bounding
   b. Thready
   c. Strong
   d. Normal

7. A nurse is caring for a client who got lost while skiing on a mountain. The nurse should assess the client for which symptom of hypothermia?
   a. Increased metabolic demand
   b. Irregular breathing rhythm
   c. Above-normal pulse rates
   d. Impaired muscle coordination

8. A nurse is caring for an adult client with a body temperature of 103.4°F. What would be an appropriate nursing intervention for this client?
   a. Provide fluids
   b. Provide aspirin
   c. Provide physical cooling
   d. Suggest rest

9. A nurse is caring for a client with dyspnea. When seeking a cause for the dyspnea, the nurse checks:
   a. The amount and type of activity performed by the client
   b. The eating habits of the client
   c. The regularity with which the dyspnea occurs
   d. The hours the client sleeps

10. A nurse uses the aneroid manometer to check the blood pressure of a client. How should the nurse check the equipment prior to measuring the blood pressure?
    a. Make sure the needle on the gauge is positioned at zero
    b. Make sure the gauge reading is the same as the client's body temperature
    c. Ensure that the gauge is connected to an electric outlet
    d. Ensure that the inflatable bladder is the correct size

11. A nurse is caring for a client whose blood flow in the arteries is very low. The nurse uses the Doppler ultrasound device to detect the movement of blood through peripheral blood vessels. Order the steps in the most likely sequence in which they would occur in this procedure.
    a. Move the probe at an angle over the skin
    b. Count the pulsating sound
    c. Document the assessment site rate
    d. Apply conductive gel over the arterial site
    e. Note the "D" for Doppler device

12. A nurse is measuring the blood pressure of a client from a site other than the brachial artery. In which examples would this be appropriate? Select all that apply.
    a. When the client's arms are missing
    b. When both breasts have been removed
    c. When a client has had vascular surgery
    d. When the client has hypothermia
    e. When the client is moderately hyperthermic

13. A nurse is caring for a client with low blood pressure. Which situations could cause this condition? Select all that apply.
    a. Increasing age
    b. Sleeping at night
    c. Lying down posture
    d. Client is a female
    e. Exercise and activity

14. A nurse needs to assess the blood pressure of a senior client. Order the steps in the most likely sequence in which they would occur.
    a. Have the client assume a sitting position
    b. Assist the client to stand and check the pressure
    c. Assess the blood pressure with the client in the supine position
    d. Deflate and leave the blood pressure cuff in place
    e. Check the client's blood pressure

15. A nurse is measuring the Korotkoff sound in a client and notes a muffled, less distinct, and softer sound with a blowing quality. Which phase of Korotkoff sounds is occurring?
    a. Phase I
    b. Phase II
    c. Phase III
    d. Phase IV

SECTION IV: REVIEWING WHAT YOU HAVE LEARNED

Activity H *Fill in the blanks by choosing the correct word from the options given in parentheses.*

1. Various anatomic and physiologic adaptations keep human body temperature within a narrow stable range regardless of environmental temperature; hence, humans are _____. (heterothermic, homeothermic, poikilothermic)

2. Prolonged _____ leads to brain damage or death. (apnea, dyspnea, orthopnea)

3. _____ is a heart rate below 60 bpm. (Bradycardia, Palpitation, Tachycardia)

4. _____ sounds are located normally in the periphery of all the lung fields. (Bronchial, Bronchovesicular, Vesicular)

5. The _____ is the brain's temperature-regulating center that initiates processes that promote heat conservation and production. (cerebellum, hypothalamus, medulla)

Activity I *Mark each statement as either T (True) or F (False). Correct any false statements.*

1. T F For every degree of Fahrenheit that temperature is elevated, heart and pulse rates increase 15 bpm.

2. T F The apical heart rate can be counted by listening at the chest with a stethoscope.

Activity J *Write the correct term for each description below.*

1. A handheld probe used during an ultrasonography to project sound through the body's surface _____

2. Rapid or deep breathing, or both, affecting the volume of air entering and leaving the lungs _____

Activity K *Differentiate between fever and hyperthermia.*
1. Definition
2. Complications or Concerns

Activity L *Consider the following figure.*

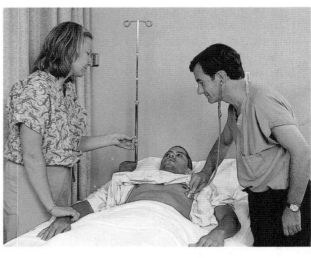

1. Identify the figure shown above.

   _____

   _____

   _____

2. Which of the two methods for assessing the pulse rate is more accurate? Why?

   _____

   _____

   _____

Activity M *Answer the following questions.*

1. What are the phases of a fever?

   _____

   _____

   _____

2. What is postural or orthostatic hypotension?

   _____

   _____

   _____

Activity N *Give a rationale for the following question.*
Why is it important for a nurse to measure a client's vital signs at regular intervals?

   _____

   _____

   _____

Activity O *Answer the following questions focusing on nursing roles and responsibilities.*

A nurse caring for a newborn at a health care facility is required to measure and document the baby's temperature at regular intervals.

1. Which are the preferred routes for measuring the temperature of newborns or infants?

_____

_____

_____

2. Why do newborns and young infants tend to experience temperature fluctuations?

_____

_____

_____

Activity P *Think over the following questions. Discuss them with your instructor or peers.*

A nurse employed in the rehabilitative care unit of a health care facility is required to measure the blood pressure of a severely obese client who is recovering from a motor vehicle collision. The client's right arm is in a cast. They have just returned to their room after actively exercising by ambulating in the hall.

1. Should the nurse assess blood pressure soon after the client has exercised?

_____

_____

_____

2. What factors should be considered when using a sphygmomanometer to assess blood pressure in this client?

_____

_____

_____

SECTION V: GETTING READY FOR NCLEX

Activity Q *Answer the following questions.*

1. During the physical assessment of a client, the nurse listens to lung sounds. How should the nurse document squeaking sounds caused by air moving through a narrowed passage in the lung?
   a. Crackle
   b. Gurgle
   c. Rub
   d. Wheeze

2. A fever generally goes through four distinct phases. Arrange the phases in the order in which they occur. Use all the options.
   a. Stationary
   b. Defervescence
   c. Invasion
   d. Prodromal

3. A nurse is assigned to measure and document the vital signs of a client recovering from an accident. The client is receiving intravenous medication in the right arm. The left arm and left lower leg are severely injured. What would be the best site for measuring the client's blood pressure?
   a. Right lower arm
   b. Right upper arm
   c. Left thigh
   d. Right thigh

4. While taking a client's vital signs, the nurse identifies that the pulse is difficult to feel and easily obliterated with slight pressure. How would the nurse document this finding?
   a. Thready
   b. Bounding
   c. Full
   d. Strong

CHAPTER 13

Physical Assessment

Learning Objectives

- List the purposes of a physical assessment.
- Name assessment techniques.
- List the items needed when performing a basic physical assessment.
- Describe the criteria for an appropriate assessment environment.
- Identify assessments that can be obtained during the initial survey of clients.
- State the reasons for draping clients.
- Differentiate between a head-to-toe and a body-systems approach to physical assessment.
- List the ways in which the body may be divided for organizing data collection.
- Identify self-examinations that nurses should teach their adult clients.

SECTION I: ASSESSING YOUR UNDERSTANDING

Activity A FILL IN THE BLANKS

1. The overall goal of a physical assessment is to gather _____ data about a client.

2. A(n) _____ is an instrument used to examine structures in the eye.

3. A(n) _____ is a professional trained to test hearing with standardized instruments.

4. _____ is an exaggerated natural lumbar curve of the spine.

5. _____ is excessive fluid within tissue and signifies abnormal fluid distribution.

6. The yellowish brown, waxy secretion produced by glands within the ear is called _____.

7. A(n) _____ chart is a visual assessment tool with small print.

8. The _____ test is an assessment technique for comparing air versus bone conduction of sound.

9. _____ is a combination of the elastic quality of the skin and the pressure exerted on it by fluid within.

10. A(n) _____ test is an assessment technique for determining equality or disparity of bone-conducted sound.

Activity B *Consider the following figures.*

1. Identify and label the figure.

_____

_____

_____

2. How is a taste assessment done?

_____

_____

_____

3. How does the nurse ensure valid results when assessing taste in a client?

_____

_____

_____

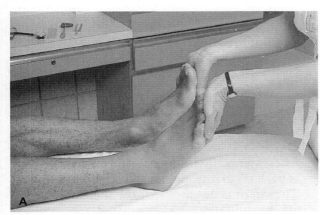

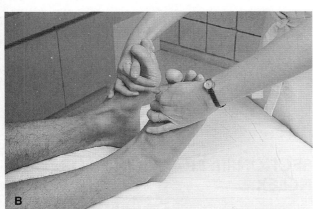

4. Identify the figure.

_____

_____

_____

5. How is this procedure performed? How would the nurse test the strength in a client's upper extremities?

_____

_____

_____

Activity C *Match the terms related to assessment of the eye in Column A with their descriptions in Column B.*

Column A

____ **1.** Visual acuity

____ **2.** Normal vision

____ **3.** Consensual response

____ **4.** Visual field examination

____ **5.** Accommodation of pupils

Column B

a. Ability to read printed letters at a distance of 20 feet without prescription lenses

b. Assessment of peripheral vision and continuity in the visual field

c. Ability to see both far and near

d. Ability to constrict when looking at a near object and dilate when looking at an object in the distance

e. Brisk, equal, and simultaneous constriction of both pupils when one eye, and then the other eye, is stimulated with light

Activity D *Presented here, in random order, are steps occurring during the assessment of pupillary response. Write the correct sequence in the boxes provided.*

1. Repeat the assessment by directly stimulating the opposite eye

2. Ask the client to look at a finger or object approximately 4 inches from their face

3. Bring a narrow beam of light from a penlight, from the temple toward the eye

4. Tell the client to look from the near object to another that is more distant

5. Dim the lights in the examination area and instruct the client to stare straight ahead

6. Observe the pupil of the stimulated eye as well as the unstimulated pupil

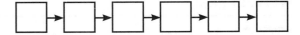

Activity E *Briefly answer the following questions.*

1. What is the purpose of a physical assessment?

   _____

   _____

   _____

2. What are the basic requirements of an examination room for assessing clients?

   _____

   _____

   _____

3. Why is it important to document the client's weight and height during an initial assessment?

   _____

   _____

   _____

4. How should the nurse assess a client's hair?

   _____

   _____

   _____

5. Why is it important for the nurse to document any unusual characteristics of the nails or surrounding tissues?

   _____

   _____

   _____

6. What equipment would the nurse need for a basic physical assessment?

   _____

   _____

   _____

SECTION II: APPLYING YOUR KNOWLEDGE

Activity F *The first step in the nursing process is assessment. The overall goal of physical assessment is to gather objective data about a client. Answer the following questions,* which involve the nurse's role in the physical assessment of clients.

A nurse is caring for a client with an abdomen that appears unusually enlarged. The nurse is assessing the bowel as part of the physical assessment.

1. In what order should the nurse use the assessment techniques?

   _____

   _____

   _____

2. How should the nurse measure the abdominal girth of the client?

   _____

   _____

   _____

A nurse is caring for a middle-aged client at the health care facility. During the physical assessment, the nurse asks the client to perform a regular testicular self-examination. The client is not aware of the method of self-examination.

3. What should the nurse tell the client with regard to the procedure for testicular self-examination?

   _____

   _____

   _____

SECTION III: PRACTICING FOR NCLEX

Activity G *Answer the following questions.*

1. A nurse, when conducting a physical assessment for a client, observes several lesions on the skin that are elevated, with irregular borders and no free fluid. The client informs the nurse that these lesions erupted after having shellfish. How should the nurse document this observation?
   a. Macules
   b. Papules
   c. Wheals
   d. Vesicles

2. A nurse is assessing the skin turgor of a client during a regular physical assessment. What technique would the nurse use?
   a. Gently pinch the area over the sternum or below the clavicle
   b. Gently pinch the area at the back of the hand
   c. Forcefully grasp the area on the forearm or upper arm
   d. Grasp and slightly twist the area on the lower leg

3. When listening to the lung sounds of a client, the nurse hears adventitious sounds that are intermittent, high-pitched, popping sounds during inspiration. As what does the nurse document these?
   a. Rubs
   b. Wheezes
   c. Gurgles
   d. Crackles

4. A nurse is caring for a client with pneumonia at a community health care facility. What intervention should the nurse take if adventitious sounds are heard upon lung assessment?
   a. Assist the client to a supine position
   b. Assess the appearance of raised sputum
   c. Move the diaphragm from the base of the lung to the top
   d. Listen for one complete inspiration or expiration

5. The nurse is examining a client with complaints of pain in the abdomen. The nurse applies pressure in the abdominal region with the fingertips and the palm of the hand to check for tenderness or unusual vibrations. What physical assessment technique is the nurse using?
   a. Inspection
   b. Percussion
   c. Palpation
   d. Auscultation

6. A nurse at the health care facility is examining a client during a routine checkup. What action should the nurse take to ensure accuracy when obtaining the client's weight?
   a. Check to see that the scale is calibrated at zero
   b. Ask the client to remove their shoes and provide the client with light slippers
   c. Move the heavier weight across the calibrations
   d. Position the lighter weight in a calibrated groove of the scale arm

7. When performing a physical assessment for a client, a nurse should also assess the mental status of the client. In which cases should the nurse perform an in-depth objective assessment? Select all that apply.
   a. Clients with head injury
   b. Clients with psychiatric diagnoses
   c. Clients with impaired visual acuity
   d. Clients who are being treated with nonsteroidal antiinflammatory drugs (NSAIDs)
   e. Clients who took an overdose of drugs

8. A nurse is caring for a child with complaints of pain in the right ear. Which action should the nurse perform when examining the child's ear?
   a. Place the vibrating tuning fork behind the head to assess hearing
   b. Pull the ear down and back to straighten the ear canal
   c. Move the external ear to determine any tenderness
   d. Position the client in front of a diffused lamp for examination

9. During a routine physical examination, the nurse inspects the skin of the client. The nurse observes purple patches of skin on the legs of the client. How should the nurse document this finding?
   a. Pallor
   b. Erythema
   c. Cyanosis
   d. Ecchymosis

10. During a visit to the health care facility, a client in her mid-30s asks the nurse for information about breast self-examination (BSE). Which point should the nurse include in the teaching plan?
   a. Perform self-examination once every 2 months
   b. Place the hand alongside the side to be examined
   c. Squeeze the nipple gently to determine whether there is any discharge
   d. Perform the entire examination while lying down

11. During a routine physical assessment of a pregnant client, the nurse observes edema on the client's feet. How should the nurse document the edema if a 4-mm pit is observed with a fairly normal contour?
   a. 1+ pitting edema
   b. 2+ pitting edema
   c. 3+ pitting edema
   d. 4+ pitting edema

12. A nurse is assessing the sensory skin perception of a client. What action should the nurse perform to test the client's ability to identify fine touch?
    a. Place the stem of a vibrating tuning fork against the wrist
    b. Touch the client with pointed and curved ends of a safety pin
    c. Stroke the skin at various areas with a cotton ball
    d. Touch the skin at various areas with warm and cold containers

13. A nurse is caring for a client with complaints of abdominal pain. The nurse auscultates the abdomen and feels for palpable masses. How should the nurse document the shape and consistency of an abdominal mass that resembles an egg and feels firm to the touch?
    a. Round and nodular
    b. Ovoid and nodular
    c. Ovoid and hard
    d. Round and hard

14. A nurse is assessing a client who has been having irregular bowel movements. The client also complains of heaviness and uneasiness in the abdomen. What action should the nurse perform when assessing the abdomen for bowel sounds?
    a. Warm the diaphragm of the stethoscope before the procedure
    b. Listen for 1 minute in each quadrant
    c. Listen for bowel sounds in one upper and one lower quadrant
    d. Explain the procedure to the client during the assessment

15. A nurse is assessing the heart sounds of a 35-year-old client with a possible heart condition. What is a normal heart sound heard upon auscultation?
    a. The "lub" sound louder at the mitral area
    b. The "lub-dub-dub" sounds
    c. The "lub-lub-dub" sounds
    d. The soft "dub" sound over the aortic area

SECTION IV: REVIEWING WHAT YOU HAVE LEARNED

Activity H *Fill in the blanks by choosing the correct word from the options given in parentheses.*

1. A/n _____ is a crack in the skin, especially in or near mucous membranes. (abrasion, fissure, laceration)

2. _____ sounds are located normally in the periphery of all the lung fields. (Bronchial, Bronchovesicular, Vesicular)

Activity I *Mark each statement as either T (True) or F (False). Correct any false statements.*

1. T F The nurse performs light palpation by depressing tissue approximately 1 inch (2.5 cm) with the forefingers of one or both hands.

2. T F Lordosis causes an increased curve in the thoracic area.

Activity J *Write the correct term for each description below.*

1. A pronounced lateral curvature of the spine _____

2. An assessment technique used to listen to body sounds _____

Activity K *Differentiate between the head-to-toe and the body-systems approaches to physical assessment.*

1. Definition

2. Advantages

3. Disadvantages

Activity L *Answer the following questions.*

1. Why is a physical assessment of the client upon admission to the health care facility important?

   _____

   _____

   _____

2. What is a Snellen eye chart?

   _____

   _____

   _____

Activity M *Give rationales for the following questions.*

1. Why should the nurse drape the client during physical examinations?

_____

_____

_____

2. Why is it better to assess skin turgor in the area over the chest in a senior client?

_____

_____

_____

Activity N *Think over the following questions. Discuss them with your instructor or peers.*

A nurse performs routine mental status assessments of clients being admitted to a health care facility.

1. What is the purpose of the assessments?

_____

_____

_____

2. What information should be documented for each client assessed?

_____

_____

_____

3. Which clients would require a detailed assessment with more objective data documented?

_____

_____

_____

SECTION V: GETTING READY FOR NCLEX

Activity O *Answer the following questions.*

1. During the physical assessment of a client, the nurse listens to lung sounds. How should the nurse document squeaking sounds caused by air moving through a narrowed passage in the lung?
   a. Crackle
   b. Gurgle
   c. Rub
   d. Wheeze

2. During a physical assessment, the nurse taps the fingers against the client's abdomen. Which technique involves tapping or striking fingers on the client's body?
   a. Auscultation
   b. Palpation
   c. Percussion
   d. Observation

CHAPTER 14

Special Examinations and Tests

Learning Objectives

- Differentiate between an examination and a test.
- Identify word endings and their meanings that provide clues as to how tests or examinations are performed.
- Discuss factors to consider when performing examinations and tests on older adults.
- List general nursing responsibilities related to assisting with special examinations and tests.
- Name positions commonly used during tests or examinations.
- List commonly performed categories of tests or examinations.
- Explain what is involved during a pelvic examination and a Pap test.
- Describe the following procedures: paracentesis, lumbar puncture, throat culture, and measurement of capillary blood glucose.

SECTION I: ASSESSING YOUR UNDERSTANDING

Activity A   FILL IN THE BLANKS

1. A consent form contains three elements: capacity, comprehension, and _____.

2. The _____ position is a reclining position with the feet in metal supports called *stirrups*.

3. _____ are samples of tissue or body fluids that are collected during an examination or test.

4. During an X-ray, the actual film image is technically called a(n) _____.

5. During a radionuclide examination, the nurse should ask clients about their allergy history because _____ is used commonly during this examination.

6. _____ is a form of radiography that displays an image in real time and is used to observe the movement of contrast media.

7. Visual examination of internal structures using optical scopes is known as _____.

8. Endoscopic examinations that produce discomfort or anxiety are performed under a light, short-acting form of _____, sometimes referred to as *conscious sedation*.

9. Barium retention can lead to _____ and bowel obstruction.

10. Ultrasonography, a soft tissue examination that uses sound waves in ranges beyond human hearing, is also known as _____.

Activity B *Consider the following figures.*

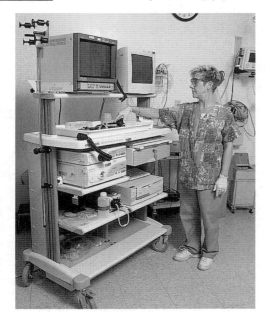

1. Identify the figure.

_____

_____

2. What care should the nurse perform before the examination?

_____

_____

_____

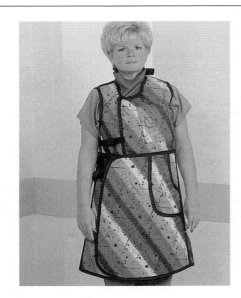

3. Identify the figure.

_____

_____

4. What is the use of the objects in the figure?

_____

_____

_____

Activity C *Match the examinations in Column A with their descriptions in Column B.*

Column A

_____ 1. Computed tomography

_____ 2. Radionuclides

_____ 3. Magnetic resonance imaging

_____ 4. Echogram

_____ 5. Cold spot

Column B

a. Elements with molecular structures that are altered to produce radiation

b. Technique for producing an image by using atoms subjected to a strong electromagnetic field

c. Area with little radionuclide concentration

d. Form of roentgenography that shows planes of tissues

e. Can be viewed in real time on a monitor and recorded for future analysis

Activity D *Presented here, in random order, are steps to collect specimens during an examination or test. Write the correct sequence in the boxes provided.*

1. Label the specimen container with the correct information

2. Collect the specimen in an appropriate container

3. Ensure that the specimen does not decompose before it can be examined

4. Deliver the specimen to the laboratory as soon as possible

5. Attach the proper laboratory request form

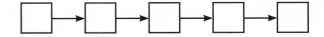

Activity E *Briefly answer the following questions.*

1. What is a diagnostic examination?

   _____

   _____

   _____

2. What is a culture?

   _____

   _____

   _____

3. What is a contrast medium?

   _____

   _____

   _____

4. How is a lumbar puncture performed?

   _____

   _____

   _____

5. What other information, in addition to a written account of the examination, should a nurse report?

   _____

   _____

   _____

6. What care should a nurse take when attending to a client undergoing a diagnostic procedure?

   _____

   _____

   _____

SECTION II: APPLYING YOUR KNOWLEDGE

Activity F *Nursing responsibilities for a client examination include gathering information from the client before an examination and providing instructions for the client to follow after the examination. Answer the following questions, which involve the nurse's responsibilities while helping a client undergo radionuclide imaging.*

An adult client needs to undergo radionuclide imaging as a part of their diagnosis.

1. What questions should the nurse ask the client before the examination?

   _____

   _____

   _____

2. What instructions should the nurse provide the client after the examination?

   _____

   _____

   _____

SECTION III: PRACTICING FOR NCLEX

Activity G *Answer the following questions.*

1. A client visits the health care agency for a scheduled checkup. In which position would the nurse place the client for examination of prostate gland?
   a. Dorsal recumbent position
   b. Lithotomy position
   c. Genupectoral position
   d. Sims position

2. A physician advises a client to undergo a physical inspection of the vagina and cervix and the nurse has been directed to collect a specimen of cervical secretions. Which test is being performed?
   a. Pap smear
   b. Radiography
   c. Fluoroscopy
   d. Endoscopy

3. A client is scheduled to undergo a procedure in which an endoscope is inserted into the upper airway. What nursing responsibility is appropriate when preparing this client for the procedure?
   a. If topical anesthesia is used, withhold food or fluids for 6 hours after the procedure
   b. Do not use ice chips or gargles to relieve a client's sore throat after the procedure

c. Confirm that bowel preparation has been completed for all endoscopic procedures

d. Withhold food and fluids for at least 6 hours before the procedure

4. A client with frequent complaints of pain in the lower abdomen has been ordered to undergo an endoscopy. The client is administered conscious sedation during the procedure. What common effect of conscious sedation would the nurse expect following the procedure?

a. The client may not recall having had the test

b. The client's breathing will be affected

c. The client will be under heavy sedation

d. The client may have a sore throat

5. A nurse is preparing a client for an endoscopic procedure of the lower intestine. What should the nurse confirm before this procedure is performed?

a. The client has not had any food for the past 2 hours

b. Bowel preparation using enemas has been completed

c. The client drank six to eight glasses of water before the examination

d. The client has good swallow, cough, and gag reflexes

6. In addition to a written account of the client's examination, what other primary information should the nurse record to share with the other nursing team members?

a. Where and how the specimen was transported

b. The client's reactions during and immediately after the procedure

c. Where the test was performed and who performed it

d. Type and quantity of the specimen obtained from the client

7. The nurse is assisting a client who is to undergo a paracentesis procedure. Why should the nurse encourage the client to empty the bladder just before the procedure?

a. To prevent any accidental puncture

b. To pool the fluids in the lower area of the abdomen

c. To displace the intestines posteriorly

d. To prevent contaminating the physician's sterile gloves

8. A client has been ordered an examination of the anal region. Which of the following positions should the nurse ask the client to maintain during the examination?

a. Dorsal recumbent position

b. Sims position

c. Genupectoral position

d. Modified standing position

9. For which procedure is the nurse preparing the client if the nurse requests the client to remove all metal items (such as religious medals or clothing that contains metal objects) before the examination?

a. Radiography

b. Endoscopy

c. Paracentesis

d. Electrocardiography (ECG or EKG)

10. During the pelvic examination of a client, the nurse folds back the drape just before the examination begins. What is the rationale for this nursing action?

a. To maintain the client's modesty and privacy

b. To reduce anxiety

c. To expose the genitalia, minimizing exposure

d. To illuminate the area, facilitating examination

11. A client has to undergo an examination of the energy emitted by the brain. The nurse instructs the client that they will need to be awake after midnight before the examination can take place. This action is required when performing:

a. Electroencephalography (EEG)

b. Electrocardiography (ECG)

c. Electromyography (EMG)

d. Placement of electrodes

12. A nurse is caring for a client with a respiratory disorder resulting from a collection of fluid in the lungs. For which procedure would the nurse expect to assist?

a. Lumbar puncture

b. Pelvic examination

c. Throat culture

d. Paracentesis

13. A pregnant client visits the health agency for a scheduled checkup. In which position will the nurse place the client?

a. Dorsal recumbent position

b. Lithotomy position

c. Sims position

d. Knee–chest position

14. A client with complaints of irritation and itching in the vaginal area visits the health agency. Which test should be ordered to determine the cause of this condition?
    a. Blood test
    b. Ultrasound
    c. Papanicolaou test
    d. Microorganisms analysis

15. A nurse teaches a diabetic client to measure their own glucose level daily. What time would the nurse tell the client is the best time to determine their blood glucose level?
    a. 30 minutes before eating and before bedtime
    b. 30 minutes after eating and before bedtime
    c. 30 minutes before eating and after waking up
    d. 30 minutes after eating and after waking up

16. A client has been ordered to have a laboratory test. What nursing actions should the nurse perform when preparing the client for this test? Select all that apply.
    a. The nurse should schedule the procedures before the client consumes the herbal medicine
    b. The nurse should know the client's previous results of the test as a baseline for comparison
    c. The nurse should inform the client when to stop consuming the prescribed medication
    d. The nurse must assess the blood pressure of older clients before the procedure
    e. The nurse should provide older adults with additional clothing to keep them warm

17. A frail senior client has to undergo a gastrointestinal examination and an examination to check blood sugar levels, which requires the client to fast for some time. The client is diabetic and also has a breathing problem. What special care should the nurse take when scheduling the tests for this client? Select all that apply.
    a. Suggest the client fasts for 8 hours before the tests
    b. Eliminate long periods of fasting during the tests
    c. Suggest the client fasts for 12 hours before the tests
    d. Offer food and fluid after the tests
    e. Provide a bedside commode if necessary

18. What measures should the nurse take when sending a stool sample, collected from a client, to the laboratory for testing? Select all that apply.
    a. Label the specimen container with the correct information
    b. Send it to the laboratory at the earliest possible moment before it decomposes
    c. Keep changing the container so that it does not decompose
    d. Store the specimen in a refrigerator
    e. Attach the proper laboratory request form

19. A nurse is caring for a client who visits the health agency for a prostate gland examination as a part of annual checkup. Order the tasks in the most likely sequence in which the nurse would have performed them while caring for the client.
    a. The nurse helps the client to a position of comfort
    b. The nurse directs the client to dress in their own clothing
    c. The nurse provides instructions for follow-up care
    d. The nurse checks the client's vital signs to verify that their condition is stable
    e. The nurse escorts the client to the discharge area
    f. The nurse cleans any substances from the client that caused soiling

20. A physician needs to examine an arthritic client with complaints of pain in the vagina. The nurse helps the client to get into the Sims position for the examination. Which positions should the nurse help the client to assume? Select all that apply.
    a. The client lies on her left side with her chest leaning forward
    b. The client's right knee is bent toward her head
    c. The client rests on her knees and chest supported by a pillow
    d. The client's head is supported on a small pillow, to one side
    e. The client's left arm is extended behind the body

SECTION IV: REVIEWING WHAT YOU HAVE LEARNED

Activity H   *Fill in the blanks by choosing the correct word from the options given in parentheses.*

1. _____ is a procedure for withdrawing fluid from the abdominal cavity. (Fluoroscopy, Paracentesis, Roentgenography)

2. _____ is a procedure involving the insertion of a needle between lumbar vertebrae in the spinal canal but below the spinal cord itself. (Spinal tap, Ultrasonography, Endoscopy)

Activity I   *Mark each statement as either T (True) or F (False). Correct any false statements.*

1. T F   A developing fetus is at increased risk for cellular damage from X-rays.

2. T F   Electroencephalography is an examination of the energy produced by stimulated muscles.

Activity J   *Write the correct term for each description below.*

1. Using atoms subjected to a strong electromagnetic field to produce an image _____

2. A handheld probe used during an ultrasonography to project sound through the body's surface _____

Activity K   *Consider the following figure.*

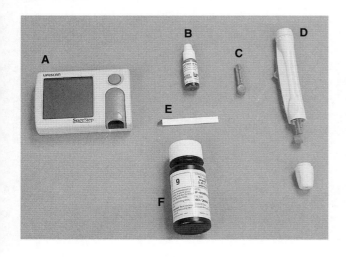

1. Identify the figure shown above.

_____

_____

_____

2. What is this equipment used for?

_____

_____

_____

Activity L   *Answer the following questions.*

1. How is a culture performed?

_____

_____

_____

2. What is the purpose of a lumbar puncture or a spinal tap?

_____

_____

_____

SECTION V: APPLYING YOUR KNOWLEDGE

Activity M   *Give a rationale for the following question.*

Why should the nurse ensure that the client's garments are free of all metallic objects, such as hooks or medals, before a radiographic examination?

_____

_____

Activity N   *Answer the following questions focusing on nursing roles and responsibilities.*

A client at the health care facility is ready to give birth. A nurse is preparing to assist the obstetrician.

1. What steps should the nurse follow before the procedure?

_____

_____

_____

2. What is the purpose of the previous steps?

_____

_____

_____

A nurse is caring for a client who is to undergo an electrocardiography (ECG).

3. How should the nurse explain to the client what to expect during the procedure?

_____

_____

_____

4. What are the nursing responsibilities for a client undergoing an ECG?

_____

_____

_____

SECTION VI: GETTING READY FOR NCLEX

Activity O *Answer the following question.*

A nurse is caring for a client scheduled for electromyography (EMG). What should the nurse tell the client about the procedure?

a. You will need to stay awake after midnight before the examination

b. You must avoid cola beverages for 8 hours before the procedure

c. Pain will be felt if the electrode touches a terminal nerve in the area

d. Your physician may withhold scheduled medications

CHAPTER 15

Nutrition

Learning Objectives

- Define nutrition and malnutrition.
- List components of basic nutrition.
- Identify five factors that influence nutritional needs.
- Explain protein complementation.
- Discuss the purpose and components of the MyPlate food guidelines.
- Describe the facts available on nutritional labels.
- Identify objective assessments for determining a person's nutritional status.
- Discuss the purpose of a diet history.
- List common problems that can be identified from a nutritional assessment.
- Plan nursing interventions for resolving problems caused or affected by nutrition.
- Describe common hospital diets and their characteristics.
- Discuss nursing responsibilities for meeting clients' nutritional needs.
- Identify facts a nurse must know about a client's diet.
- Describe and demonstrate techniques for feeding clients.
- Explain how to meet the nutritional needs of clients with dysphagia, visual impairment, and dementia.
- Discuss unique aspects of nutrition that apply to older adults.

SECTION I: ASSESSING YOUR UNDERSTANDING

Activity A FILL IN THE BLANKS

1. _____ is a condition resulting from lack of proper nutrients in the diet.

2. The energy, or heat equivalent, of food is measured in _____.

3. _____ is the amount of heat that raises the temperature of 1 kg water by 1°C.

4. Cholesterol absorbs fatty acids and binds them to molecules of protein referred to as _____.

5. Carbohydrates contain _____, an indigestible fiber in the stems, skins, and leaves of fruits and vegetables, which forms intestinal bulk to promote bowel elimination.

6. _____ help to regulate many of the body's chemical processes such as blood clotting and conduction of nerve impulses.

7. _____ amino acids are protein components that must be obtained from food because the body cannot synthesize them.

8. _____ fats are the predominate type of fat in fish, poultry, nuts, and most plant oils, such as corn, safflower, olive, peanut, and soybean.

9. _____ is a condition associated with Alzheimer disease and refers to the deterioration of previous intellectual capacity.

10. _____ is gas formed in the intestine and released from the rectum when eructation does not occur.

Activity B   *Consider the following figure.*

Nutrition Facts

Serving Size 1/2 cup (114g)
Servings Per Container 4

Amount Per Serving

Calories 90	Calories from Fat 30

	% Daily Value*
Total Fat 3 g	5
Saturated Fat 0 g	0
Trans Fat 1 g	
Cholesterol 0 mg	0
Sodium 300 mg	13
Total Carbohydrate 13 g	4
Dietary Fiber 3 g	12
Sugars 3 g	
Protein 3 g	

Vitamin A	80%	•	Vitamin C	60%
Calcium	4%	•	Iron	4%

* Percent Daily Values are based on a 2,000 cal diet. Your daily values may be higher or lower depending on your caloric needs:

	Calories	2,000	2,500
Total Fat	Less than	65 g	80 g
Sat Fat	Less than	20 g	25 g
Cholesterol	Less than	300 mg	300 mg
Sodium	Less than	2,400 mg	2,400 mg
Total Carbohydrate		300 g	375 g
Fiber		25 g	30 g

Calories per gram:
Fat 9 • Carbohydrate 4 • Protein 4

1. Identify the figure.

   _____

   _____

   _____

2. What does the figure display?

   _____

   _____

   _____

3. What are daily values (DVs)?

   _____

   _____

   _____

Activity C   *Match the food nutrients in Column A with their descriptions and functions in Column B.*

Column A

____ 1. Vitamins

____ 2. Minerals

____ 3. Cholesterol

____ 4. Fats

____ 5. Carbohydrates

Column B

a. Noncaloric substances in food that help regulate many of the body's cellular functions

b. Chemical substances necessary in minute amounts for normal growth, maintenance of health, and functioning of the body

c. Chief component of most diets and the body's primary source for quick energy

d. Absorbs fatty acids and binds them to molecules of protein referred to as lipoproteins

e. Concentrated energy source supplying more than twice the calories per gram than proteins

Activity D   *Presented here, in random order, are steps followed for measuring midarm circumference. Write the correct sequence in the boxes provided.*

1. Find the midpoint of the upper arm between the shoulder and elbow

2. Record the circumference in centimeters

3. Mark the midarm location

4. Use the nondominant arm

5. Position the arm loosely at the client's side

6. Encircle the arm with a tape measure at the marked position

☐ → ☐ → ☐ → ☐ → ☐ → ☐

Activity E   *Briefly answer the following questions.*

1. What are the parameters for nutritional needs?

   _____

   _____

   _____

2. How do water-soluble vitamins differ from fat-soluble vitamins?

_____

_____

_____

3. What factors influence an individual's eating habits?

_____

_____

_____

4. What should the nurse check for during the physical assessment of a client?

_____

_____

_____

5. What measures should the nurse take when feeding a visually impaired client?

_____

_____

_____

6. What are the various factors that reduce appetite and nutritional intake in older adults?

_____

_____

_____

SECTION II: APPLYING YOUR KNOWLEDGE

Activity F *Nurses use various assessment techniques and equipment to perform physical assessment. The environment must facilitate accurate data collection and be conducive to the client's privacy and comfort. Answer the following question, which involves the nurse's role in feeding, assessment, and planning for the client.*

A nurse is caring for a client with dysphagia who has undergone a surgery for a cataract in their left eye.

1. What care should the nurse take when feeding this client?

_____

_____

_____

SECTION III: PRACTICING FOR NCLEX

Activity G *Answer the following questions.*

1. During the assessment of a client's diet a nurse notes that the client's diet lacks adequate sources of complete protein. What food would the nurse recommend to help correct this deficiency?
   a. Poultry
   b. Beans
   c. Nuts
   d. Grains

2. A nurse is physically assessing a client with malnutrition who belongs to an affluent family in the United States. What could be a probable reason for the client's malnutrition, taking into consideration that the client belongs to an affluent family?
   a. Eating disorders
   b. Religious beliefs
   c. History of malnutrition
   d. Emotional disorders

3. A nurse is caring for a client diagnosed with deficiency of water-soluble vitamins. Which vitamin should the nurse recommend as a supplement?
   a. Vitamin A
   b. Vitamin C
   c. Vitamin D
   d. Vitamin E

4. A nurse is assessing the body mass index of four clients diagnosed with risk of weight-related problems. Which of these clients can be categorized as obese?
   a. Client A, who has a body mass index of 30.2 kg/m^2
   b. Client B, who has a body mass index of 28.6 kg/m^2
   c. Client C, who has a body mass index of 29 kg/m^2
   d. Client D, who has a body mass index of 29.5 kg/m^2

5. A nurse is caring for a client who has been diagnosed with a blood clot in their lower left leg. What would the nurse recommend adding to the diet to regulate the blood-clotting processes in the client's body?
   a. Proteins
   b. Fats
   c. Carbohydrates
   d. Minerals

6. When assessing the client's dietary intake, the nurse notes that the client's daily diet exceeds 2,000 calories. What should the nurse recommend changing in the client's diet?
   a. Unsaturated fats
   b. Vitamins
   c. Cholesterol
   d. Minerals

7. A nurse is analyzing the eating habits of a female client who works in a high-profile law firm in the city. The nurse notes that the client does not include any meat or dairy products in her diet. Which factor could be influencing the client's eating habits?
   a. Access to food markets
   b. Vegetarianism
   c. Veganism
   d. Pregnancy

8. A nurse is assessing the diet of a vegan client. What nutrient does the nurse observe is lacking in this diet?
   a. Fats
   b. Vitamin C
   c. Protein
   d. Minerals

9. A nurse is recording the objective data of a vegetarian client. What should the nurse measure to obtain anthropometric data of the client?
   a. Height
   b. Biceps skin thickness
   c. Chest width
   d. Wrist diameter

10. A nurse is recording the dietary history of a client to obtain facts about their eating habits. What factor will the nurse note when obtaining this history?
    a. The timing of meals
    b. The protein intake
    c. The amount of cholesterol level
    d. The intake of unsaturated fats

11. A nurse is conducting a physical assessment of a client who has been admitted to the health care facility. What factor should the nurse check during the physical assessment?
    a. Height
    b. Diet
    c. Skin
    d. Weight

12. The nurse is caring for a visually impaired client at the health care facility. What should the nurse do when feeding a visually impaired client?
    a. Request a full liquid diet or a mechanically soft diet
    b. Provide small, frequent meals if eating efforts tire the client
    c. Determine whether the client has swallowed the food before offering another mouthful
    d. Arrange to have finger food prepared for the client

13. After completing the physical assessment of a client, the nurse notices a gag reflex in the client. What does the finding indicate?
    a. Dysphagia
    b. Nausea
    c. Eructation
    d. Xerostomia

14. Which observation made during the physical assessment of a client indicates obesity in the client?
    a. A body mass index of 15 or more and a triceps skinfold measurement of more than 15 mm
    b. A body mass index of 25 or more and a triceps skinfold measurement of less than 15 mm
    c. A body mass index of 30 or more and a triceps skinfold measurement of more than 15 mm
    d. A body mass index of 35 or more and a triceps skinfold measurement of more than 15 mm

15. A nurse is caring for a client with a body mass index of 37. How can the nurse help the client to lose weight safely?
    a. Reducing the diet by 200 calories/day
    b. Reducing the diet by 1,200 calories/day
    c. Reducing the diet by 1,500 calories/day
    d. Reducing the diet by 800 calories/day

16. A nurse is assisting a client with dementia. How can the nurse ensure that the client eats the food that they have been served? Select all that apply.
    a. Communicate visually and spatially that the client should eat the food
    b. Inform the client about the kind of food you are offering with each mouthful

c. Ensure that the client is able to see another person eating in the vicinity

d. Be firm with the client and insist that the client eats the food

e. Provide small, frequent meals if efforts to eat and swallow tire the client

17. A nurse is assessing the diet of a client diagnosed with a fat-soluble vitamin deficiency. Which vitamin supplements might the nurse recommend to cover this deficiency? Select all that apply.
a. Vitamin A
b. Vitamin B
c. Vitamin C
d. Vitamin D
e. Vitamin E
f. Vitamin K

18. During the physical assessment of a client, the nurse notes that the client appears exhausted and devoid of energy. The medical records indicate that the client's diet lacks carbohydrates. What can the nurse change in the diet to cover the lack of carbohydrates? Select all that apply.
a. Increase quantity of cereals
b. Increase quantity of grains
c. Increase quantity of egg
d. Increase quantity of yolk
e. Increase quantity of meat

19. A nurse is caring for an older client with complaints of dental pain. What measures can the nurse take to remedy the oral problems that interfere with nutritional intake? Select all that apply.
a. Get dental care every 6 months
b. Practice good dental hygiene daily
c. Encourage drinking noncaffeinated beverages
d. Encourage over-the-counter, herbal therapies
e. Increase caloric intake in the diet

20. During the physical assessment of a client, the nurse records the weight of the client as 185 lb and the height as 5 feet 4 inches. What is the body mass index of the client?
a. 26.3
b. 28.2
c. 27.4
d. 29.0

SECTION IV: REVIEWING WHAT YOU HAVE LEARNED

Activity H *Fill in the blanks by choosing the correct word from the options given in parentheses.*

1. _____ is a loss of appetite associated with illness, altered taste and smell, oral problems, or tension and depression. (Anorexia, Cachexia, Nausea)

2. _____, which commonly accompanies nausea, is the loss of stomach contents through the mouth. (Emesis, Regurgitation, Retching)

Activity I *Mark each statement as either T (True) or F (False). Correct any false statements.*

1. T F Flatus is a discharge of gas from the stomach through the mouth.

2. T F Fat-soluble vitamins (A, D, E, and K) are stored in the body as reserves for future needs.

Activity J *Write the correct term for the description below.*

Anthropometric measurement that helps to determine a client's skeletal muscle mass

_____

Activity K *Match the terms related to nutritional sources in Column A with their descriptions in Column B.*

Column A	Column B
____ 1. Proteins	a. Noncaloric substances in food that are essential to all cells
____ 2. Carbohydrates	b. Nutrients that contain glyceride molecules and are collectively known as lipids
____ 3. Minerals	c. Nutrients composed of amino acids (chemical compounds containing nitrogen, carbon, hydrogen, and oxygen)
____ 4. Fats	d. Nutrients that include sugars and starches

Activity L   *Answer the following questions.*

1. What are the six nutritional components in food?

_____

_____

_____

2. What are the seven common hospital diets?

_____

_____

_____

SECTION V: APPLYING YOUR KNOWLEDGE

Activity M   *Give a rationale for the following question.*

1. Why is high-density lipoprotein (HDL) referred to as "good cholesterol?"

_____

_____

_____

Activity N   *Answer the following questions focusing on nursing roles and responsibilities.*

1. A nurse at an extended care facility is caring for a client having difficulty chewing and swallowing food.
   a. What kind of a diet is likely to be offered to this client?

   _____

   _____

   _____

b. What interventions should the nurse perform when feeding the client?

_____

_____

_____

SECTION VI: GETTING READY FOR NCLEX

Activity O   *Answer the following question.*

A client who has been hospitalized and is recuperating from pneumonia is complaining of stomach gas. Which of the following interventions should the nurse perform? Select all that apply.
a. Encourage walking if possible
b. Suggest drinking carbonated beverages
c. Provide a straw for drinking
d. Ask the client to avoid chewing gum
e. Remind the client to eat with the mouth closed

CHAPTER 16

Fluid and Chemical Balance

Learning Objectives

- Name the components of body fluid.
- List physiologic transport mechanisms for distributing fluid and its constituents.
- Name assessments that provide data about a client's fluid status.
- Explain the purpose for assessing intake and output and circumstances when it is warranted.
- Describe methods for maintaining or restoring fluid volume.
- Describe methods for reducing fluid volume.
- List reasons for administering intravenous (IV) fluids.
- Differentiate between crystalloid and colloid solutions and give examples of each.
- Explain the terms "isotonic," "hypotonic," and "hypertonic" when used in reference to IV solutions.
- List factors that affect the choice of tubing used to administer IV solutions.
- Name techniques for infusing IV solutions.
- Discuss criteria for selecting a vein when administering IV fluid.
- List complications associated with IV fluid administration.
- Discuss purposes for inserting an intermittent venous access device.
- Name the types of transfusion reactions.
- Explain the concept of parenteral nutrition.
- Identify differences between administering blood and crystalloid solutions.

SECTION I: ASSESSING YOUR UNDERSTANDING

Activity A   FILL IN THE BLANKS

1. _____ is the escape of intravenous fluid into the tissue.

2. Fluid that represents the greatest proportion of water in the body is present inside the cells and is called _____ fluid.

3. Fluid present outside the cells is called _____ fluid.

4. Fluid in the tissue space between and around the cells is called _____ fluid.

5. _____ are neurologic infectious microorganisms that cause various brain disorders.

6. _____ are substances that carry either a positive or negative electrical charge.

7. A fluid deficit in both extracellular and intracellular compartments causes _____.

8. _____ tubing is necessary for administering solutions packaged in rigid glass containers.

9. _____ devices are used to access the venous system by piercing a vein with a needle.

10. _____ or the inflammation of a vein is a complication associated with the infusion of intravenous solutions.

Activity B *Consider the following figure.*

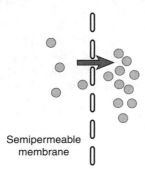

Semipermeable
membrane

1. Identify the type of distribution mechanism.

   _____

   _____

   _____

2. How does this method help regulate the distribution of water in the body?

   _____

   _____

   _____

3. How do colloids affect this distribution mechanism?

   _____

   _____

   _____

Activity C *Match the terms related to fluids and chemical balance in Column A with their description in Column B.*

Column A

_____ **1.** Filtration

_____ **2.** Hydrostatic pressure

_____ **3.** Passive diffusion

_____ **4.** Electrochemical neutrality

_____ **5.** Facilitated diffusion

Column B

a. Physiologic process in which dissolved substances move from an area of higher concentration to an area of lower concentration

b. Identical balance of cations with anions

c. The process in which certain dissolved substances require the assistance of a carrier

molecule to pass from one side of a cellular membrane to the other

d. Regulates the movement of water and substances from a compartment where the pressure is higher to one where pressure is lower

e. Pressure exerted against a membrane

Activity D *Presented here, in random order, are mechanisms that maintain a match between fluid intake and output. Write the correct sequence in the boxes provided.*

1. Stimulates the person to drink.

2. Kidneys excrete water to maintain proper balance.

3. The brain triggers the sensation of thirst.

4. Fluid volume expands.

5. Body fluid becomes concentrated.

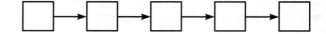

Activity E *Briefly answer the following questions.*

1. What is body fluid made of? What are the sources of body water?

   _____

   _____

   _____

2. What is donated blood tested for?

   _____

   _____

   _____

3. What is the importance of electrolytes?

   _____

   _____

   _____

4. Who are universal donors and recipients? Which are the blood groups that come under this category?

_____

_____

_____

5. What is the importance and role of nonelectrolytes?

_____

_____

_____

6. What are the differences between donor blood and blood recipient?

_____

_____

_____

SECTION II: APPLYING YOUR KNOWLEDGE

Activity F *Fluid deficit occurs when there is a low volume in the extracellular fluid compartments. Fluid deficit leads to dehydration, which can be mild, moderate, or severe. Answer the following questions, which involve the nurse's role in the physical assessment of clients.*

A client is admitted to the health agency with complaints of dizziness and weakness. The client complains that they lack the energy to perform daily activities. The physician, on examining them, directs the nurse to put them on glucose drips.

1. What are the other symptoms that the nurse should observe in this client?

_____

_____

_____

2. What nursing intervention should the nurse perform to ensure that the client's condition improves?

_____

_____

_____

SECTION III: PRACTICING FOR NCLEX

Activity G *Answer the following questions.*

1. A client with severe leg injury from an accident has been brought to the health agency. The client has lost a lot of blood and needs a transfusion. The client's blood group is A, Rh negative. Which blood group could be considered for use in this client (apart from A, Rh negative)?
   a. A, Rh positive
   b. O, Rh negative
   c. AB, Rh negative
   d. B, Rh positive

2. A nurse is caring for several clients at the health care facility. Which client requires fluid volume assessment?
   a. Client with tonsillitis
   b. Client with diarrhea
   c. Client with viral infection
   d. Client with jaundice

3. A client has been admitted to the health agency with complaints of loose bowel movements and vomiting that has persisted for more than a week. The client has become weak and exhausted. Which one of the following is a cause the nurse should suspect?
   a. Hypervolemia
   b. Edema
   c. Hypovolemia
   d. Hypoalbuminemia

4. During the initial assessment of a client who has been admitted to the health agency as a result of dehydration, the nurse notes a 4% loss of body weight. How should the nurse document the client's level of dehydration?
   a. Moderate dehydration
   b. Severe dehydration
   c. Total dehydration
   d. Mild dehydration

5. A nurse is caring for an older client with a cardiovascular disorder. What should the nurse do to avoid the fluid and electrolyte imbalances that may result from the administration of diuretic medication to this client?
   a. Encourage noncaffeinated beverages
   b. Encourage consumption of more food
   c. Offer caffeinated beverages every 3 hours
   d. Avoid intake of salt in food

6. A client who has been diagnosed with hypovolemic shock is being treated with plasma expanders to increase blood volume and raise blood pressure. Which one of the following might the nurse use?
   a. Dextran 40
   b. Perfluorocarbons
   c. Microencapsulated hemoglobin
   d. Hemosol

7. A client is diagnosed with body fluid in excess of 3 L. The physician directs the nurse to reduce the client's fluid intake and to administer medication that would promote urine elimination in the client. How should the nurse note the client's condition in their medical record?
   a. Edema
   b. Hypervolemia
   c. Hypovolemia
   d. Hypoalbuminemia

8. The nursing care plan states that a client is to be weighed regularly. Which guideline should the nurse consider when weighing the client?
   a. Should be weighed wearing light clothes daily
   b. Should be weighed at the same time of day daily
   c. Should be weighed on a different scale to avoid discrepancy
   d. Should be weighed three times a week at the same time

9. A client with symptoms of edema has been brought to the health agency for treatment. Which intervention is appropriate for this client?
   a. Increasing the infusing volume
   b. Increasing fluid intake
   c. Restricting salt intake
   d. Reducing sugar intake

10. A client is being treated for swelling in their tissues and fluid accumulation in the body cavity. Per the direction of the physician, the nurse administers albumin by intravenous infusion. What is an appropriate nursing action for this client?
    a. Infuse fluids at smaller volumes at rapid rates
    b. Monitor the client for signs of circulatory overload
    c. Infuse fluids at smaller volumes at slower rates
    d. Monitor the client for signs of dehydration

11. A client has been diagnosed with albumin deficiency in the blood. The physician directs the nurse to administer albumin by intravenous infusion to the client. For what potential problem would the nurse monitor the client?
    a. Heart disease
    b. Dehydration
    c. Peritoneum infection
    d. Liver disease

12. When administering lipid emulsions to a malnourished client, the nurse observes a certain adverse reaction in the client resulting from the administration of the medication. What is the related symptom?
    a. Cyanosis
    b. Cardiac arrest
    c. Gallbladder enlargement
    d. Anemia

13. A physician directs the nurse to administer isotonic solution to a client who is dehydrated. Under what condition is an isotonic solution administered to the client?
    a. The client's fluid losses exceed fluid intake
    b. The client is not able to eat or drink for a short period
    c. The client's cerebral edema has to be reduced
    d. The client is not able to urinate properly

14. A client is being treated for hypovolemic shock at the health agency. What treatment would be appropriate?
    a. D10W
    b. TPN
    c. Hespan
    d. 3% NaCl

15. A client is being administered an intravenous solution. The physician orders the nurse to monitor the client for any signs of complications. What are common complications of intravenous administration? Select all that apply.
    a. Edema
    b. Phlebitis
    c. Hypervolemia
    d. Dehydration
    e. Thrombus formation

16. A client at the health agency is receiving a blood transfusion. What nursing intervention should the nurse perform during the transfusion?
    a. Release the blood from the blood bank 5 hours prior to transfusion

b. Stay with the client for the first 15 minutes of the transfusion

c. Squeeze and turn the container before starting the transfusion

d. Avoid frequent assessment of the client during the transfusion

17. After weighing a client who uses a diaper, the nurse subtracts the weight of a similar dry item to record the total fluid output of the client on a daily basis. The nurse records the output as 0.47 kg. What is the equivalent of this output in milliliters?
a. 487 mL
b. 100 mL
c. 475 mL
d. 337 mL

18. A nurse needs to provide a client 1 tablespoon of glucose in 1 ounce of water. The nurse knows that the solution prepared is how many milliliters of glucose with 30 mL water?
a. 15
b. 20
c. 10
d. 25

19. A nurse has been directed by the physician to give 1 ounce of glucose to a client who is on an intravenous fluid intake. The nurse would need to give how many milliliters of glucose?
a. 10
b. 30
c. 20
d. 15

SECTION IV: REVIEWING WHAT YOU HAVE LEARNED

Activity H *Fill in the blanks by choosing the correct word from the options given in parentheses.*

1. Electrolytes with a positive charge are called _____. (anions, cations, ions)

2. _____ is a fluid imbalance with an increased volume of water in the intravascular fluid compartment. (Hypervolemia, Hypoalbuminemia, Hypovolemia)

Activity I *Mark each statement as either T (True) or F (False). Correct any false statements.*

1. **T F** Dehydration is a fluid deficit in both the extracellular and intracellular compartments of the human body.

2. **T F** Passive diffusion is an identical balance of cations with anions in any given fluid compartment.

Activity J *Write the correct term for the description below.*

Fluid in the tissue space between and around cells _____

Activity K *Match the terms related to body fluids and chemical balance in Column A with their descriptions in Column B.*

Column A

_____ **1.** Venipuncture

_____ **2.** Emulsion

_____ **3.** Edema

_____ **4.** Osmosis

Column B

a. Process by which body fluid is distributed from one location to another

b. Method of accessing the venous system by piercing a vein with a needle

c. Mixture of two liquids, one of which is insoluble in the other

d. Condition that develops when excess fluid is distributed to the interstitial space

Activity L *Differentiate between crystalloid and colloid solutions based on the criteria given below.*

	Crystalloid Solution	**Colloid Solution**
Definition		
Effects		
Example		

Activity M   *Answer the following questions.*

1. What is parenteral nutrition?

   _____

   _____

   _____

2. What are the reasons for administering intravenous solutions?

   _____

   _____

   _____

SECTION V: APPLYING YOUR KNOWLEDGE

Activity N   *Give a rationale for the following question.*

1. Why do the plastic bags of intravenous solutions not need vented tubing?

   _____

   _____

   _____

Activity O   *Answer the following questions focusing on nursing roles and responsibilities.*

1. A nurse is caring for a client who has been ordered intravenous therapy.
   a. What actions should the nurse perform before preparing the intravenous solution?

      _____

      _____

      _____

   b. What technique will the nurse follow to remove air bubbles from the tubing?

      _____

      _____

      _____

SECTION VI: GETTING READY FOR NCLEX

Activity P   *Answer the following question.*

Which nursing interventions are appropriate for a client who is on fluid restrictions? Select all that apply.

a. Suggest rinsing the mouth without swallowing water

b. Provide fluids in a plastic squeeze bottle or spray atomizer

c. Explain the need to restrict fluids in the diet

d. Encourage intake of food with a moderately high salt content

e. Encourage the client to suck on ice chips

CHAPTER 17

Hygiene

Learning Objectives

- Define hygiene.
- Name hygiene practices that most people perform regularly.
- Provide reasons why a partial bath is more appropriate than a daily bath for older adults.
- List advantages of towel or bag baths.
- Name situations in which shaving with a safety razor is contraindicated.
- List items recommended for oral hygiene.
- Identify methods to prevent the chief hazard when providing oral hygiene to an unconscious client.
- Describe techniques for preventing damage to dentures during cleaning.
- Describe methods for removing hair tangles.
- Name types of clients for whom nail care is provided with extreme caution.
- Identify visual and hearing devices.
- List alternatives for clients who cannot insert or care for their own contact lenses.
- Discuss reasons for sound disturbances experienced by people who wear hearing aids.
- Describe an infrared listening device.

SECTION I: ASSESSING YOUR UNDERSTANDING

Activity A   FILL IN THE BLANKS

1. _____ protects the layers and structures within the lower portions of the skin.

2. _____ is a slimy substance that keeps the membranes soft and moist.

3. As the jaw grows, the _____ teeth are replaced by permanent teeth.

4. The combination of sugar, plaque, and bacteria may eventually erode the tooth enamel and cause _____.

5. A contact lens is a small plastic disk placed directly on the _____ of the eye.

6. Oral hygiene consists of those practices used to clean the _____.

7. A podiatrist undergoes special training in caring for the _____.

8. Older adults are more susceptible to impacted _____, a common cause of hearing loss.

9. A(n) _____ is a person who prescribes corrective lenses.

10. The _____ layer separates the skin from skeletal muscles.

Activity B   *Consider the following figures.*

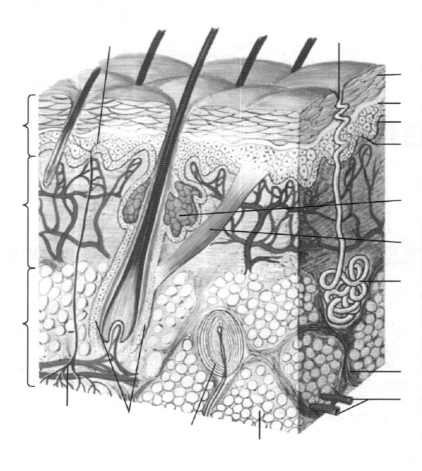

1. Identify and label the figure.

   _____

   _____

   _____

2. What are the functions of the various layers in the figure?

   _____

   _____

   _____

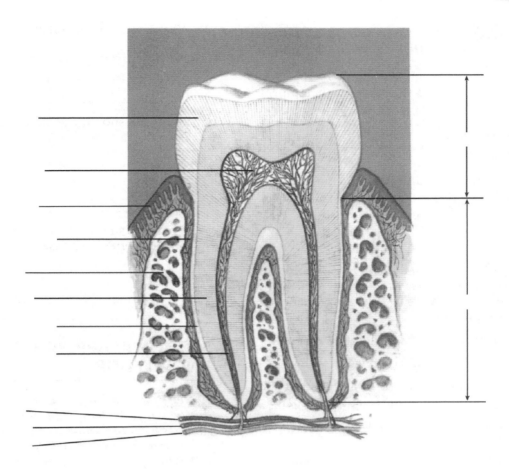

3. Identify and label the figure.

_____

_____

_____

4. List three common problems associated with this part of the body.

_____

_____

_____

Activity C *Match the terms related to hygiene in Column A with their functions in Column B.*

Column A

_____ **1.** Contact lenses

_____ **2.** Bathing

_____ **3.** Flossing

_____ **4.** Skin

_____ **5.** Shaving

Column B

a. Regulates body temperature

b. Reduces the potential of getting infected

c. Removes unwanted body hair

d. Placed directly on the cornea

e. Removes plaque

Activity D *Presented here, in random order, are steps that a nurse takes when providing nail care for clients. Write the correct sequence in the boxes provided.*

1. Push cuticles downward with a soft towel.

2. Soak the hands or feet in warm water.

3. Use a handheld electric rotary file to reduce the length of long fingernails or toenails.

4. Clean under the nails with a wooden orange stick.

5. Check with the client's physician before cutting fingernails or toenails.

☐ → ☐ → ☐ → ☐ → ☐

Activity E *Briefly answer the following questions.*

1. How should the nurse provide oral care for an unconscious client?

_____

_____

_____

2. What is a partial bath?

_____

_____

_____

3. What are the four important functions of the skin?

_____

_____

_____

4. What care should the nurse take when grooming a client's hair?

_____

_____

_____

5. What care should the nurse take when caring for the client's eyeglasses?

_____

_____

_____

SECTION II: APPLYING YOUR KNOWLEDGE

Activity F *Bathing is a hygienic practice during which a cleaning agent (such as soap) is used to remove sweat, oil, dirt, and microorganisms from the skin. Answer the following questions, which involve the nurse's role in assisting clients with bathing.*

A nurse is caring for a senior client who has undergone rectal surgery. The client is averse to bathing daily. The nurse needs to ensure that body areas subject to greatest soiling or that are sources of body odor are cleaned and infections do not occur.

1. What kind of bath should the nurse suggest to the client?

_____

_____

_____

2. What care should the nurse take when providing perineal care to the client?

_____

_____

_____

SECTION III: PRACTICING FOR NCLEX

Activity G *Answer the following questions.*

1. A nurse is assisting a client to clean a prosthetic eye. How will the nurse remove the eye for cleaning?
   a. Depress the lower eyelid to remove the artificial eye
   b. Place an ophthalmic suction cup on the eye
   c. Extend the eyelid to remove the prosthetic eye
   d. Irrigate the eye socket

2. A nurse is providing personal hygiene for a 71-year-old client with acute arthritis. What kind of bath should the nurse consider for this client?
   a. Bed bath
   b. Towel bath
   c. Partial bath
   d. Shower

3. A client is new to wearing soft contact lenses. They are nervous and need help to remove the lenses. How should the nurse remove the lenses?
   a. Remove the lens from the cornea to the sclera by sliding it into position
   b. Remove the lens by depressing the lower eyelid to allow the lens to slide free
   c. Place the thumb on the upper lid and use the other finger to remove the lens
   d. Press the upper lid and ask the client to blink to separate the lens

4. A nurse is caring for a client with a high fever. What type of bath is best for this client?
   a. Sitz
   b. Sponge
   c. Medicated
   d. Whirlpool

5. A nurse is caring for a young woman with a severe hearing impairment, who needs a new hearing aid. The woman travels and meets clients as part of her work. What kind of hearing aid should the nurse suggest for this client?
   a. Behind-the-ear device
   b. Infrared listening device
   c. Body aid device
   d. Canal aid

6. A nurse is caring for a senior client with reduced mobility. The nurse cleans the client's glasses by running tepid water over both sides of the glass. What would the nurse use to dry them?
   a. Woolen cloth
   b. Soft handkerchief
   c. Paper tissues
   d. Dryer

7. A nurse is caring for a client who has been diagnosed with cancer. The client is undergoing chemotherapy. What precaution should the nurse take when grooming their hair?
   a. Use a wide-tooth comb
   b. Ask the client to keep their hair short
   c. Brush their hair from the crown
   d. Brush their hair vigorously

8. A nurse is caring for a client who is in a coma. What care should the nurse take with regard to the client's oral hygiene?
   a. The nurse should use waxed floss
   b. The nurse should use sterile solution
   c. The nurse should use liquid oral hygiene
   d. The nurse should use oral swabs

9. A nurse is caring for a senior client with limited mobility resulting from arthritis. How should the nurse assist the client to take care of their dentures?
   a. Clean the dentures with hot water and antiseptic solution
   b. Store the dentures in a bowl of warm water
   c. Use cotton swabs to clean the dentures
   d. Use a clean facecloth to free the dentures from the mouth

10. A senior client needs assistance in bathing. The client refuses to have a partial bath and insists on a shower. How should the nurse help the client?
    a. Provide nonskid mat on floor
    b. Give them a towel bath
    c. Give them a bag bath
    d. Insist on a partial bath

11. A nurse is caring for a diabetic client with thick and discolored nails. How should the nurse help this client with regard to nail care?
    a. Clean the nails with warm water
    b. File and trim the client's nails
    c. Clean under the nails with a clean towel
    d. Request the services of a podiatrist

12. A nurse is caring for a client with impaired skin on the feet. What should the nurse suggest to this client with regard to care of the skin?
    a. Instruct the client to wear leather slippers
    b. Instruct the client to wear flip-flops
    c. Instruct the client to wear sturdy slippers
    d. Instruct the client to wear heeled shoes

13. A nurse is assessing an older client with brown, flat patches on the face, hands, and forearms. How should the nurse document this finding?
    a. Seborrheic keratoses
    b. Senile lentigines
    c. Scleroderma
    d. Acne

14. A nurse is caring for a client with long hair who fractured their arm. How should the nurse care for their hair? Select all that apply.
    a. Brush the hair for a longer time
    b. Tie the hair into a bun
    c. Use a wide-tooth comb
    d. Brush the hair slowly and carefully
    e. Start combing the hair from the crown

15. A nurse is assisting a client in cleaning their eyeglasses. Arrange the tasks in the most likely sequence in which the nurse should perform them when caring for the client's eyeglasses.
    a. Wash the lenses with soap or detergent
    b. Rinse with running tap water
    c. Hold the eyeglasses by the nose or ear braces
    d. Run tepid water over both sides of the lenses
    e. Dry with a clean, soft cloth such as a handkerchief

16. A client who has just started wearing soft contact lenses needs some help in removing them. Arrange the tasks in the most likely sequence in which the nurse should perform them when removing the client's contact lenses.
    a. Remove the lenses using the thumb and forefinger
    b. Place a towel on the client's chest
    c. Compress the lid margins together
    d. Elevate the client's head
    e. Move the contact lens from the cornea to the sclera

SECTION IV: REVIEWING WHAT YOU HAVE LEARNED

Activity H   *Fill in the blanks by choosing the correct word from the options given in parentheses.*

1. _____ can result from a combination of sugar, plaque, and bacteria eroding the tooth enamel. (Caries, Gingivitis, Tartar)

2. A/an _____ treats eye disorders medically and surgically. (ophthalmologist, optometrist, podiatrist)

Activity I   *Mark each statement as either T (True) or F (False). Correct any false statements.*

1. T F   The cells in the epidermis are shed continuously and replaced from the dermis.

2. T F   The contraction of small arrector pili muscles around hair follicles is commonly described as goosebumps.

Activity J   *Write the correct term for each description below.*

1. Practices that promote health through personal cleanliness _____

2. Dried crusts containing mucus, microorganisms, and epithelial cells shed from the mucous membrane _____

Activity K   *Consider the Following Figure*

1. Identify and label the figure.

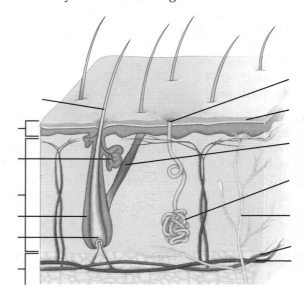

Activity L *Answer the following questions.*

1. What is an infrared listening device?

_____

_____

_____

2. How should the nurse care for a client's dentures?

_____

_____

_____

SECTION V: APPLYING YOUR KNOWLEDGE

Activity M *Give a rationale for the following question.*

Why is it important for the nurse to consult the client regarding a convenient time for a bath?

_____

_____

_____

Activity N *Answer the following questions focusing on nursing roles and responsibilities.*

1. A nurse is providing oral care for a client in a coma.
   a. What risks are involved in giving oral care to this client?
   b. What precautions should the nurse take when providing oral care for the client?

2. A nurse is preparing to provide perineal care to a client who has given birth vaginally.
   a. What precautions should the nurse take when providing perineal care to the client?
   b. For what reasons would a sitz bath be beneficial to this client?

Activity O *Consider the following questions. Discuss them with your instructor or peers.*

A nurse is caring for an older adult client with Alzheimer disease at an extended care facility. Sometimes the client is alert and oriented; at other times, they are agitated or unaware of their surroundings. During periods of confusion and disorientation, the client needs assistance with activities of daily living and hygiene.

a. How should the nurse assist the client with activities of daily living?

b. What actions should the nurse take with respect to the client's hygiene?

SECTION VI: GETTING READY FOR NCLEX

Activity P *Answer the following question.*

Which measure is most appropriate when cleaning plastic eyeglasses?
a. Use paper tissue to clean the lenses
b. Rinse the lenses with running tap water
c. Immerse the lenses in hot soapy water
d. Allow the lenses to air-dry

CHAPTER 18

Comfort, Rest, and Sleep

Learning Objectives

- Differentiate between comfort, rest, and sleep.
- Describe ways to modify the client environment to promote comfort, rest, and sleep.
- List standard furnishings in each client room.
- State the functions of sleep.
- Describe the phases of sleep and their differences.
- Describe the general trend in sleep requirements as a person ages.
- Identify factors that affect sleep.
- List categories of drugs that affect sleep.
- Name techniques for assessing sleep patterns.
- Describe categories of sleep disorders.
- Discuss techniques for promoting sleep.
- Plan nursing measures that promote relaxation.
- Discuss unique characteristics of sleep among older adults.

SECTION I: ASSESSING YOUR UNDERSTANDING

Activity A   FILL IN THE BLANKS

1. _____ is the ability to maintain stable body temperature.

2. The rapid eye movement (REM) phase of sleep is referred to as _____ sleep.

3. _____ are conditions associated with activities that cause arousal or partial arousal usually during transitions in non-REM (NREM) periods of sleep.

4. _____ are a class of drugs that excite structures in the brain and cause wakefulness.

5. _____ means difficulty falling asleep, awakening frequently during the night, or awakening early.

6. _____ is a technique used to treat the suppression of melatonin caused by seasonal affective disorder, by stimulating light receptors in the eye.

7. _____ refers to the waking state characterized by reduced activity and mental stimulation.

8. The onset of disorientation as the sun sets generally seen in older adults is referred to as _____ syndrome.

9. _____ is a sleep disorder characterized by feeling sleepy despite getting normal sleep.

Activity B *Consider the following figures.*

Awake:
low-voltage, fast

Awake eyes closed:
alpha-waves, 8–12 cps

NREM:
Stage 1:
theta-waves, 3–7 cps

Stage 2:
sleep spindles, 12–14 cps;
K-complex

sleep spindle
K-complex

Stages 3 and 4:
delta-waves, 0.5–2 cps

REM:
low-voltage mixed frequency
sawtoothed waves

sawtooth

1. Identify the figure.

   _____

   _____

   _____

2. Explain the phases of sleep.

   _____

   _____

   _____

Pineal
gland

☽ = ↑ Melatonin

☀ = ↓ Melatonin

3. Identify the figure.

   _____

   _____

   _____

4. Explain the role of phototherapy in the sleep–
   wake cycle.

   _____

   _____

   _____

Activity C *Match the types of parasomnias in Column A with their descriptions in Column B.*

Column A

_____ 1. Nocturnal enuresis

_____ 2. Somnambulism

_____ 3. Bruxism

_____ 4. Restless legs syndrome

Column B

a. Condition in which the individual walks in their sleep

b. Condition in which the individual grinds their teeth during sleep

c. Movement, typically in the legs, to re-lieve disturbing skin sensations

d. Also known as bed-wetting

Activity D *Briefly answer the following questions.*

1. What are the functions of sleep?

   _____

   _____

   _____

2. What is progressive relaxation?

_____

_____

_____

3. What are the factors that affect sleep?

_____

_____

_____

4. What is nocturnal polysomnography?

_____

_____

_____

5. What is seasonal affective disorder?

_____

_____

_____

SECTION II: APPLYING YOUR KNOWLEDGE

Activity E   *Answer the following questions that involve the nurse's role in the physical assessment of clients with sleep apnea.*

A client is admitted to the health care facility with a diagnosis of sleep apnea. The nurse understands that the condition can be life-threatening at times.

1. What are the risks associated with sleep apnea?

_____

_____

_____

2. What nursing interventions should the nurse implement to promote sleep in the client?

_____

_____

_____

SECTION III: PRACTICING FOR NCLEX

Activity F   *Answer the following questions.*

1. A nurse is caring for a client diagnosed with somnambulism. Which activity should the nurse include in the plan of care for this client?
   a. Keep the client restrained
   b. Lock the stair gates and doors
   c. Keep a call bell within reach of the client
   d. Administer sedatives if prescribed

2. A client is admitted to the health care facility after getting a plaster cast put on a fractured tibia. Which bed accessory should the nurse use to provide comfort to the fractured leg?
   a. Mattress
   b. Blanket
   c. Pillows
   d. Headboard

3. A nurse is performing cardiopulmonary resuscitation (CPR) on a client experiencing an acute myocardial infarction. Which room furnishing would the nurse use to facilitate this procedure?
   a. Over-the-bed table
   b. Side stand
   c. Bedside chair
   d. Headboard

4. A nurse is caring for a client who is bedridden as a result of a spinal cord injury. Which intervention would the nurse implement to keep the client's skin intact?
   a. Place an extra draw sheet
   b. Provide extra pillows
   c. Place a mattress overlay
   d. Provide a soft mattress

5. A nurse finds that a client with leg ulcers has swelling resulting from infection. Which intervention would the nurse initiate immediately to reduce the swelling?
   a. Elevate the limb with pillows
   b. Immobilize the affected limb
   c. Change the wound dressing
   d. Restrict fluid intake

6. A client has been diagnosed with urinary incontinence. Which intervention would be

appropriate to prevent the frequent changing of bed linens?
a. Restricting the amount of fluid intake by the client
b. Placing an absorbent pad between the client and the bottom sheet
c. Providing an extra bottom sheet to the client
d. Adding an extra draw sheet on the bed of the client

7. A nurse is examining the mastectomy site in a female client a week after breast surgery. Which intervention would help to maintain the dignity of the client?
a. Provide an explanation for the procedure
b. Draw the privacy curtain around the client
c. Place the client in a comfortable position
d. Use soft strokes when palpating the site

8. A nurse is caring for a client who has sleep apnea. What intervention would the nurse perform to prevent hypoxia in this client?
a. Provide a special breathing mask
b. Encourage physical exercises
c. Provide milk before sleeping
d. Provide a back massage before sleep

9. A client visits the health care facility with complaints of sleeplessness. During the interview, the client tells the nurse that they awaken very early in the morning and then is unable to get any more sleep. Which nursing action would be most beneficial for this client?
a. Ask the client to exercise before bedtime
b. Ask the client to engage in more diversional activities
c. Ask the client to avoid drinking alcohol before sleeping
d. Ask the client to avoid listening to music before bedtime

10. A nurse is caring for a client who is unable to get proper sleep as a result of an increased frequency in urination. Which intervention should the nurse implement to help the client?
a. Administer diuretics in the morning
b. Reduce the dose of diuretics in the evening
c. Get a physician's order for catheterization
d. Restrict fluid intake for the client

11. A nurse is preparing a discharge teaching plan for a client with narcolepsy. Which activity should the nurse suggest the client avoid?
a. Driving motor vehicles
b. Performing moderate exercise
c. Watching television before sleep
d. Practicing relaxation techniques

12. A client who visits the health care center complains to the nurse that they have been lacking energy while awake; however, their appetite has increased accompanied by a craving for sweets, which has led to weight gain. The client has noticed that these symptoms begin during darker winter months and disappear as daylight hours increase in the spring. Which therapy would the nurse expect to initiate for this client?
a. Tranquilizers
b. Relaxation
c. Back massage
d. Phototherapy

13. A client is admitted to the health care facility for an angiography that has been scheduled for the next day. The client tells the nurse that they are unable to sleep because the place is new to them. What nursing diagnosis is appropriate for this client?
a. Impaired bed mobility
b. Disturbed sleep pattern
c. Relocation stress syndrome
d. Impaired gas exchange

14. A nurse is providing a back massage to a client to facilitate relaxation. What is a recommended technique?
a. Perform circular strokes
b. Omit stimulating strokes
c. Ask the client to take shallow breaths
d. Perform firm strokes

15. A senior client is admitted to the health care unit with insomnia. Which nursing interventions should the nurse implement to promote sleep in the client? Select all that apply.
a. Promote physical exercise.
b. Administer sedatives.
c. Provide milk before sleeping.
d. Provide a warmer environment.
e. Encourage relaxation techniques.

16. A client visits their primary health care facility with complaints of difficulty in falling asleep. Which food items should the nurse tell the client to avoid before bedtime? Select all that apply.
    a. Coffee
    b. Cola
    c. Chocolate
    d. Fish
    e. Legumes

SECTION IV: REVIEWING WHAT YOU HAVE LEARNED

Activity G   *Fill in the blanks by choosing the correct word from the options given in parentheses.*

1. _____ is a waking state characterized by reduced activity and decreased mental stimulation. (Comfort, Rest, Sleep)

2. _____ refers to disturbances in the sleep–wake cycle in which there is arousal or partial arousal, usually during transitions in NREM periods of sleep. (Hypersomnia, Insomnia, Parasomnia)

Activity H   *Mark each statement as either T (True) or F (False). Correct any false statements.*

1. **T F**   Sedatives produce a relaxing and calming effect in older clients, thus promoting rest.

2. **T F**   The EEG waves produced during REM sleep appear similar to those produced during wakefulness.

Activity I   *Write the correct term for the description below.*

1. Hormone secreted by the pineal gland in the absence of bright light _____

Activity J   *Answer the following questions.*

1. What are the benefits of sleep?

_____

_____

_____

2. What are the four categories of drugs that promote or interfere with sleep?

_____

_____

_____

SECTION V: APPLYING YOUR KNOWLEDGE

Activity K   *Give rationales for the following questions.*

1. Why are diuretics administered early in the morning?

_____

_____

_____

2. Why should the nurse suggest that the client with a disturbed sleep pattern reduce or eliminate caffeine intake?

_____

_____

_____

Activity L   *Answer the following questions, focusing on nursing roles and responsibilities.*

1. A nurse is caring for a client with a disturbed sleep pattern who cannot sleep for more than 4 hours most nights.
   a. What measures could the nurse take to promote the client's sleep?
   b. What methods could the nurse use to promote relaxation of the sleep-disturbed client's muscles and improve blood circulation?

Activity M   *Consider the following questions. Discuss them with your instructor or peers.*

1. A nurse is caring for a client who is to undergo surgery the following day. The client is anxious and cannot sleep.
   a. What interventions should the nurse perform to help the client relax?
   b. How can the nurse ensure that the client gets adequate sleep?

SECTION VI: GETTING READY FOR NCLEX

Activity N *Answer the following question.*

A client with hypersomnolence related to seasonal affective disorder has been prescribed phototherapy. Which point should the nurse include in client teaching?

a. Wear eyeglasses or contact lenses with ultraviolet filters
b. Sit 5 feet from the artificial light during phototherapy
c. Look at the artificial light continuously
d. Repeat exposure to artificial light up to 3 to 6 hours a day

Safety

Learning Objectives

- Discuss the purpose of the National Patient Safety Goals (NPSGs) and methods for implementing them.
- Give an example of one common injury that predominates during each developmental stage (infancy through older adulthood).
- Name injuries that result from environmental hazards.
- Identify methods for reducing latex sensitization.
- Discuss measures for preventing burns.
- List areas of responsibility incorporated in most fire plans.
- Describe the indications for using each class of fire extinguishers.
- Name common causes of asphyxiation.
- Discuss methods for preventing drowning.
- Explain why humans are susceptible to electrical shock.
- Discuss methods for preventing electrical shock.
- Name common substances associated with poisoning.
- Discuss methods for preventing poisonings.
- Explain why older adults are prone to falling.
- Discuss the benefits and risks of using physical restraints.
- Explain the basis for enacting restraint legislation and the Joint Commission's accreditation standards.
- Identify criteria for applying a physical restraint.
- Differentiate between a restraint and a restraint alternative.
- Describe two areas of concern during an accident.

SECTION I: ASSESSING YOUR UNDERSTANDING

Activity A   FILL IN THE BLANKS

1. A(n) _____ burn is a skin injury caused by flames, hot liquids, or steam and is the most common form of burn.

2. _____ is the inability to breathe and results from airway obstruction, drowning, or inhalation of noxious gases such as smoke or carbon monoxide.

3. _____ is a harmless distribution of low-amperage electricity over a large area of the body.

4. _____ are used to restrict a person's freedom of movement, physical activity, or normal access to their body.

5. _____ dermatitis refers to a delayed localized skin reaction that occurs within 6 to 48 hours and lasts several days.

6. A(n) _____ is a substance that facilitates the flow of electrical current.

7. A _____ is a plan or set of steps to follow when implementing an intervention.

8. _____ refers to the loss of bone mass, which increases the risk for fractures, especially in older women.

9. A _____ diverts leaking electrical energy to the earth.

10. A _____ is low-voltage but high-amperage electricity.

Activity B *Consider the following figures.*

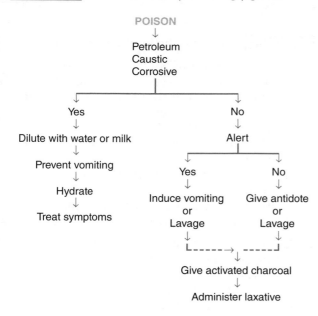

1. Identify the figure.

_____

_____

_____

2. Explain the management of accidental poisoning.

_____

_____

_____

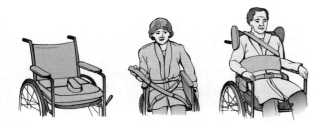

3. Identify the figure.

_____

_____

_____

4. Differentiate between restraints and restraint alternatives.

_____

_____

_____

Activity C *Match the type of extinguisher in Column a with the type of substances it is used for in Column B.*

Column A

____ **1.** Class A

____ **2.** Class B

____ **3.** Class C

____ **4.** Class ABC

Column B

a. Gasoline, oil, paint, grease, and other flammable liquids

b. Electrical fires

c. Fires of any kind

d. Burning paper, wood, cloth

Activity D *Presented here, in random order, are the steps to be taken during fire management. Write the correct sequence in the boxes provided.*

1. Rescue

2. Confine the fire

3. Alarm

4. Extinguish

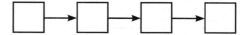

Presented here, in random order, are the steps to be taken during the management of accidental poisoning resulting from the consumption of sedatives. Write the correct sequence in the boxes provided.

1. Check for vital signs.

2. Administer laxatives.

3. Give activated charcoal.

4. Induce vomiting.

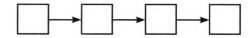

Activity E *Briefly answer the following questions.*

1. What are the types of latex reaction?

_____

_____

_____

2. What are the methods used to prevent thermal burns?

_____

_____

_____

3. What is meant by carbon monoxide poisoning?

_____

_____

_____

4. What measure should be practiced to prevent drowning?

_____

_____

_____

5. What is meant by restraint alternatives?

_____

_____

_____

SECTION II: APPLYING YOUR KNOWLEDGE

Activity F *In health care agencies, fall prevention measures may include the use of physical and chemical restraints, which are methods of restricting a person's freedom of movement, physical activity, or normal access to his or her body. The use of restraints, however, is closely regulated. Answer the following questions, which involve the nurse's role in the use of restraints.*

A nurse is caring for a senior client who is confused but has a steady gait. Repeatedly, the client tries to get out of their room. The nurse plans to restrain the client to prevent them from walking off the premises.

1. What kind of alternative restraint should the nurse use on the client?

_____

_____

_____

2. What are the disadvantages of conventional restraints?

_____

_____

_____

SECTION III: PRACTICING FOR NCLEX

Activity G *Answer the following questions.*

1. A nurse is planning discharge teaching for a senior client with cognitive impairment. Which intervention should the nurse adopt to ensure that the client does not take an accidental overdose of medicines?
   a. Write the medication order on a piece of paper
   b. Prefill separate containers for the medicines
   c. Instruct the client to see the blister pack
   d. Explain the drug regimen to the client

2. A 4-year-old child with accidental poisoning resulting from the consumption of sedative medications is brought to the health care facility. Which action should be the first priority of the nurse?
   a. Take a detailed history
   b. Induce vomiting in the child
   c. Assess breathing and cardiac function
   d. Give gastric lavage

3. A nurse finds that a client in the psychiatric nursing unit is looking frightened and expresses that they are feeling out of control. Which nursing intervention is the most appropriate?
   a. Restrain the client on the bed
   b. Isolate the client in a time-out room
   c. Administer the prescribed antianxiety medication
   d. Move the client to a quiet room and talk to them

4. A nurse is preparing discharge teaching for the mother of a 10-month-old baby. Which teaching point should the nurse include to prevent accidental falls in the infant?
   a. Educate the parents to restrain the infant in automobiles
   b. Avoid making the baby sit on a chair or bed
   c. Keep the baby restrained while feeding
   d. Prevent the baby from moving around

5. A nurse is providing health education in a pediatric clinic about the prevention of accidental poisoning in toddlers. Which activity should the nurse encourage parents to perform?
   a. Avoid keeping any cleaning solutions at home
   b. Educate kids about the consequences of poisoning
   c. Label poisonous substances
   d. Keep cleaning solutions locked

6. A nurse prepares a plan of care for a client who is restrained due to a psychiatric condition. Which nursing diagnosis should be a priority in the client?
   a. Impaired mobility
   b. Risk for injury
   c. Impaired sensory perception
   d. Altered consciousness

7. A nurse-in-charge is educating team members about electrical safety and the prevention of electrical hazards in the nursing unit. Which safety factor should the nurse emphasize the most?
   a. Unplug the equipment after use
   b. Put electrical cords under the carpet
   c. Use grounded equipment
   d. Avoid operating devices with wet hands

8. A toddler is admitted to the health care facility for a diagnostic test scheduled the next day. Which nursing action should be the highest priority?
   a. Protect the toddler from injury
   b. Befriend the toddler for confidence
   c. Adapt the toddler to hospital routines
   d. Prepare for the diagnostic test

9. A nurse is caring for a senior client who is disoriented and has been restrained. On reassessment, the nurse finds that the client has improved, but the restraint order is for another 2 hours. What is the most appropriate action?
   a. Wait for the physician to inspect the client and revise the order
   b. Remove the restraint, even if the order has not expired
   c. Continue the restraint until the order has expired
   d. Loosen the restraint to allow limited movement

10. An industrial health nurse is preparing a health education class about the management of carbon monoxide poisoning. Which interventions are appropriate to manage carbon monoxide poisoning? Select all that apply.
    a. Remove the person from the site
    b. Check for vital signs
    c. Administer oxygen inhalation
    d. Keep the doors and windows closed
    e. Reorient the client

11. Upon entering a client's room, a nurse finds that there is an outbreak of fire from an electrical point. Which nursing action should be the highest priority?
    a. Call for the electrician
    b. Raise the alarm for help
    c. Extinguish the fire
    d. Evacuate the client

12. A nurse gets an order to restrain a client for 2 hours with a restraint alternative. Which alternatives would be appropriate? Select all that apply.
    a. Tilt wedges
    b. Vest restraint
    c. Seat belts with Velcro
    d. Harnesses with buckles
    e. Elbow restraints

13. A nurse is preparing discharge teaching for a 5-year-old client admitted with accidental drowning. Which teaching points should be included in the plan to prevent further incidences of drowning? Select all that apply.
    a. Never let the child swim alone
    b. Provide life jackets when swimming
    c. Let the child swim with his or her friends
    d. Keep the swimming pool fenced
    e. Let the child swim alone to gain confidence

14. A nurse is caring for a client who is repeatedly trying to take out the endotracheal tube that facilitates breathing. What would be an appropriate action taken by the nurse to prevent the client from removing the endotracheal tube?
    a. Apply elbow restraints to the client
    b. Tell a family member to sit with the client
    c. Take a restraint order from a physician by telephone
    d. Apply waist restraints to the client

15. A 10-year-old child is brought to the primary health center with wounds on their knees. Based on their age, what would be a likely cause of the injury?
    a. Play-related activities
    b. Automobile accident
    c. A fall from a bed
    d. A fall down the stairs

16. A nurse is caring for a client who develops contact dermatitis on exposure to latex. What interventions should the nurse implement to protect the client from latex exposure? Select all that apply.
    a. Attach an allergy-alert ID bracelet to the client
    b. Stock the client's room with latex-free equipment
    c. Communicate with other personnel to use nonlatex equipment
    d. Wash hands before wearing gloves to provide care to the client
    e. Instruct the client to wash the area in contact with latex immediately

17. An empty client room has caught fire. The nurse takes all measures according to the fire plan of the health care facility. The nurse finds that the smoke is escaping from the room into the corridors. What measure should the nurse implement to prevent smoke escaping from the room?
    a. Close the door of the room on fire
    b. Place a moist blanket at the thresholds of the doors
    c. Switch on the fans in the corridors to spread the smoke
    d. Wait for the firemen to come and handle it

18. A nurse is planning discharge teaching for a senior client. Which teaching point should the nurse include to prevent falls for this client?
    a. Wear slippers at home
    b. Walk with a supporting cane
    c. Call for assistance to ambulate
    d. Avoid using area rugs

SECTION IV: REVIEWING WHAT YOU HAVE LEARNED

Activity H   *Fill in the blanks by choosing the correct word from the options given in parentheses.*

1. _____ can result from airway obstruction, drowning, or inhalation of noxious gases such as smoke or carbon monoxide. (Asphyxiation, Macroshock, Poisoning)

2. A(n) _____ is a substance that confines electrical currents so that they do not scatter. (conductor, ground, insulator)

Activity I   *Mark each statement as either T (True) or F (False). Correct any false statements.*

1. **T F**   Carbon dioxide is an odorless gas released during the complete combustion of fossil fuels commonly used to heat homes.

2. **T F**   A person with intact skin usually does not feel microshock.

Activity J   *Write the correct term for the description below.*

1. A condition in which fluid occupies the airway and interferes with ventilation _____

Activity K   *Answer the following questions.*

1. What is a thermal burn?

2. What are environmental hazards? Give examples.

SECTION V: APPLYING YOUR KNOWLEDGE

Activity L   *Give a rationale for the following question.*

1. Why are victims of cold-water drowning more likely to be resuscitated?

_____

_____

_____

Activity M   *Answer the following question, focusing on nursing roles and responsibilities.*

A nurse is caring for a client who keeps tugging at the line being used for intravenous therapy.

a. What should the nurse do before considering the use of any restraint?

_____

_____

_____

b. What are the nurse's responsibilities if a restraint is applied to the client?

_____

_____

_____

Activity N *Think over the following question. Discuss them with your instructor or peers.*

A fire erupts in the storeroom of the health care facility following an electrical short circuit. The storage area contains papers, books, and gauze dressing supplies. The fire spreads quickly toward other client rooms.

a. How can the nurse ensure client safety in this situation?

b. What are the nurse's responsibilities during a fire?

SECTION VI: GETTING READY FOR NCLEX

Activity O *Answer the following question.*

During a routine well-child visit, a nurse needs to teach parents safety measures to prevent childhood poisoning. What teaching point is appropriate?

a. Discard old medications in the wastebasket

b. Tell the child that medication is sweet to help them take it

c. Keep the home ventilated when using aerosol sprays

d. Carry regular medications in purses

CHAPTER 20

Pain Management

Learning Objectives

- Give a general definition of pain.
- List phases in the pain process.
- Explain the difference between pain perception, pain threshold, and pain tolerance.
- List pain theories.
- Describe the gate-control theory and how it applies to methods for reducing the perception and intensity of pain.
- Explain how endogenous opioids reduce pain transmission.
- Name types of pain.
- Differentiate the characteristics of acute pain from those of chronic pain.
- List components of a basic pain assessment.
- Identify occasions when it is essential to perform a pain assessment and document assessment findings.
- Name common pain intensity assessment tools used by nurses.
- Name physiologic mechanisms for managing pain.
- Give categories of drugs used alone or in combination to manage pain.
- Identify surgical procedures used when other methods of pain management are ineffective.
- List complementary and alternative medical (CAM) therapies for managing pain.
- Define addiction.
- Discuss how fear of addiction affects pain management.
- Discuss the most common reason why clients request frequent administrations of pain-relieving drugs.
- Define placebo and explain the basis for its positive effect.

SECTION I: ASSESSING YOUR UNDERSTANDING

Activity A FILL IN THE BLANKS

1. The American Pain Society has called pain assessment the _____vital sign; therefore, the nurse checks and documents the client's pain every time they assess the client's temperature, pulse, respirations, and blood pressure.

2. _____ is the last phase of pain impulse transmission in which the brain interacts with the spinal nerves in a downward fashion to subsequently alter the pain experience.

3. _____ pain lasts longer than 6 months.

4. The surgical process _____ prevents sensory impulses from entering the spinal cord and traveling to the brain.

5. Using the procedure known as _____, a client learns to control or alter a physiologic phenomenon as an adjunct to traditional pain management.

6. _____ is the intentional diversion of attention to switch a person's focus from an unpleasant sensory experience to one that is neutral or more pleasant.

7. _____ refers to the conversion of chemical information at the cellular level into electrical impulses that move toward the spinal cord.

8. _____ are a type of sensory nerve receptors activated by around 20 neuropeptides and noxious chemicals released from damaged tissue, which is metabolized into prostaglandin, acetylcholine, and others.

9. _____ drugs relieve pain by altering neurotransmission peripherally at the site of injury.

10. _____ is a pain management technique in which long, thin needles are inserted into the client's skin.

Activity B *Consider the following figure.*

1. Identify the image.

_____

_____

_____

2. What are the advantages of this mechanism?

_____

_____

_____

Activity C *Match the pain management techniques in Column A with their descriptions in Column B.*

Column A

____ 1. Thermal therapy

____ 2. Transcutaneous electrical nerve stimulation (TENS)

____ 3. Acupressure

____ 4. Percutaneous electrical nerve stimulation (PENS)

____ 5. Hypnosis

Column B

a. Passing of an electrical stimulus through tiny needles inserted within the soft tissue

b. Compression of tissues to prevent or relieve pain

c. Applications of hot or cold packs on the affected body part to relieve pain

d. Initiating a person to enter a trancelike state, resulting in an alteration in perception and memory

e. Delivers bursts of electricity to the skin and underlying nerves

Activity D *Presented here, in random order, are the four phases in which people experience pain. Write the correct sequence in the boxes provided.*

1. Modulation

2. Transmission

3. Transduction

4. Perception

☐ → ☐ → ☐ → ☐

Activity E *Briefly answer the following questions.*

1. How does transmission of pain occur?

_____

_____

_____

2. What is acute pain?

_____

_____

_____

3. What is transduction and when does it begin?

_____

_____

_____

4. In what type of research trials has PENS been successful on clients?

_____

_____

_____

5. How can placebos help a client to relieve pain?

_____

_____

_____

6. What are the factors that influence pain tolerance in clients?

_____

_____

_____

SECTION II: APPLYING YOUR KNOWLEDGE

Activity F   _When caring for clients in pain, the most important nursing process is pain assessment. Nurses should thoroughly document the client's pain to gather objective data about a client. Answer the following questions which involve the nurse's role in the pain assessment of clients._

A nurse is caring for a senior client at the health care facility. During the pain assessment, the nurse asks the client about their pain and the names and dosages of pain medicine they have been taking. The client informs the nurse that they are in great pain and unable to recollect the name and dosage of their medication.

1. What interventions should the nurse follow when conducting pain assessments?

_____

_____

_____

2. What kinds of behavioral signs should the nurse observe when assessing pain in clients?

_____

_____

_____

SECTION III: PRACTICING FOR NCLEX

Activity G   _Answer the following questions._

1. Per the direction of the physician, the nurse needs to administer pain medication to a senior client who complains of acute abdominal pain. What route of administration should the nurse use to achieve effective absorption of the medication?
  a. Rectal route
  b. Oral route
  c. Nasal route
  d. Intramuscular route

2. For which client would the nurse anticipate a nonopioid drug to be prescribed?
  a. A client with a migraine
  b. A client with an injury
  c. A client with muscle weakness
  d. A client with pain related to inflammation of a wound

3. A physician orders an EMG machine for a senior client with pain from a recent surgery. How would the nurse describe the effect of the biofeedback to the client?
  a. The machine produces signals correlating to your heart rate, skin temperature, or muscle tension
  b. The machine produces signals correlating with your pain
  c. The machine produces signals correlating with your age and intramuscular tension
  d. The machine produces signals correlating with your age and body mass index

4. A nurse is conducting the initial interview of a client who has been admitted to the health care facility with chronic back pain. What is a priority question related to pain assessment that the nurse should ask during the interview?
  a. "Do you ever take pain medications in the morning?"
  b. "What are the names and dosages of pain medicine you take?"
  c. "Does your daily diet contain any calcium supplements?"
  d. "Are you able to do strenuous activities despite the pain?"

5. A nurse is caring for a client with complaints of severe backache who has been prescribed TENS as a pain management technique. Which candidates would the nurse counsel to

seek medical advice before opting for TENS? Select all that apply.
a. Clients involved in sports activities
b. Clients who are pregnant
c. Clients with cardiac pacemakers
d. Clients prone to irregular heartbeats
e. Clients who are young adults

6. A client with acute spinal cord pain has been prescribed an intraspinal analgesia. How much intraspinal analgesia would the nurse administer to the client?
a. Several times a day or as a continuous low-dose infusion
b. Once a day with high-dose infusion
c. Twice a day with low-dose infusion
d. Once in 6 months with continuous low-dose infusion

7. A nurse is caring for a 3-year-old client who is in pain. Which pain scale would the nurse use to assess this client?
a. Numeric scale
b. Word scale
c. Linear scale
d. FACES scale

8. A nurse is caring for a senior client who has been complaining of back pain for the past 8 months. The client's daughter informs the nurse that lately the client gets angry over minor issues. Which statements describe a common reaction of persons associated with clients in chronic pain? Select all that apply.
a. They suggest that the pain has a psychological basis
b. They suggest that the client is addicted to pain medication
c. They say that the client uses drugs as a crutch
d. They say that they pay close attention to the client's concerns
e. They say they are eager to hear about the client's pain

9. A client whose left limb has been amputated after an accident 2 months earlier complains to the nurse that they experience a burning, itching, and deep pain in the amputated limb, as if it were still attached. How would the nurse respond?
a. "Somatic pain may occur in the affected limb"
b. "You are experiencing chronic pain in the affected limb"
c. "Many times acute pain exists that simulates the amputated limb"
d. "You are experiencing neuropathic pain, which feels like the limb still exists"

10. A nurse is caring for a client with acute abdominal pain. The physician directs the nurse to administer dosages of meperidine. What routes of administration are appropriate for this drug? Select all that apply.
a. Oral route
b. Sublingual route
c. Rectal route
d. Intramuscular route
e. Transdermal route

11. A client is taking antidepressant drugs prescribed by the physician. What therapeutic effect would the nurse anticipate?
a. Increase in norepinephrine and serotonin levels
b. Regulation of inhibitory neurotransmitter γ-aminobutyric acid
c. Blockage of the release of substance P and other inflammatory chemicals
d. Stimulation of the body of the client to release endogenous opioids

12. A nurse is caring for a client who has been prescribed several drugs to treat chronic back pain. The client asks for nondrug and non-surgical interventions in pain management. What treatments might the nurse recommend? Select all that apply.
a. TENS
b. Cordotomy
c. Meditation
d. Hypnosis
e. Acupressure

13. A senior client is being treated for pain in the joints for several months. Initially, the client used to obtain some relief. Now, however, they tell the nurse that despite taking the prescribed medicine, the pain continues to persist. What would the nurse suspect as the most likely reason for this reaction?
a. The client's body may have developed a drug tolerance to the prescribed dose
b. The physician may have prescribed a lower dosage
c. The nurse may have administered lower levels of the prescribed drug
d. The client's body may be absorbing the drug quickly

14. A nurse is caring for a client with under-treated pain. The client complains that their bowel motility has reduced considerably. What other autonomic nervous system responses would the nurse observe in this client related to the undertreated pain?
    a. Dilated pupils
    b. Dehydration
    c. Reduced glucose level
    d. Convulsions

15. A nurse is caring for a client who has developed somatic pain after a road accident. What would the nurse suspect as the cause of the client's pain?
    a. Irritation to the dermis and epidermis
    b. Traumatic injury to the head and neck
    c. Injury to muscles, tendons, and joints
    d. Effect of opioids and opiate analgesics

16. A client with acute upper abdominal pain has been admitted to the health care facility. Per The Joint Commission's pain assessment standards, what is the appropriate nursing intervention when caring for this client?
    a. Assess the client's pain after checking the medical history
    b. Assess the client's pain once per shift
    c. Assess the client's pain and refer elsewhere
    d. Assess the client's pain on an hourly basis

17. After being administered a dosage of codeine sulfate for their knee pain, a senior man complains of an uneasy sensation. What other symptoms should the nurse note that the client could experience after taking opioid drugs? Select all that apply.
    a. Sedation
    b. Nausea
    c. Diarrhea
    d. Respiratory depression
    e. Dilated pupils

18. A nurse is assessing a client with acute pain. Which condition should the nurse document when assessing the client?
    a. The client's discomfort has lasted longer than 6 months
    b. The client's discomfort originates at the skin level
    c. The client's discomfort reduces gradually with medicine
    d. The client is not showing autonomic nervous system responses

SECTION IV: REVIEWING WHAT YOU HAVE LEARNED

Activity H   *Fill in the blanks by choosing the correct word from the options given in parentheses.*

1. _____ is the conversion of chemical information at the cellular level into electrical impulses that move toward the spinal cord. (Perception, Transduction, Transmission)

2. _____ pain is discomfort arising from diseased or injured internal organs. (Cutaneous, Neuropathic, Visceral)

3. _____ is the intentional diversion of attention from an unpleasant sensory experience to one that is neutral or more pleasant. (Distraction, Imagery, Meditation)

Activity I   *Mark each statement as either T (True) or F (False). Correct any false statements.*

1. T F   Sedatives produce a relaxing and calming effect in older clients, thus promoting rest.

2. T F   The Wong–Baker FACES scale can be used to assess pain in clients with language barriers.

3. T F   Adjuvant drugs are used as a first-line treatment for pain.

Activity J   *Write the correct term for each description below.*

1. An inactive substance that resembles medication and can relieve symptoms, like pain, despite the absence of any active chemicals _____

2. Sensory nerve receptor activated by noxious stimuli _____

3. Naturally produced morphine-like chemicals that reduce pain _____

Activity K   *Differentiate between acute and chronic pain based on the criteria given below.*

Duration

Cause

Site of pain

Relief of pain

Activity L *Answer the following questions.*

1. Which two surgical procedures may be used when other methods of pain management are ineffective?

_____

_____

_____

2. What is addiction?

_____

_____

_____

Activity M *Give a rationale for the following question.*

Why should the nurse administer analgesic drugs on a scheduled basis rather than whenever pain occurs?

_____

_____

_____

Activity N *Think over the following question. Discuss it with your instructor or peers.*

1. A nurse is caring for a client who has undergone an amputation of the left leg and is complaining of pain at the severed site.

_____

_____

_____

2. What methods should the nurse use to divert the client's attention from the pain?

What actions should the nurse perform when administering ordered drugs for pain relief?

_____

_____

_____

SECTION V: GETTING READY FOR NCLEX

Activity O *Answer the following question.*

A client with cancer is receiving patient-controlled analgesia (PCA). Which teaching point should the nurse make during client teaching about the equipment?

a. Pain relief is slow and long lasting.

b. PCA requires less drug overall to control pain

c. Ambulation may be difficult

d. Complications from immobility may arise

CHAPTER 21

Oxygenation

Learning Objectives

- Explain the difference between ventilation and respiration.
- Differentiate between external and internal respiration.
- Name methods for assessing the oxygenation status of clients at the bedside.
- List signs of inadequate oxygenation.
- Name nursing interventions that can be used to improve ventilation and oxygenation.
- Name sources for supplemental oxygen.
- Identify items that may be needed when providing oxygen therapy.
- List common oxygen delivery devices.
- Discuss hazards related to the administration of oxygen.
- Describe additional therapeutic techniques that relate to oxygenation.
- Discuss facts concerning oxygenation that affect the care of older adults.

SECTION I: ASSESSING YOUR UNDERSTANDING

Activity A FILL IN THE BLANKS

1. _____ results from pressure changes within the thoracic cavity produced by the contraction and relaxation of respiratory muscles.

2. _____ occurs when there is insufficient oxygen within arterial blood.

3. The _____ position allows room for maximum vertical and lateral chest expansion and provides comfort while resting or sleeping.

4. _____ breathing, which involves taking in a large volume of air, fills alveoli to a greater capacity, thus improving gas exchange.

5. A _____ is a gauge used to regulate the amount of oxygen delivered to the client and is attached to the oxygen source.

6. A _____ is a device that produces small water droplets and is used during oxygen administration because oxygen is drying to the mucous membranes.

7. A _____ mask mixes a precise amount of oxygen and atmospheric air.

8. A _____ collar delivers oxygen near an artificial opening in the neck.

9. As a client grows older, the chest walls become stiffer as a result of _____ of the intercostal muscles.

10. During _____, the dome-shaped diaphragm contracts and moves downward in the thorax.

Activity B *Consider the following figure.*

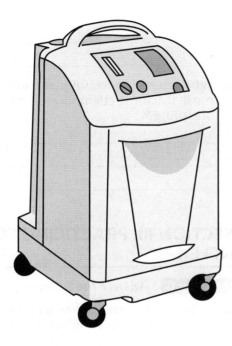

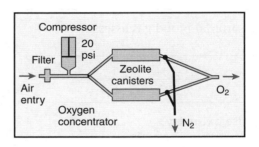

1. Identify the figure.

_____

_____

_____

2. What are the advantages of this equipment?

_____

_____

_____

____ 3. Partial rebreather mask

____ 4. Pursed-lip breathing

____ 5. Incentive spirometry

c. A technique for deep breathing, using a calibrated device

d. Measures the percentage of oxygen delivered to the client

e. A form of controlled ventilation in which the client consciously prolongs the expiration phase of breathing

Activity C *Match the terms related to oxygenation in Column A with their description in Column B.*

Column A

____ 1. Oxygen analyzer

____ 2. Nasal cannula

Column B

a. Hollow tube with half-inch prongs placed into the client's nostrils

b. Oxygen delivery device through which a client inhales a mixture of atmospheric air, oxygen from its source, and oxygen contained within a reservoir bag

Activity D *Presented here, in random order, are steps occurring during ventilation. Write the correct sequence in the boxes provided.*

1. The thoracic cavity expands.

2. Air is pulled in through the nose, filling the lungs.

3. The intercostal muscles move the chest outward by elevating the ribs and sternum.

4. Pressure within the lungs falls below pressure in the atmosphere.

☐ → ☐ → ☐ → ☐

Activity E   *Briefly answer the following questions.*

1. How does a nurse physically assess a client for oxygenation?

   _____

   _____

   _____

2. What is an arterial blood gas assessment?

   _____

   _____

   _____

3. What is pulse oximetry?

   _____

   _____

   _____

4. What is oxygen therapy?

   _____

   _____

   _____

5. What are the disadvantages of an oxygen concentrator?

   _____

   _____

   _____

6. What is a non-rebreather mask?

   _____

   _____

   _____

SECTION II: APPLYING YOUR KNOWLEDGE

Activity F   *Many factors affect ventilation and, subsequently, respiration. Positioning and teaching breathing techniques are two nursing interventions frequently used to promote oxygenation. Answer the questions related to nursing intervention to promote oxygenation.*

A nurse is caring for a client who is brought to the health care facility with breathing difficulty. The client is diagnosed with hypoxia.

1. In what position should the nurse place the client to promote better breathing?

   _____

   _____

   _____

2. What breathing techniques could the nurse teach the client to ensure efficient breathing?

   _____

   _____

   _____

SECTION III: PRACTICING FOR NCLEX

Activity G   *Answer the following questions.*

1. A client has been ordered an arterial blood gas test as part of assessing the quality of oxygenation. What data do the arterial blood gas test provide?
   a. It measures the partial pressure of oxygen dissolved in plasma
   b. It measures the blood pressure of the client
   c. It monitors the oxygen saturation in the blood
   d. It monitors the level of consciousness of the client

2. A nurse is caring for a client who has been diagnosed with emphysema. Which breathing technique is most appropriate for this client to improve gas exchange?
   a. Deep breathing
   b. Incentive spirometry
   c. Pursed-lip breathing
   d. Nasal strips

3. A client at the health care facility is provided with a liquid oxygen unit to keep the blood adequately saturated with oxygen. What information should the nurse include in the teaching plan regarding the potential problems related to the liquid oxygen unit? Select all that apply.
   a. Frozen moisture may occlude the outlet
   b. It may leak during warm weather
   c. It is more expensive than other portable sources
   d. It produces an unpleasant odor
   e. It increases the electricity bill

4. A nurse is caring for a client who has been put on a ventilator in the ICU of the health care facility. Which device would the nurse use to check whether the client is getting the prescribed amount of oxygen?
   a. Flowmeter
   b. Oxygen analyzer
   c. Humidifier
   d. Nasal cannula

5. Which oxygen delivery device would be the best choice for a claustrophobic client with facial burn injuries from a barbecue fire?
   a. Nasal cannula
   b. Face tent
   c. Tracheostomy collar
   d. T-piece

6. A nurse is caring for a 2-year-old client with symptoms of bronchitis. The nurse notices that the client is less active and is having difficulty breathing. Which device should the nurse use to deliver oxygen to the client to facilitate efficient breathing?
   a. Nasal catheter
   b. Oxygen tent
   c. Transtracheal catheter
   d. Continuous positive airway pressure (CPAP) mask

7. A nurse is caring for a client who is being administered oxygen through a transtracheal catheter. What precaution should the nurse take when cleaning the opening and the tube?
   a. Administer oxygen with a nasal cannula
   b. Administer oxygen with a Venturi mask
   c. Administer oxygen with a face tent
   d. Administer oxygen with a partial breather mask

8. A nurse is caring for a client with labored breathing. The client has been prescribed supplemental oxygen by the physician. When administering oxygen to the client, the nurse needs to be aware of oxygen toxicity. Which situation could lead to oxygen toxicity in the client?
   a. Administration of 35% oxygen concentration for 24 hours
   b. Administration of 50% oxygen concentration for 36 hours
   c. Administration of 25% oxygen concentration for 48 hours
   d. Administration of 60% oxygen concentration for 48 hours

9. A nurse is treating a client for carbon monoxide poisoning. Which oxygenation technique is the best choice?
   a. Water-seal chest tube drainage
   b. Hyperbaric oxygen technique
   c. Liquid oxygen unit
   d. Oxygen concentrator

10. A 65-year-old client is being treated at the health care facility for a respiratory-related disorder. Which age-related structural change that affects the respiratory systems in older clients should the nurse consider?
    a. Alveolar walls become thicker
    b. Lungs become more elastic
    c. More breathing occurs from the mouth
    d. Chest walls become stiffer

11. A nurse is caring for a 45-year-old client with lowered respiratory function at a health care facility. What is the best suggestion the nurse could make to improve the client's long-term breathing?
    a. Avoid strenuous exercise
    b. Use a nasal strip
    c. Drink fluids liberally
    d. Maintain proper skin care

12. A nurse is caring for an older client who requires administration of supplemental oxygen. The nurse uses a T-piece to administer oxygen to the client. What point should the nurse remember when using a T-piece to administer oxygen?
    a. It interferes with eating
    b. It creates a feeling of suffocation
    c. It delivers an inconsistent amount of oxygen
    d. It needs to be drained regularly

13. Arrange the following steps in the order that they occur during the process of expiration.
    a. Thoracic cavity decreases
    b. Intrathoracic pressure increases
    c. Respiratory muscles relax
    d. Lung tissue recoils
    e. Air exits the respiratory tract

14. Place the following steps in the order in which the nurse should teach a client to breathe using the pursed-lip technique.
    a. Contract the abdominal muscles
    b. Inhale slowly through the nose while counting to three
    c. Exhale through the pursed lips for a count of six or more
    d. Purse the lips as though to whistle

15. An oxygen tent is being used to administer oxygen to a 2½-year-old client with bronchiolitis. What care should the nurse take when using an oxygen tent for the client? Select all that apply.
    a. Tuck the edges securely beneath the mattress
    b. Limit the opening of the zippered access port
    c. Monitor oxygen levels regularly with an analyzer
    d. Regulate the amount of oxygen delivered if inconsistent
    e. Provide proper skin care to avoid problems as a result of trapped moisture

SECTION IV: REVIEWING WHAT YOU HAVE LEARNED

Activity H   *Fill in the blank by choosing the correct word from the options given in parentheses.*

1. Insufficient oxygen in the arterial blood is called _____. (hypocarbia, hypoxemia, hypoxia)

Activity I   *Mark each statement as either T (True) or F (False). Correct any false statements.*

1. T F   Carbon dioxide is an odorless gas released during the complete combustion of fossil fuels commonly used to heat homes.

2. T F   Pursed-lip breathing is a form of controlled ventilation in which the client consciously prolongs the expiration phase.

3. T F   Oxygen toxicity is lung damage that develops when oxygen concentrations of more than 20% are administered for longer than 24 hours.

Activity J   *Write the correct term for the description below.*

1. Fluid in the tissue space between and around cells _____

Activity K   *Differentiate between inspiration and expiration based on the criteria given below.*

a. Definition
b. Process
c. Additional muscles involved

Activity L   *Incentive spirometry, a technique for deep breathing using a calibrated device, encourages clients to reach a goal-directed volume of inspired air. Write down in the boxes below the correct sequence for using an incentive spirometer.*

a. Hold the breath for 3 to 6 seconds.
b. Sit upright unless contraindicated.
c. Insert the mouthpiece, sealing it between the lips.
d. Exhale normally.
e. Relax and breathe normally before the next breath with the spirometer.
f. Identify the mark indicating the goal for inhalation.
g. Remove the mouthpiece and exhale normally.
h. Inhale slowly and deeply until the predetermined volume has been reached.

☐ → ☐ → ☐ → ☐ → ☐ → ☐ → ☐ → ☐

Activity M   *Answer the following question.*

1. Why are adhesive nasal strips used?

_____

_____

_____

Activity N   *Give rationales for the following question.*

1. Why is it important to use a humidifier when administering 4 or more liters of oxygen?

_____

_____

_____

Activity O *Give a rationale for the following question.*

A client has been instructed to perform diaphragmatic breathing to reduce respiratory effort and relieve rapid, ineffective breathing. How should the nurse instruct this client to perform diaphragmatic breathing?

_____

_____

_____

Activity P *Consider the following questions. Discuss them with your instructor or peers.*

During assessment of an adolescent in her first trimester of pregnancy, the nurse learns that the client smokes regularly. The client plans to care for the baby herself.

a. What are the possible implications for the client's respiratory health and the health of the pregnancy?
b. What client teaching should the nurse provide?

SECTION V: GETTING READY FOR NCLEX

Activity Q *Answer the following question.*

A nurse is caring for a client with hypoxia. What position should the nurse assist the client to assume to best facilitate improved breathing?
a. Lie flat on the back
b. Sit with the bed inclined 15 degrees
c. Lie on the left side
d. Lean forward over the bedside table

CHAPTER 22

Infection Control

Learning Objectives

- Define infectious diseases.
- Differentiate between infection and colonization.
- List the stages in the course of an infectious disease.
- Define infection control measures.
- Name two major techniques for infection control.
- Identify the elements of standard precautions.
- Discuss situations in which nurses use standard precautions and transmission-based precautions.
- Describe the rationale for using airborne, droplet, and contact precautions.
- Explain the purpose of personal protective equipment (PPE).
- Discuss the rationale for removing PPE in a specific sequence.
- Explain how nurses perform double bagging.
- List psychological problems common among clients with infectious diseases.
- Provide teaching suggestions for preventing infections.
- Discuss unique characteristics of older adults in relation to infectious diseases.

SECTION I: ASSESSING YOUR UNDERSTANDING

Activity A FILL IN THE BLANKS

1. _____ is a condition that results when microorganisms cause injury to a host.

2. _____ is a condition during which microorganisms are present, but the host does not manifest any signs or symptoms of infection.

3. Nurses should remove their _____ and wash their hands immediately before caring for another client.

4. _____ waste containers are emptied at the end of each shift.

5. Maintaining _____ skin is an excellent first-line defense against acquiring nosocomial infections.

6. The incidence of _____ infection for senior citizen community living is twice that of the general population.

7. The use of standard precautions reduces the potential for transmitting _____ pathogens from moist body substances.

8. Symptoms of infections tend to be _____ among senior clients.

9. Diseases that spread from one person to another are also called _____ or communicable diseases.

10. _____ trash is refuse that will decompose naturally into less complex compounds.

Activity B   *Consider the following figure.*

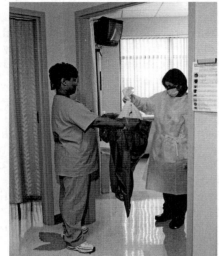

1. Identify the image.

_____

_____

_____

2. What are the advantages of this technique?

_____

_____

_____

Activity C   *Match the stages of infectious diseases in Column A with their characteristics in Column B.*

Column A

____ **1.** Incubation period

____ **2.** Prodromal stage

____ **3.** Acute stage

____ **4.** Convalescent stage

____ **5.** Resolution

Column B

a. Host overcomes the infectious agent

b. Symptoms become severe and specific

c. Initial symptoms are vague and nonspecific

d. Infectious agent reproduces and exits host

e. The pathogen is destroyed. Health improves or is restored

Activity D   *Presented here are steps in random order. They are steps that occur during the removal of personal protective equipment worn by nurses. Write the correct sequence in the boxes provided.*

1. Roll up the gown and discard it in the waste container.

2. Remove the gown without touching the frontside.

3. Fold the soiled side of the gown to the inside.

4. Untie the mask and discard without touching the facial portion.

5. Remove the gloves and discard them in a lined waste container.

6. Untie the neck and waist closure of the gown.

□→□→□→□→□→□

Activity E   *Briefly answer the following questions.*

1. How can nurses promote social interaction for infectious clients?

_____

_____

_____

2. Why are senior clients more susceptible to infections?

_____

_____

_____

3. What are the three types of transmission-based precautions?

_____

_____

_____

4. What is meant by the terms *direct* and *indirect contact* in contact precautions?

_____

_____

_____

5. Which items are included in personal protective equipment?

_____

_____

_____

6. Why are soiled dressings wrapped before being destroyed?

_____

_____

_____

SECTION II: APPLYING YOUR KNOWLEDGE

Activity F *Infectious diseases spread from one person to another, so prevention and proper infection control are the best ways to approach interaction with infectious diseases. Answer the following questions regarding the nurse's role in infection control.*

A nurse is caring for a senior client with influenza at the health care facility. The client does not show any major symptoms of the infection. The client's family members have come to visit them at the health care facility because they are a long-term resident.

1. What precautions should the nurse take to avoid the transmission of pathogens?

_____

_____

_____

2. Why do symptoms of infections tend to be more subtle among senior clients?

_____

_____

_____

SECTION III: PRACTICING FOR NCLEX

Activity G *Answer the following questions.*

1. A nurse is caring for a senior client who has been prescribed an indwelling catheter. What measure should the nurse take to prevent urinary tract infections?
   a. Place the catheter tubing lower than the client's bladder
   b. Clean the client's urinary and rectal area
   c. Clean the indwelling catheter every week
   d. Bend the catheter tubing slightly toward the bladder

2. A client with pulmonary tuberculosis is returning to their private room from the X-ray department. What is an appropriate nursing action to prepare the room for their return?
   a. Obtain a second sheet to cover the client's body
   b. Line the edge of the client's bed with a clean sheet
   c. Spray the X-ray department with disinfectant after the client leaves
   d. Deposit the soiled linen in the linen hamper in the client's room

3. A nurse needs to collect contaminated material from the room of a client with pulmonary tuberculosis. Which infection control measure should the nurse employ when disposing of the articles?
   a. Collect articles in a sturdy bag without contaminating the outside of the bag
   b. Place bulkier items in a trash bag and remove them from the room
   c. Place biodegradable trash in a plastic biohazard bag and destroy it in an incinerator
   d. Wear a nonsterile gown and spray disinfectant on the contaminated material

4. A nurse has finished cleaning the infectious warts of a client and needs to apply the prescribed medicine to the infected area. What precaution should the nurse take when caring for the client?
   a. Remove the contaminated cover gown before leaving the client's room
   b. Change gloves between tasks when caring for the client
   c. Wash hands thoroughly after leaving the client's room
   d. Make contact between two contaminated surfaces or two clean surfaces

5. A group of nurses are caring for victims of bioterrorism. What type of respirator mask should the nurses wear when caring for these clients?
   a. Atomizer
   b. N-95 respirator
   c. Drinker respirator
   d. Powered air-purifying respirator

6. A nurse needs to administer an intravenous drug to a client with chickenpox and the common cold. Which special precautions should the nurse follow before entering the client's room? Select all that apply.
   a. Standard
   b. Contact
   c. Airborne
   d. Droplet
   e. Basic

7. A nurse observes that a client with full-blown AIDS looks very frightened and refuses to meet anybody. Which of the following is the most appropriate nursing diagnosis for the client?
   a. Risk of infection
   b. Social isolation
   c. Ineffective protection
   d. Powerlessness

8. Two nurses are bagging contaminated material from the room of a client using the double-bagging method. Which action is appropriate when performing this procedure?
   a. Biodegradable waste is collected in two plastic bags
   b. Contaminated material is disposed of in two separate bags
   c. One bag of contaminated items is placed within another
   d. Soiled linen is wrapped at the end of the shift

9. After taking standard precautions, a nurse starts cleaning the infected wound of a client. Which bodily substances related to this client require this type of precaution? Select all that apply.
   a. Blood of the infected client
   b. Sweat of the infected client
   c. Mucous membranes of the client
   d. Nonintact skin of the infected client
   e. Breath of the infected client

10. A nurse used droplet precautions for 2 weeks when caring for a client with acute rheumatic fever. The nurse knows that transmission-based precautions depend mostly on which factor?
    a. The nature of the infecting microorganisms
    b. The route of transmission of the pathogen
    c. The stage of the infection in the client
    d. The treatment available for the infection

11. A nurse is cleaning a client's infected wound that is partially healed. When will the nurse discontinue transmission-based precautions?
    a. When culture findings are positive
    b. When a lesion stops draining
    c. When the client shows drug-resistant strains
    d. When the blood around the wound dries

12. A nurse needs to collect urine and stool specimens of a client with acute meningococcal meningitis. Which precaution should the nurse take when delivering the specimens to the laboratory?
    a. Leave some air gap in the container after collecting the specimens
    b. Wear new gloves when collecting the specimens from the client
    c. Collect and deliver the specimens in a plastic biohazard bag
    d. Collect the specimens in sealed containers and place them in a plastic biohazard bag

13. A nurse is caring for a client with tuberculosis, who is admitted to a private room in the health care facility. Which infection control measures are appropriate for this client? Select all that apply.
    a. Close the doors and windows to control air currents
    b. Allow only one visitor at any given time to meet the client
    c. Ask housekeeping to clean the infectious client's room last
    d. Use only disposable linen and medical equipment for the infectious client
    e. Post an instruction card on the door or nearby at eye level

14. A nurse is using droplet precaution measures when caring for a client with streptococcal pharyngitis. The nurse knows that the droplet precaution will reduce pathogen transmission from the client to the nurse up to how many feet?
    a. Less than 10 feet
    b. Less than 3 feet
    c. Less than 5 feet
    d. Less than 8 feet

15. A nurse is cleaning the room of a client who has open tuberculosis. The nurse has collected the soiled dressings of the client. Which substance can be safely disposed of in landfills?
    a. Autoclaved items
    b. Unused syringes
    c. Wrapped dressings
    d. Sealed containers

16. In the health care facility, a nurse is caring for a long-term senior client with chronic asthma and skin infections. This client is at higher risk for which infectious diseases? Select all that apply.
    a. Pneumonia
    b. Influenza
    c. Urinary tract infection
    d. AIDS
    e. Glanders

17. A nurse needs to fix a respirator mask on the face of a bearded client with tuberculosis. Which of the following respirator masks would be the best choice?
    a. N-95 respirator
    b. Powered air-purifying respirator
    c. Ultrasonic nebulizer
    d. Nebulizer

SECTION IV: REVIEWING WHAT YOU HAVE LEARNED

Activity H   *Fill in the blank by choosing the correct word from the options given in parentheses.*

1. A caregiver should use _____ to avoid infectious diseases transmitted by direct contact with a client's body, blood, or body substances. (gloves, hand lotion, towels)

Activity I   *Mark each statement as either T (True) or F (False). Correct any false statements.*

1. T F   Infection control precautions are physical measures designed to curtail the spread of contagious diseases.

2. T F   When preparing to assist with a surgical or obstetric procedure, the nurse should perform a surgical scrub before applying a mask and hair cover.

Activity J   *Answer the following question.*

1. What are the uses and common characteristics of medical cover gowns?

_____
_____
_____

Activity K   *Give a rationale for the following question.*

1. What is the purpose for implementing contact precautions during client care?

_____
_____
_____

Activity L   *Answer the following question.*

1. A nurse at an extended-care facility is using transmission-based precautions while caring for a client with acute diarrhea caused by an infectious microorganism.
    a. What transmission-based precautions should the nurse take when caring for this client?

    _____
    _____
    _____

    b. What actions should the nurse perform when discarding biodegradable trash from this client and their room?

    _____
    _____
    _____

Activity M   *Consider the following questions. Discuss them with your instructor or peers.*

1. A nurse is required to clean and dress pressure ulcers on the feet of a client with restricted mobility.
    a. What actions should the nurse take to promote healing of the pressure ulcers?
    b. What precautions should the nurse take when changing this client's bed linens that contain serous drainage?

    _____
    _____
    _____

SECTION V: GETTING READY FOR NCLEX

Activity N   *Answer the following question.*

1. A nurse is caring for a client recovering from tuberculosis. What infection control interventions should the nurse follow? Select all that apply.
   a. Ask family members and friends to obtain a tuberculosis skin test
   b. Ask the client to use paper tissues when coughing and then dispose of them
   c. Keep the client's wheelchair or stretcher covered with a clean sheet
   d. Read and analyze the client's latest skin test report for tuberculosis
   e. Wear a particulate air filter respirator during client care

Body Mechanics, Positioning, and Moving

Learning Objectives

- Identify characteristics of good posture in a standing, sitting, or lying position.
- Describe principles of correct body mechanics.
- Explain the purpose of ergonomics.
- Give examples of ergonomic recommendations in the workplace.
- Describe common client positions.
- Describe different positioning devices used for safety and comfort.
- Discuss advantages of three different pressure-relieving devices.
- Identify types of transfer devices.
- Outline general guidelines that apply to transferring clients.
- Describe signs or symptoms associated with the disuse syndrome.

SECTION I: ASSESSING YOUR UNDERSTANDING

Activity A FILL IN THE BLANKS

1. The consequences of inactivity are collectively referred to as the _____ syndrome.

2. Good posture distributes _____ through the center of the body over a wide base of support.

3. Muscle _____ occur more often when muscles are strained and forced to work beyond their capacity.

4. _____ is a specialty field of engineering science devoted to promoting comfort, performance, and health in the workplace.

5. Placing a bed in a slight _____ position may help keep the client from sliding down toward the foot of the bed.

6. _____ refers to moving a client from the bed to a chair, toilet, or stretcher and back to the bed again.

7. _____ are the bony protrusions at the head of the femur near the hip.

8. Foot drop hinders _____ because it interferes with a person's ability to place the heel on the floor.

Activity B *Consider the following figures.*

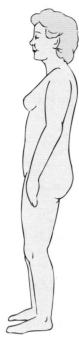

1. Identify the figure.

_____

_____

2. What are its benefits?

_____

_____

_____

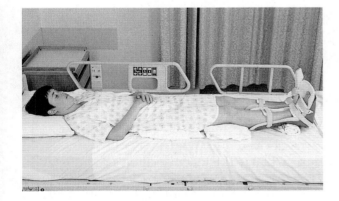

3. Identify the figure.

_____

_____

_____

4. What is this device used for?

_____

_____

_____

Activity C *Match the specialty beds in Column A with their descriptions in Column B.*

Column A

____ **1.** Low air loss bed

____ **2.** Air-fluidized bed

____ **3.** Oscillating support bed

____ **4.** Circular bed

Column B

a. Contains a collection of tiny beads within a mattress cover

b. The client is sandwiched between the anterior and posterior frames in a 180-degree arc

c. Contains inflated air sacs within the mattress

d. Slowly and continuously rocks the client from side to side in a 124-degree arc

Activity D *Presented here, in random order, are steps in using a transfer board to transfer a client from a bed to a chair. Write the correct sequence in the boxes provided.*

1. Angle the transfer board from the client's buttocks and hips down toward the seat of the chair.

2. Slide the client down the transfer board into the seat of the chair at an agreed-upon signal.

3. Remove an arm from the wheelchair and slide the client to the edge of the bed.

4. Support and brace the client's knee with your knees while maintaining proper body mechanics.

5. Position the transfer board beneath the client.

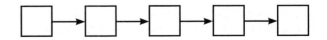

Activity E *Briefly answer the following questions.*

1. How is a good sitting posture maintained?

   _____

   _____

   _____

2. What are the benefits of maintaining good body mechanics?

   _____

   _____

   _____

3. What causes ergonomic hazards to health care workers?

   _____

   _____

   _____

4. What are the potential problems of an air-fluidized bed?

   _____

   _____

   _____

5. What are the effects of immobility faced by older adults?

   _____

   _____

   _____

SECTION II: APPLYING YOUR KNOWLEDGE

Activity F *Nursing care activities such as positioning, moving, and transferring clients reduce the potential for disuse syndrome. Nurses can become injured if they fail to use good posture and body mechanics while performing these activities. Answer the following questions, which involve the nurse's role in preventing work-related injuries.*

A nurse is caring for a senior client with a fractured leg following a fall. When caring for this client, the nurse should take precautions to prevent injuries to themselves.

1. What care should the nurse take before planning to turn and move the client?

   _____

   _____

   _____

2. What should the nurse do as part of planning to move the client?

   _____

   _____

   _____

SECTION III: PRACTICING FOR NCLEX

Activity G *Answer the following questions.*

1. A nurse is aware of the importance of maintaining a good standing posture to promote efficient use of the musculoskeletal system. What is a step the nurse would take to attain this posture?
   a. Keep feet about 2 to 3 inches apart
   b. Avoid bending the knees
   c. Maintain hips at an even level
   d. Hold the chest slightly backward

2. A nurse is working at a health care facility where client data are recorded on a computer. What action would the nurse take when using ergonomics correctly?
   a. Use dim lights
   b. Flex elbows at 120 degrees
   c. Use a low chair
   d. Use wrist rests

3. A nurse is caring for an inactive client. Which principles of positioning should the nurse follow? Select all that apply.
   a. Raise the bed to the height of the caregiver's elbow
   b. Remove the pillows and positioning devices
   c. Change the inactive client's position at least every 2 hours
   d. Turn the upper part of the client's body and then the lower part
   e. Lift and drag the client when transferring to a stretcher

4. A nurse is caring for a senior client with restricted movement. In what position would the nurse avoid placing the client for long

periods of time due to the risk of skin breakdown at the end of the spine?
a. Prone
b. Supine
c. Lateral
d. Sims

5. A nurse is caring for a client with dyspnea.
In which position would the nurse place the
client to allow for the exchange of a greater
volume of air?
a. Supine
b. Sims
c. Fowler
d. Lateral

6. When caring for a client at their home, the
nurse uses pillows to provide comfort and elevate a body part. What might the nurse use
to elevate the upper part of the body if an adjustable bed is not available?
a. Oversized pillows
b. Contour pillows
c. Triangular wedges
d. Bolsters

7. A nurse is caring for a client who had a stroke
and has restricted mobility of their right arm.
Why should the nurse use hand rolls for this
client?
a. To prevent contractures of the fingers
b. To hold the fingers in a tight fist
c. To keep the fingers and thumb together
d. To prevent the wrist from turning outward

8. A team of nurses is using a roller sheet to
turn a client who is in the supine position
to the lateral position. What consideration
is imperative when using the roller sheet
ergonomically?
a. Lift the client to change position
b. Avoid stooping when turning the client
c. Place the sheet away from the client
d. Keep the sheet rolled on the bed after use

9. A nurse is caring for a client whose right leg
has been amputated after a motor vehicle
accident. Which device should the nurse provide to help the client move about in bed?
a. Footboard
b. Bed board
c. Trochanter roll
d. Trapeze

10. A nurse is caring for a senior client who has
undergone surgery for cataracts. Which device should the nurse use on the client's bed?
a. Side rails
b. Cradle
c. Transfer handles
d. Transfer board

11. A nurse is caring for a client who is confined
to bed at their home. The client uses a water
mattress to prevent pressure ulcers. What is
a characteristic of these mattresses?
a. They distribute water cyclically
b. They contain inflated air sacs
c. They require much time to refill
d. They drain excretions away from the
body

12. Nurses at a health care facility are required
to use assistive devices whenever they care
for immobile clients. What is a benefit for
the nurse of using an assistive device?
a. Maintains dignity and self-esteem
b. Reduces musculoskeletal injuries
c. Relieves anxiety concerning safety
d. Promotes faster recovery

13. Two nurses are using a roller sheet to move
a client. Which step is appropriate for this
procedure?
a. Stand on the same side of the client
b. Lower the bed to waist level
c. Face each other on opposite sides of the
bed
d. Place the sheet beneath the shoulders
and buttocks

14. A nurse is caring for a client whose level
of functional status is indicated as 4 in the
health record. What does a functional status
of level 4 indicate?
a. Needs total assistance
b. Needs total supervision
c. Needs assistive device
d. Needs minimal help

15. A nurse is caring for a client with severe
burn injuries. The client requires frequent
dressing changes and topical applications.
Which pressure-relieving device should the
nurse provide for this client?
a. Oscillating support bed
b. Foam mattress
c. Gel cushion
d. Circular bed

SECTION IV: REVIEWING WHAT YOU HAVE LEARNED

Activity H   *Fill in the blanks by choosing the correct word from the options given in parentheses.*

1. The force of _____ pulls objects toward the center of the earth. (density, energy, gravity)

2. Permanent shortening of muscles that resist stretching is called a _____. (contraction, contracture, fracture)

Activity I   *Mark each statement as either T (True) or F (False). Correct any false statements.*

1. T F   The ability of the muscles to respond to stimulation is referred to as strength.

2. T F   A trapeze is a rectangular piece of metal hung by a chain over the foot of the bed.

Activity J   *Write the correct term for the description below.*

Field of engineering science devoted to promoting comfort, performance, and health in the workplace _____

Activity K   *Match the common body positions in Column A with their descriptions in Column B.*

Column A

___ 1. Supine position

___ 2. Lateral position

___ 3. Prone position

___ 4. Sims position

___ 5. Fowler position

___ 6. Lateral oblique position

Column B

a. Semi-prone with the right knee drawn toward the chest

b. Semi-sitting

c. Side-lying with the hip and knee of the top leg in flexion

d. Back-lying

e. Abdomen-lying

f. Side-lying

Activity L   *A trochanter is the bony protrusion at the head of the femur near the hip. Trochanter rolls prevent the legs from turning outward. Write in the boxes provided below the correct sequence for using trochanter rolls.*

1. Roll the sheet around the blanket so that the end of each roll is underneath.

2. Fold a sheet lengthwise in half or in thirds and place it under the client's hips.

3. Secure the rolls next to each hip and thigh.

4. Permit the leg to rest against the trochanter roll.

5. Place a rolled-up bath blanket under each end of the sheet that extends on either side of the client.

□ → □ → □ → □ → □

Activity M   *Answer the following questions.*

1. How can one maintain a good standing posture?

_____
_____
_____

2. What methods are used to prevent foot drop?

_____
_____
_____

Activity N   *Give rationales for the following questions.*

1. Why should the nurse encourage a client who is being fitted with a prosthetic limb to lie supine or prone periodically during the day?

_____
_____
_____

2. Why is Fowler position helpful for clients with dyspnea?

_____
_____
_____

Activity O *Answer the following question, focusing on nursing roles and responsibilities.*

A nurse is preparing to transfer a senior client from bed to a chair. What general guidelines should the nurse follow when assisting with this client transfer?

_____

_____

_____

Activity P *Consider the following questions. Discuss them with your instructor or peers.*

A nurse is providing care for a client with paraplegia who requires assistance with activities of daily living.

a. How can the nurse help to prevent disuse syndrome?

_____

_____

_____

b. What positioning devices might be considered for this client?

_____

_____

_____

SECTION V: GETTING READY FOR NCLEX

Activity Q *Answer the following question.*

The nurse is caring for a client with impaired mobility who is to be moved to another unit of the health care facility. What principles of body mechanics should the nurse follow to avoid self-injury when transferring the client to a wheelchair? Select all that apply.

a. Stretch the muscles as far as possible

b. Keep feet apart for a broad base of support

c. Rest between periods of exertion

d. Keep the knees bent

e. Avoid contracting the abdominal muscles

Therapeutic Exercise

Learning Objectives

- List benefits of regular exercise.
- Define fitness.
- Identify factors that interfere with fitness.
- Name methods of fitness testing.
- Describe how to calculate a person's target heart rate.
- Define metabolic energy equivalent.
- Differentiate fitness exercise from therapeutic exercise.
- Differentiate isotonic exercise from isometric exercise.
- Give examples of isotonic, isometric, and isokinetic exercises.
- Differentiate between active exercise and passive exercise.
- Discuss how and why range-of-motion exercises are performed.
- Provide suggestions for helping older adults become or stay physically active.

SECTION I: ASSESSING YOUR UNDERSTANDING

Activity A FILL IN THE BLANKS

1. _____ or purposeful physical activity is beneficial to people of all age groups.

2. Body _____ is the amount of body tissue that is lean versus the amount that is fat.

3. The validity of _____ tests is less reliable than results obtained through ECG testing.

4. _____ heart rate means the goal for heart rate during exercise.

5. _____ energy equivalent is the measure of energy and oxygen consumption during exercise.

6. _____ exercise involves rhythmically moving all parts of the body at a moderate to slow speed without hindering the ability to breathe.

7. _____ exercise is therapeutic activity that the client performs independently after proper instruction.

Activity B   *Consider the following figures.*

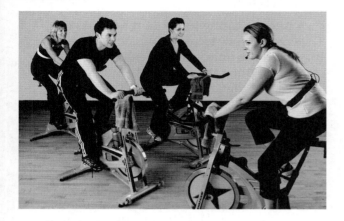

1. Identify the figure.

    _____

    _____

    _____

2. What is the benefit of this type of activity?

    _____

    _____

    _____

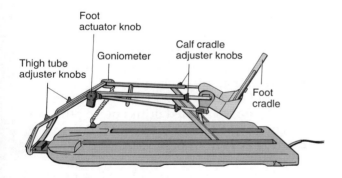

Foot
actuator knob

Calf cradle
adjuster knobs

Goniometer

Thigh tube
adjuster knobs

Foot
cradle

3. Identify the figure.

    _____

    _____

    _____

4. What is this device used for?

    _____

    _____

    _____

Activity C   *Match the positions in Column A with their descriptions in Column B.*

Column B

____ **1.** Hyperextension

____ **2.** Abduction

____ **3.** Rotation

____ **4.** Pronation

____ **5.** Inversion

Column A

a. Turning downward

b. Increasing the angle between two adjoining bones more than 180 degrees

c. Turning the sole of the foot toward the midline

d. Turning from side to side, as in an arc

e. Moving away from the midline

Activity D   *Briefly answer the following questions.*

1. What are the factors that can affect a client's fitness and stamina?

    _____

    _____

    _____

2. Why are fitness tests important?

    _____

    _____

    _____

3. What is recovery index?

    _____

    _____

    _____

4. How is a walk-a-mile test conducted?

    _____

    _____

    _____

5. How is the maximum heart rate calculated?

    _____

    _____

    _____

SECTION II: APPLYING YOUR KNOWLEDGE

Activity E *Nurses are responsible for assessing each client's fitness level before initiating an exercise program with the client. Exercise must be individualized per the need and fitness ability of the client. Answer the following questions, which involve the nurse's role in assisting the client in a safe exercise program.*

1. What are the initial requirements for starting an exercise program that the nurse should explain to the client?

   _____

   _____

   _____

2. What kind of activities should the nurse suggest for a client with a metabolic energy equivalent to 6 to 7 METs?

   _____

   _____

   _____

SECTION III: PRACTICING FOR NCLEX

Activity F *Answer the following questions.*

1. A nurse is assisting an immobile client to perform ROM exercises. What techniques should the nurse keep in mind when performing ROM exercises? Select all that apply.
   a. Raise the level of the bed
   b. Repeat each exercise five times
   c. Avoid forceful joint movements
   d. Begin with foot exercises and work upward
   e. Move the client closer to the edge of the bed

2. A nurse is caring for a client who has been prescribed isometric exercises. What is one benefit of isometric exercises?
   a. Preserving muscle mass
   b. Preventing joint deformities
   c. Preventing stiffness of joints
   d. Preventing skin breakdown

3. A client has been recommended isotonic exercises by the health care provider. What exercise would the nurse suggest?
   a. Bodybuilding
   b. Weight lifting
   c. Holding a yoga position
   d. Aerobics

4. A nurse is caring for a client who has undergone a mastectomy. Which exercises should the nurse recommend to the client to strengthen the arm on the surgical side? Select all that apply.
   a. Squeezing a softball
   b. Combing the hair
   c. Swimming
   d. Finger climbing
   e. Rotating the arm

5. Before starting the client on a suitable exercise routine, the nurse is required to assess the client's fitness. Which assessment technique will provide reliable results for fitness levels?
   a. Walk-a-mile test
   b. Step test
   c. ECG
   d. Aerobic fitness

6. A nurse is caring for a senior client with diabetes who has been asked to exercise on a regular basis. Which exercise would be ideal for this client?
   a. Walking
   b. Cycling
   c. Running
   d. Jogging

7. What is an appropriate teaching point for a nurse to make when preparing a safe exercise regimen for an older client?
   a. Avoid drinking water just before exercising
   b. Take sips of aerated drinks during the exercise program
   c. Balance periods of physical activity with periods of rest
   d. Wear shoes with a smooth sole for easy walking

8. A nurse is assessing a client for unilateral neglect. Which client response would confirm this condition?
   a. The client constantly ignores objects placed on the right side
   b. The client differentiates warm and cold on both sides
   c. The client combs their hair well on both sides
   d. The client observes objects on the table on either side

9. A client who has undergone knee replacement therapy has been ordered the use of a passive motion machine as a substitute for

manual ROM exercise. What precautionary measures should the nurse take when caring for this client? Select all that apply.
a. Provide pain medication after exercise is completed
b. Instruct the client on techniques for relaxation
c. Compare assessment findings with the unaffected extremity
d. Assess vital signs and mobility of the affected extremity
e. Adjust the machine to the prescribed rate and degree of flexion

10. When caring for a client with unilateral neglect, the client is only aware of activities on the left-hand side. Which of the following interventions should the nurse follow?
a. Suggest that the client view the environment from one side
b. Place the signal cord on the right side of the client
c. Avoid asking the client to participate in self-care for the left side
d. Always approach the client from the left side

11. A nurse is assisting a client in performing ROM exercises. The nurse assists the client to move the arm in a full circle. Which movement is the nurse providing?
a. Flexion
b. Extension
c. Circumduction
d. Hyperextension

12. A client is to undergo an ambulatory ECG to record heart rate and rhythm continuously during normal activity. What instruction should the nurse give the client?
a. Wear the Holter monitor for 12 hours
b. Walk slowly first on a flat treadmill
c. Measure peripheral oxygenation
d. Avoid the use of electric blankets

13. A client has been ordered a step test, which is a submaximal fitness test involving a timed stepping activity. Which statement describes a factor involved in this testing?
a. The platform height is 30 inches for men
b. The platform height is 16 inches for men
c. A step up and down together is one step
d. The exercise involves about 76 steps/minute

14. A nurse is caring for a client whose cardiovascular endurance fitness level is 60. How would the nurse classify this fitness level?
a. Poor
b. Below average
c. Average
d. Good

15. A nurse is assisting a client to perform ROM exercises. What action would the nurse perform in this procedure?
a. Provide the client with pillows
b. Move each joint until there is pain
c. Support the joint being exercised
d. Follow a different pattern each time

SECTION IV: REVIEWING WHAT YOU HAVE LEARNED

Activity G *Fill in the blanks by choosing the correct word from the options given in parentheses.*

1. _____ exercises are stationary movements performed against a resistive force. (Dangling, Isometric, Isotonic)

2. The capacity to which a person can exercise is called _____. (fitness, power, strength)

3. The range-of-motion exercise that involves spreading the fingers and thumb as widely as possible is called _____. (abduction, adduction, flexion)

Activity H *Mark each statement as either T (True) or F (False). Correct any false statements.*

1. T F The ability of the muscles to respond to stimulation is referred to as strength.

2. T F Target heart rate means the goal for heart rate during exercise.

Activity I *Differentiate between active exercise and passive exercise based on the criteria given below.*

	Active Exercise	Passive Exercise
Definition		
Uses		
Examples		

Activity J   *Answer the following question.*

What are the seven factors that may compromise a client's fitness and stamina?

_____

_____

_____

Activity K   *Give rationales for the following question.*

Why is a continuous passive motion machine used for the rehabilitation of clients who have undergone hip replacement surgery?

_____

_____

_____

Activity L   *Answer the following questions, focusing on nursing roles and responsibilities.*

1. A nurse is caring for an obese client with cardiovascular symptoms. The physician has ordered a balanced diet and exercise program aimed at weight reduction for the client.
   a. What methods can the nurse use to assess the client's fitness level?

   _____

   _____

   _____

   b. How is the client's target heart rate calculated, and how does the client's fitness influence the prescription of a metabolic energy equivalent?

   _____

   _____

   _____

2. A nurse is caring for older clients at an extended care facility who can maintain some regular activity and exercise.
   a. How can the nurse help to ensure that fluid intake is appropriate for these clients?

   _____

   _____

   _____

   b. How can the nurse help these clients stay physically active?

   _____

   _____

   _____

Activity M   *Consider the following questions. Discuss them with your instructor or peers.*

A nurse is working with a client who has lost movement on one side of their body following a cerebrovascular accident. What interventions can the nurse perform to maintain or restore functional use when caring for this client?

CHAPTER 25

Mechanical Immobilization

Learning Objectives

- List purposes of mechanical immobilization.
- Name types of splints.
- Discuss why slings and braces are used.
- Explain the purpose of a cast.
- Name types of casts.
- Describe nursing actions that are appropriate when caring for clients with casts.
- Discuss how casts are removed.
- Explain what traction implies.
- List types of traction.
- Explain principles that apply to maintaining effective traction.
- Describe the purpose for an external fixator.
- Identify the rationale for performing pin site care.

SECTION I: ASSESSING YOUR UNDERSTANDING

Activity A **FILL IN THE BLANKS**

1. A _____ cast encircles one or both arms or legs and the chest or the trunk.

2. A _____ is a cloth device used to elevate, cradle, and support parts of the body.

3. _____ are custom-made or custom-fitted devices designed to support weakened structures such as weak muscles or unstable joints.

4. A _____ cast encircles an arm or leg and leaves the toes or fingers exposed.

5. _____ is a pulling effect exerted on a part of the skeletal system.

6. An external _____ is a metal device inserted into and through one or more broken bones to stabilize fragments.

7. _____ fractures are common, especially in postmenopausal women who are not treated for osteoporosis.

8. _____ traction is most often used briefly to realign a broken bone as also to replace a dislocated bone into its original position within a joint.

9. The pull of the traction generally is offset by the _____ from the client's own body weight.

10. A light-cured _____ cast requires exposure to ultraviolet light to harden.

Activity B *Consider the following figures.*

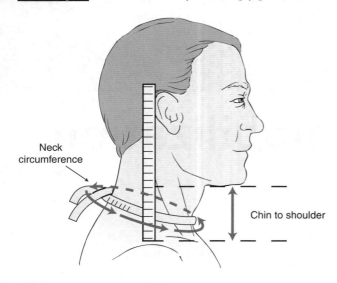

Neck circumference

Chin to shoulder

1. Identify and label the image.

_____

_____

_____

2. What is this procedure used for?

_____

_____

_____

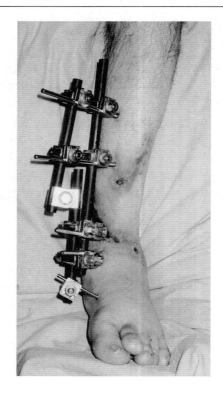

3. Identify the image.

_____

_____

_____

4. What is the use of the metal device in this image?

_____

_____

_____

Activity C *Match the mechanical immobilization devices in Column A with their features in Column B.*

Column B

_____ **1.** Thomas splint

_____ **2.** Makeshift splint

_____ **3.** Pelvic belt

_____ **4.** Ice pack

Column A

a. Applied to the lower extremity

b. Pulling effect on the skeletal system

c. Applied to alleviate pain or swelling

d. Board, broom, handle, or golf club

Activity D *Presented here, in random order, are the steps to be taken when applying an arm sling. Write the correct sequence in the boxes provided.*

1. Position the forearm across the client's chest with the thumb upward.

2. Slip the flexed arm into the canvas sling so that the elbow fits flush.

3. Tighten the strap to keep the elbow flexed and the wrist elevated.

4. Assess the skin color and temperature of the injured arm.

☐ → ☐ → ☐ → ☐

Activity E *Briefly answer the following questions.*

1. What are the disadvantages of plaster of Paris casts?

_____

_____

_____

2. What is the purpose of mechanical immobilization?

_____

_____

_____

3. What is the function of splints?

_____

_____

_____

4. What are gerontologic considerations when caring for an older adult with an immobilization device?

_____

_____

_____

5. Why is care at the pin site essential?

_____

_____

_____

6. What skin care needs to be taken after removing a cast?

_____

_____

_____

SECTION II: APPLYING YOUR KNOWLEDGE

Activity F   *External fixators are inserted into and through one or more broken bones to stabilize fragments during healing. Although the external fixator immobilizes the area of injury, the client is encouraged to be active and mobile. During recovery, the nurse provides care for the pin sites. In conjunction with an external fixator and skeletal traction, pin site care is essential to prevent infection. Answer the following questions, which involve the nurse's role in caring for a client with an external fixator.*

A nurse is taking care of a client with pin sites. A culture from a specimen taken at a pin site reveals that the pin site is infected with *Staphylococcus aureus.*

1. What nursing actions are required for contact precautions to control transmission of the pathogen?

_____

_____

_____

2. How should the nurse assess a client with pin site insertion in their body?

_____

_____

_____

SECTION III: PRACTICING FOR NCLEX

Activity G   *Answer the following questions.*

1. A nurse has finished applying a cast to a client. What action would the nurse perform to reduce the pain and swelling?
   a. Elevate the cast on pillows or other supports
   b. Administer pain-relief medication
   c. Provide written instructions on cast care
   d. Place the bed at a comfortable height

2. A nurse is caring for a client with injury to their right leg. Which immobilization devices are most suitable for short-term duration? Select all that apply.
   a. Pneumatic splints
   b. Immobilizers
   c. Thomas splints
   d. Molded splints
   e. Russell traction

3. A nurse is assessing a client with a pin inserted in a fractured femur. The client's pin insertion site shows no evidence of purulent drainage. What other signs should the nurse look for to check for pin site infection?
   a. Check whether the pin is bent
   b. Check white blood cell count
   c. Check for dry skin
   d. Check the client's pulse rate

4. A nurse has applied a molded splint to the sprained ankle of a client. What are the desired outcomes of applying a molded splint? Select all that apply.
   a. Reduce the load-bearing force on the cervical spine
   b. Maintain the body part in a functional position
   c. Prevent contractures and muscle atrophy during immobility
   d. Immobilize the injured structure and align it

5. A nurse is trimming a cast in the anal and genital area so that the client can eliminate urine and stool. What type of cast is the nurse trimming?
   a. Cylinder cast
   b. Spica cast
   c. Bivalved cast
   d. Body cast

6. A nurse is caring for a senior client with musculoskeletal injury near the hip. What action should the nurse take to promote the quick healing of a musculoskeletal injury?
   a. Encourage the client to have a diet rich in protein, calcium, and zinc
   b. Encourage the client to protect him or herself from exposure to sun
   c. Ask the client to avoid taking supplements of vitamin D
   d. Encourage the client to perform isometric exercise daily

7. A nurse has removed the cast applied to the forearm of a client. What condition would the nurse most likely assess after removal of the cast?
   a. Joints have better flexibility
   b. Skin appears pale and waxy
   c. Unexercised muscles appear bigger
   d. Major swelling appears on the affected area

8. A nurse needs to apply Buck traction to a client with severe muscle spasms in their leg. Which action would the nurse perform?
   a. A pulling effect caused by the use of the hands and muscular strength
   b. A pulling effect caused on the skeletal system by devices
   c. A pulling exerted directly by devices through bone
   d. A pulling effect caused by a metal device inserted into broken bone

9. A nurse is caring for an older client with a fractured hip. What factor predisposes seniors to hip fractures?
   a. Weakness of bone
   b. Poor diet
   c. Reduced synovial fluid
   d. Flexible joints

10. A nurse is applying a custom-made leg brace to the client. What will happen if it is an ill-fitting brace or it is applied improperly? Select all that apply.
    a. Causes discomfort
    b. Causes skin ulcerations
    c. Causes deformity
    d. Causes permanent stiffness
    e. Causes muscle contractures

11. A client whose neck has been in traction for 10 minutes tells the nurse that they feel exhausted. What nursing action would be appropriate for this client?
    a. Avoid giving a pillow to the client
    b. Reduce the amount of weights
    c. Use a pressure-relieving device
    d. Change the position of the client

12. A nurse is caring for a client who has an injured elbow. What should the nurse do to facilitate circulation?
    a. Slip the flexed arm in the canvas sling
    b. Avoid more than 90 degrees of flexion
    c. Position the triangle apex under the elbow
    d. Position the knot near the neck side

13. Per the physician's orders, a nurse is prematurely removing the cast of a client with a fractured arm. Under what circumstance is it appropriate to remove a cast prematurely?
    a. When complications develop
    b. When the injury is healed sufficiently
    c. When the cast edges become soft
    d. When there is a need for hygiene

14. A nurse is assisting a client with a hip spica cast during elimination. What action will the nurse take to protect it from being soiled?
    a. Tuck in an adult diaper
    b. Provide a bedpan
    c. Insert a catheter
    d. Use a plastic wrap

15. A nurse is assisting a physician in applying a pneumatic splint to the severely injured leg of a client. How will the nurse know

the point up to which the pneumatic splint needs to be inflated with air?
   a. Ask the client if the splint feels heavy
   b. Touch the splint and determine whether it is cold
   c. Determine whether the splint can be indented a half inch
   d. Push a fingertip between the splint and leg

16. A nurse is administering prescribed medicine to an older client with a fractured hip. Which effects of narcotic analgesics are visible in senior adults? Select all that apply.
   a. Pale skin
   b. Dilated pupils
   c. Constipation
   d. Depressed respiration
   e. Mental changes

17. A client accidentally pours a glassful of water on the cast. The nurse quickly dries the cast using a blow dryer set on a cool setting. What other basic care should the nurse provide when caring for a client with a cast?
   a. Keep clients from writing anything on the cast
   b. Avoid elevating the cast on a pillow or support
   c. Apply heat packs to the cast at the level of injury
   d. Avoid client ambulating until the injury is healed

18. A nurse is caring for a client who is in Russell traction for long-term treatment. Which action should the nurse perform to maintain the client's personal hygiene?
   a. Clean the skin around insertion site
   b. Cover the metal pins with corks
   c. Bathe the client's back
   d. Insert padding within the slings

SECTION IV: REVIEWING WHAT YOU HAVE LEARNED

Activity H *Fill in the blanks by choosing the correct word from the options given in parentheses.*

1. A(n) _____ splint is made of rigid materials that maintain a body part in a functional position to prevent contractures and muscle atrophy during periods of immobility. (inflatable, molded, traction)

2. A _____ cast encircles one or both arms or legs and the chest or trunk. (bivalved, cylinder, spica)

Activity I *Mark each statement as either T (True) or F (False). Correct any false statements.*

1. T F Braces are custom-made or custom-fitted devices designed to support weakened structures.

2. T F A bivalved cast is cut in two pieces lengthwise from either a body or a cylinder cast.

3. T F A trapeze is a rectangular piece of metal hung by a chain over the foot of the bed.

Activity J *Write the correct term for each description below.*

1. Metal device inserted into and through one or more broken bones to stabilize fragments during healing _____

2. Large cylinder cast that encircles the trunk, rather than an extremity _____

3. Pulling effect directly exerted on a bone by attaching wires, pins, or tongs into or through it _____

Activity K *Match the types of mechanical immobilizing devices in Column A with their uses in Column B.*

Column A
____ 1. Inflatable splint
____ 2. Prophylactic brace
____ 3. Manual traction
____ 4. Cylinder cast

Column B
a. Prevents or reduces the severity of a joint injury
b. Prevents movement to maintain alignment during healing
c. Controls bleeding and swelling
d. Realigns a broken bone briefly by pulling on the body using muscular strength

Activity L   *Differentiate between plaster of Paris and fiberglass casts based on the criteria given below.*

	Plaster of Paris	Fiberglass
Application		
Cost		
Durability		
Weight		
Weight bearing		
Effect of water		

Activity M   *Answer the following questions.*

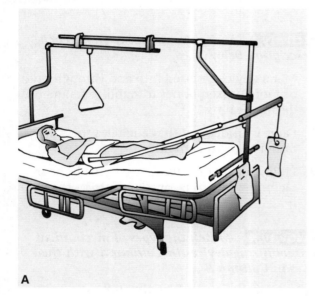

A

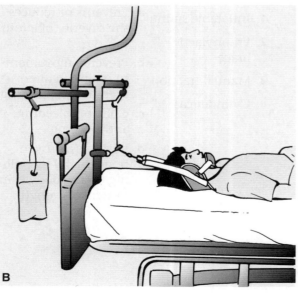

B

a. Identify the devices shown in the figure.

_____

_____

_____

b. What are they used for?

_____

_____

_____

Activity N   *Answer the following questions.*

1. What are the functions of mechanical immobilization of a body part?

_____

_____

_____

2. What is a cast? When is it used?

_____

_____

_____

3. What are common nursing diagnoses applicable to a client with an immobilizing device?

_____

_____

_____

SECTION V: APPLYING YOUR KNOWLEDGE

Activity O   *Give rationales for the following questions.*

1. Why are bedridden older adults prone to developing problems from skin pressure?

_____

_____

_____

2. Why is it important for the nurse to provide meticulous care to a pin site?

_____

_____

_____

Activity P *Answer the following questions, focusing on nursing roles and responsibilities.*

A nurse is caring for a client who has a whiplash injury.

a. How should the nurse determine the size of the cervical collar for this client?

_____

_____

_____

b. How should the nurse assess the client's neuromuscular function during recovery?

_____

_____

_____

Activity Q *Consider the following questions. Discuss them with your instructor or peers.*

A nurse is caring for a 64-year-old client with a fractured leg in a cast following a fall. The client is taking prescribed analgesics for pain. They have not been eating well, and their mobility is restricted.

a. What actions can the nurse take regarding the client's nutritional intake and use of analgesics?

_____

_____

_____

b. What are major concerns when caring for senior clients with casts?

_____

_____

_____

SECTION VI: GETTING READY FOR NCLEX

Activity R *Answer the following questions.*

1. What guidelines should the nurse follow when applying an emergency splint to a client? Select all that apply.
   a. Cover any open wounds with a clean material
   b. Swab the skin using alcohol or acetone
   c. Select rigid material to provide support
   d. Use wide tape to confine the injured part to the splint
   e. Encourage the client to exercise fingers and toes frequently

2. A nurse is caring for a client with a fractured wrist in a cylinder cast. What should the nurse do to obtain information about the client's neuromuscular function? Select all that apply.
   a. Monitor the mobility of the fingers
   b. Assess for sensation in the exposed fingers
   c. Elevate the cast on pillows or another support
   d. Apply an ice pack at the level of injury
   e. Depress nailbeds and time the color return

CHAPTER 26

Ambulatory Aids

Learning Objectives

- Name activities that prepare clients for ambulation.
- Give examples of isometric exercises that tone and strengthen lower extremities.
- Identify techniques for building upper arm strength.
- Explain the reason for dangling clients or using a tilt table.
- Name devices used to assist clients with ambulation.
- Give examples of ambulatory aids.
- Identify the most stable type of ambulatory aid.
- Describe characteristics of appropriately fitted crutches.
- Name types of crutch-walking gaits.
- Explain the purpose of a temporary prosthetic limb.
- Name four components of above-the-knee and below-the-knee prosthetic limbs.
- Describe how a prosthetic limb is applied.
- Discuss age-related changes that affect the gait and ambulation of older adults.

SECTION I: ASSESSING YOUR UNDERSTANDING

Activity A   FILL IN THE BLANKS

1. _____ exercises are used to promote muscle tone and strength.

2. _____ helps to normalize blood pressure, which may drop when the client rises from a reclining position.

3. A client who has weakness on one side of the body uses a _____, which is a handheld ambulatory device made of wood or aluminum.

4. _____ crutches are generally used by experienced clients who need permanent assistance with walking.

5. Many clients with arthritis use _____ crutches.

6. The word *point* in four-point gait refers to the _____ of the crutches and legs used when performing a gait.

7. Some clients with leg amputation ambulate with a _____ limb without the assistance of crutches or other ambulatory aids.

8. _____ crutches are used by clients who cannot bear weight with the hands and wrists.

9. As a person ages, they may develop_____ of the spine, which can alter the center of gravity and may result in an increased risk for falls.

10. Clients who need temporary assistance with ambulation are likely to use _____ crutches.

Activity B *Consider the following figure.*

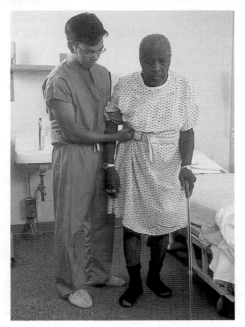

1. Identify the assistive device used to help the client ambulate.

   _____

   _____

   _____

2. How does a nurse assist the client ambulate using this assistive device?

   _____

   _____

   _____

Activity C *Match the terms in Column A with their description in Column B.*

Column A

_____ **1.** Quadriceps setting

_____ **2.** Parallel bars

_____ **3.** T-handle cane

_____ **4.** Forearm crutches

Column B

a. Used as hand rails to gain practice in ambulating

b. Have an arm cuff but do not have an axillary bar

c. An isometric exercise during which the client alternately tenses and relaxes the quadriceps muscles

d. Has a handgrip with a slightly bent shaft, offering users more stability

Activity D *Presented here, in random order, are the instructions a nurse gives to a client who uses a walker. Write the correct sequence in the boxes provided.*

1. Take a step forward.

2. Support the body weight on the handgrips when moving the weaker leg.

3. Hold on to the walker at the padded handgrips.

4. Stand within the walker.

5. Pick up the walker and advance it 6 to 8 inches (15 to 20 cm).

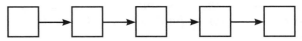

Activity E *Briefly answer the following questions.*

1. What are the techniques that a nurse can use to help a client increase muscular strength and the ability to bear weight?

   _____

   _____

   _____

2. What is the function of the quadriceps muscles?

   _____

   _____

   _____

3. What does an exercise regimen to strengthen the upper arm include?

   _____

   _____

   _____

4. What is a tilt table?

   _____

   _____

   _____

5. How is the correct height of the cane for a client achieved?

   _____

   _____

   _____

6. What is the importance of the immediate postoperative prosthesis?

_____

_____

_____

SECTION II: APPLYING YOUR KNOWLEDGE

Activity F   *A prosthetic limb allows clients with leg amputation to ambulate without the assistance of crutches or other ambulatory aids. Answer the questions related to nursing intervention for a client with prosthetic limbs.*

A nurse is caring for a client whose right leg was amputated because of gangrene. The client has been fitted with a temporary prosthetic limb immediately after the surgery.

1. What procedure should the nurse follow when fitting a client with a prosthetic limb?

_____

_____

_____

2. What are the responsibilities of the nurse to ensure that no complications develop?

_____

_____

_____

SECTION III: PRACTICING FOR NCLEX

Activity G   *Answer the following questions.*

1. A nurse is caring for a client who temporarily lost the function of their legs due to a motor vehicle accident. How can the nurse prepare the client for ambulation?
   a. By assisting the client in performing isometric exercises of the upper arms
   b. By assisting the client in walking using a supportive belt
   c. By using a tilt table to help the client stand
   d. By assisting the client in performing isotonic exercises of the lower limbs

2. A nurse needs to prepare a client whose leg is in a cast because of a hairline fracture for ambulation. Which ambulation aid would help the client to reestablish their previous ability to walk?
   a. Walking belt
   b. Isometric exercises
   c. Dangling
   d. Tilt table

3. A nurse is assisting a mid-life client who has been admitted to the facility with diarrhea. The client is weak and in the recovery stage. Why should the nurse assist the client to dangle before ambulating?
   a. To promote muscle tone and strength
   b. To improve upper arm strength
   c. To normalize the blood pressure
   d. To help the client bear weight on their feet

4. A nurse is caring for a client who is being treated at the health care facility for a torn muscle fiber in the quadriceps. The nurse understands that the quadriceps function to
   a. Aid in supporting body weight
   b. Aid in adducting the leg
   c. Aid in rotating the leg
   d. Aid in walking upright

5. A client is being treated for injury to the gluteal muscle. The physician has prescribed exercises in a gluteal setting to rehabilitate the client. How should the nurse instruct the client to exercise the gluteal muscles in a gluteal setting?
   a. By practicing ambulation with the help of handrails
   b. By performing modified hand push-ups in bed
   c. By sitting on the edge of the bed
   d. By contracting and relaxing the muscles

6. A client has been prescribed modified hand push-ups in bed to strengthen their upper arms because the client will have to use axillary crutches for a while after discharge from the facility. What should the nurse do if the mattress of the bed is too soft?
   a. Remove the mattress from the bed
   b. Replace the mattress with a firmer one
   c. Place books under the client's hand
   d. Provide the client with a sturdy armchair

7. When applying a prosthetic limb to a client at the health care facility, what instruction

should the nurse give to the client to prevent circulatory problems?
a. Ask the client to wear a nylon sheath beneath the stump sock
b. Ask the client to avoid keeping the knee naturally flexed for a prolonged period
c. Ask the client to dry the socks well before donning them
d. Ask the client to wear the prosthesis for a short period initially

8. A nurse is using a tilt table to prepare a client for ambulation. When would the nurse lower the table and return it to the horizontal position?
a. When the client appears to be dizzy
b. When the table has been tilted to 30 degrees
c. When the client is in a vertical position
d. When the device has been used for more than 10 minutes

9. When ambulating the client, the nurse notices that the client appears dizzy and is about to faint. What should the nurse do in this case? Select all that apply.
a. Slide an arm under the client's axilla
b. Balance the client on their hip
c. Slide the client down to the floor
d. Place the client on the bed
e. Provide water for the client

10. A nurse at the health care facility is caring for clients who are beginning to ambulate and may require the help of an ambulatory aid. In which case would a nurse suggest the use of a cane to a client to aid ambulation?
a. Clients who have weakness on one side of the body
b. Clients who require considerable assistance with balance
c. Clients who need brief, temporary assistance ambulating
d. Clients who need permanent assistance when walking

11. A nurse is caring for a client who has a fractured leg in a cast. Which ambulatory device should the nurse use to aid this client to ambulate?
a. Cane
b. Axillary crutch
c. Walker
d. Platform crutch

12. A nurse is caring for a client whose legs have been amputated from below the knee. Which

components form part of the below-the-knee prosthesis? Select all that apply.
a. Socket
b. Shank
c. Ankle/foot system
d. Knee system
e. Lightweight tube

13. Listed here, in random order, are the steps followed when a client with a walker has to sit down in an armchair. Arrange the steps in the proper order.
a. Release the grip of the walker
b. Grip the armrest of the chair
c. Lower him or herself in the chair
d. Grasp the opposite armrest

14. Listed here, in random order, are the steps followed when a client with a walker has to get up from the armchair. Arrange the steps in the proper order.
a. Reposition the walker
b. Push up on the armrest with both arms
c. Move to the edge of the chair
d. Use one hand to grasp the walker and place the other on the armrest

15. Which client who uses crutches to ambulate would the nurse expect to have a swing-through gait?
a. A paralyzed client with leg braces
b. An amputee learning to use prosthesis
c. A client with a severe ankle sprain
d. A client who has more strength and balance

16. An arthritic client who uses crutches to ambulate is being treated at the health care facility. Which gait would the nurse observe when this client ambulates using the crutches?
a. Four-point
b. Two-point
c. Three-point non-weightbearing
d. Three-point partial weightbearing

SECTION IV: REVIEWING WHAT YOU HAVE LEARNED

Activity H *Fill in the blanks by choosing the correct word from the options given in parentheses.*

1. _____ crutches are used by clients who cannot bear weight on their hands and wrists. (Axillary, Forearm, Platform)

2. _____ exercises are stationary movements performed against a resistive force. (Dangling, Isometric, Isotonic)

Activity I   *Mark the statement as either T (True) or F (False). Correct any false statements.*

1. **T F**   The gluteal muscles in the buttocks aid in extending, abducting, and rotating the leg.

Activity J   *Answer the following question.*

What is the purpose of a tilt table?

_____

_____

_____

SECTION V: APPLYING YOUR KNOWLEDGE

Activity K   *Give a rationale for the following question.*

Why should the nurse encourage a client who is being fitted with a prosthetic limb to lie supine or prone periodically during the day?

_____

_____

_____

Activity L   *Answer the following questions, focusing on nursing roles and responsibilities.*

1. A nurse is caring for a client who is recovering from hip surgery and is learning to ambulate with a walker.
    a. What instructions should the nurse give to the client regarding the use of the walker?

    _____

    _____

    _____

    b. How should the nurse teach this client the techniques of sitting down and rising from a chair?

    _____

    _____

    _____

2. The nurse is caring for a client who will need to use crutches to move around.
    a. How can the nurse ensure that the client will be strong enough to use crutches?

    _____

    _____

    _____

    b. What kind of push-ups should the nurse teach a client who is still in bed?

    _____

    _____

    _____

Activity M   *Consider the following questions. Discuss them with your instructor or peers.*

A nurse is caring for a 32-year-old client who is to be fitted with a prosthetic limb following a below-the-knee amputation of their right leg. The client is struggling to accept their condition.
a. What actions can the nurse take to ensure that the prosthetic limb is comfortable for the client?

_____

_____

_____

b. How can the nurse help the client to begin accepting the amputation and the need for the prosthetic limb?

_____

_____

_____

SECTION VI: GETTING READY FOR NCLEX

Activity N   *Answer the following questions.*

1. A nurse is teaching a client with a fractured right leg how to climb stairs with a pair of crutches. What instruction would the nurse give the client?
    a. Step up by raising the right leg
    b. Use the handrail if it is on the right side
    c. Grasp both crutches at the handpiece in the right hand
    d. Follow the right leg with the left leg

2. A nurse is measuring a senior client for a cane following an ankle sprain. Which nursing action would the nurse perform?
    a. Instruct the client to lean forward
    b. Have the client stand barefoot with a support
    c. Ensure 40 degrees of elbow flexion with the hand on the grip
    d. Measure from the client's wrist to the floor

CHAPTER 27

Perioperative Care

Learning Objectives

- Define perioperative care.
- Identify the phases of perioperative care.
- Differentiate inpatient from outpatient surgery.
- List advantages of laser surgery.
- Discuss methods for donating blood before surgery.
- Identify major activities that nurses perform for all clients immediately before surgery.
- Name topics to address during preoperative teaching.
- Explain the purpose of antiembolism stockings.
- Name recommended methods for removing hair when preparing the skin for surgery.
- List items that are verified on the preoperative checklist.
- Discuss the purpose and information required during a presurgical time-out according to The Joint Commission's Universal Protocol.
- Name the areas of the surgical department used during the intraoperative period.
- Describe the focus of nursing care during the immediate postoperative period.
- Give examples of common postoperative complications.
- Discuss the purpose of a pneumatic compression device.
- Describe the information included in discharge instructions for postsurgical clients.
- Discuss ways in which the surgical care of older adults differs from that of other age groups.

SECTION I: ASSESSING YOUR UNDERSTANDING

Activity A   FILL IN THE BLANKS

1. _____ surgery is the term used for procedures performed on a client who is expected to stay at the facility at least overnight and is in need of nursing care for more than 1 day after surgery.

2. _____ surgery is the term used for operative procedures performed on clients who return home the same day.

3. Receiving one's own blood is called a(n) _____ transfusion.

4. _____ technology requires unique safety precautions such as eye, fire, heat, and vapor protection.

5. Shaving causes tiny cuts, also known as _____, that provide an entrance for microorganisms.

6. A _____ bladder increases the risks of bladder trauma and may cause difficulty in performing the procedure of inserting an indwelling urinary catheter.

7. When a laser is used, it releases a _____ (a substance composed of vaporized tissue, carbon dioxide, and water), which may contain intact cells.

8. _____ preparation for surgery involves preparing the client emotionally and spiritually and should begin as soon as the client is aware that surgery is necessary.

9. A preoperative _____ identifies the status of essential presurgical activities and is completed before surgery.

10. _____ drugs are medications that counteract the effects of those used for conscious sedation.

Activity B   *Consider the following figure.*

A

B

1. Identify the image.

_____

_____

_____

2. What are the benefits of the different positions shown in the figure?

_____

_____

_____

Activity C   *Match the types of anesthesia in Column A with their description in Column B.*

Column A	Column B
____ **1.** General	**a.** Blocks sensation in a particular area without affecting consciousness
____ **2.** Regional	
____ **3.** Local	**b.** Inhibits sensation in skin and mucous membranes where applied directly
____ **4.** Topical	
____ **5.** Spinal	**c.** Eliminates sensation in the lower extremities, lower abdomen, and pelvis
	d. Blocks sensation in a circumscribed area of skin and subcutaneous tissue
	e. Eliminates all sensation and consciousness or memory of an event

Activity D   *Presented here, in random order, are the steps that occur during initial postoperative assessments. Write the correct sequence in the boxes provided.*

1. Vital signs

2. Condition of wound and dressing

3. Level of consciousness

4. Effectiveness of respirations

5. Presence of urinary catheter and urine volume

6. Location of pain and need for analgesia

☐→☐→☐→☐→☐→☐

Activity E   *Briefly answer the following questions.*

1. Why should a nurse assess a client's support system before discharge?

_____

_____

_____

2. What should a nurse do for effective wound management?

_____

_____

_____

3. When does a preoperative period start and end?

_____

_____

_____

4. What is plume?

_____

_____

_____

5. How is consent obtained if a client is under the influence of drugs?

_____

_____

_____

6. What procedure should nurses follow regarding valuables?

_____

_____

_____

SECTION II: APPLYING YOUR KNOWLEDGE

Activity F _Nurses need to insert an indwelling urinary catheter preoperatively for some surgeries, particularly of the lower abdomen. If a catheter is not inserted, the nurse instructs the client to urinate immediately before receiving preoperative medication. Answer the following questions, which involve the nurse's role in preoperative care._

A nurse is caring for a client who is scheduled for pelvic surgery. The client has undertaken skin care by cleaning the affected area with soap for several days before surgery.

1. How can the nurse ensure that the client has a clean bowel before the surgery?

_____

_____

_____

2. Why is a clean bowel important during surgery?

_____

_____

_____

SECTION III: PRACTICING FOR NCLEX

Activity G _Answer the following questions._

1. A nurse is assessing a client with a superficial cyst near the ear. What type of surgery can the removal of the cyst be classified as?
   a. Optional
   b. Elective
   c. Urgent
   d. Emergency

2. A nurse is assisting a physician during a breast biopsy. The nurse explains to the client that breast biopsy is performed for
   a. The improvement of appearance or correction of defects
   b. The removal of defective tissue to restore function
   c. The enhancement of function without cure
   d. The removal and study of tissue to make a diagnosis

3. A nurse is preparing the discharge sheet of an outpatient client. When is an outpatient client discharged? Select all that apply.
   a. When the client is awake and alert
   b. When the client is out of anesthesia
   c. When the client's oral fluids are retained
   d. When the client is able to walk independently
   e. When the client's vital signs are stable

4. A nurse is applying antiembolism stockings to a client who will undergo surgery for venous stasis ulcers. What should the nurse do?
   a. Massage the legs before applying the stockings
   b. Remove the stockings once during the day and then reapply
   c. Lower the legs before applying the stockings
   d. Turn the stockings inside out before applying

5. A directed blood donor has come to the health care facility to donate blood. Which criterion does the nurse know is applicable for directed blood donation?
   a. The donor should be at least 17 years of age
   b. The donor should have a hematocrit level within a safe range
   c. The donor should donate 3 to 40 days before date of use
   d. The donor should have received a blood transfusion within the past 6 months

6. A nurse is teaching postsurgical clients to perform forced coughing. Which clients are most appropriate for trying this technique? Select all that apply.
   a. Clients who have moist lung sounds
   b. Clients who raise thick sputum
   c. Clients with chronic back pain
   d. Clients with abdominal incisions
   e. Clients with severe muscle spasms

7. A nurse is completing the preoperative checklist of a client scheduled for a cholecystectomy. What is the main purpose of a preoperative checklist?
   a. It identifies the status of essential presurgical activities
   b. It identifies the type of surgery required for the client
   c. It prepares the client spiritually, emotionally, and physically
   d. It allows the nurse to monitor the client for complications

8. A nurse is caring for a client during the intraoperative period. Which activity would the nurse perform?
   a. Transporting the client to a receiving room, then on to the operating room
   b. Determining whether the client has developed any allergies

   c. Preparing the client psychosocially before surgery
   d. Checking for the completion of skin preparation

9. The abdominal surgery of a client has been delayed because of an incomplete preoperative checklist submitted by a nurse. What factor could be responsible for an incomplete preoperative checklist?
   a. Unavailability of surgical equipment
   b. Improper documentation of physical examination
   c. Agency policy and availability of anesthesiologist
   d. Unavailability of well-fitting dentures for the client

10. A nurse is assisting a physician who is performing laser surgery on a client with cataracts. To which other conventional surgical techniques can laser surgery be used as an alternative? Select all that apply.
    a. Reattaching the retina
    b. Revascularizing ischemic heart muscle
    c. Replacing decayed teeth
    d. Removing skin tattoos
    e. Replacing and adjusting dislocated bones

11. A physician has ordered a nurse to administer regional anesthesia to a client to clean their severely infected leg injury. What is the major advantage of regional anesthesia?
    a. Promotes relaxation without any sedative
    b. Avoids continuous monitoring
    c. Increases mobility of anesthetized area
    d. Decreases the risk of respiratory complication

12. A nurse is caring for a client who has developed a postoperative complication of airway occlusion. What nursing intervention should the nurse perform for this client?
    a. Administer prescribed intravenous fluid
    b. Place the client in the Trendelenburg position
    c. Tilt the client's head and lift the chin
    d. Insert a nasogastric tube very gently

13. A nurse is applying a pneumatic compression device to a client with impaired circulation in their lower extremity. What is the appropriate nursing action?
    a. Help the client into a lateral position
    b. Palpate the pedal pulses
    c. Secure the air pump above the bed
    d. Stack and compress the air tubes

14. A nurse is writing discharge instructions for a client who has undergone exploratory laparoscopy. Which teaching point should be addressed in the discharge instructions?
    a. How to identify purulent drainage
    b. How to assess level of pain
    c. How to care for the incision site
    d. How to ensure a patent airway

15. A nurse is administering prescribed preoperative medications to a client. What precautions should the nurse take before administering these medications? Select all that apply.
    a. Check the client's ID bracelet
    b. Allay the client's fears about the surgery
    c. Explain the process of surgery
    d. Obtain and record vital signs
    e. Ask about allergies, if any

16. A nurse is assessing the condition of an older client scheduled for surgery. What is a common preoperative consideration for an older client that the nurse should address?
    a. May be prone to allergies
    b. May be susceptible to urinary tract infection
    c. May be on anticoagulation therapy
    d. May have impaired circulation and oxygenation

17. A nurse is assisting a physician during laser surgery. What precautions should they take? Select all that apply.
    a. Use alcohol and acetone during surgery
    b. Ensure that black-coated surgical instruments are used
    c. Ensure that the client's teeth are covered with plastic
    d. Remove all the jewelry and metal from body
    e. Avoid using prescription glasses with shields

18. A nurse needs to perform presurgical skin preparation on a mid-life adult client scheduled for rectal surgery. Which action should the nurse perform as part of presurgical skin preparation?
    a. Apply moisturizer to the skin
    b. Use electric hair clippers
    c. Use a depilatory agent
    d. Assess the condition of the hair

SECTION IV: REVIEWING WHAT YOU HAVE LEARNED

Activity H *Fill in the blanks by choosing the correct word from the options given in parentheses.*

1. A stationary blood clot in the veins is called a(n) _____. (embolus, thrombophlebitis, thrombus)

2. Surgery that removes or replaces defective tissue to restore function is called _____. (curative, exploratory, palliative)

Activity I *Mark each statement as either T (True) or F (False). Correct any false statements.*

1. T F   The care that clients receive before, during, and after surgery is called perioperative care.

2. T F   A wound is damaged skin or soft tissue that results from trauma.

Activity J *Write the correct term for each description below.*

1. A physician who administers chemical agents that temporarily eliminate sensation and pain _____

2. Blood donors chosen from among the client's relatives and friends _____

Activity K *Coughing is the natural method of clearing secretions from the airways. Write in the boxes provided below the correct sequence of performing forced coughing.*

1. Take a slow deep breath through the nose.

2. Exhale slowly through the mouth.

3. Sit upright.

4. Lean slightly forward.

5. Pull the abdomen inward.

6. Make the lower abdomen rise to the maximum.

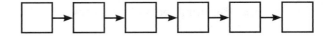

Activity L *Answer the following questions.*

1. What is a pneumatic compression device?

_____

_____

_____

2. What are the three methods for preparing the skin for surgery?

_____

_____

_____

SECTION V: APPLYING YOUR KNOWLEDGE

Activity M *Answer the following questions.*

1. Why are volatile substances such as alcohol and acetone avoided around lasers?

_____

_____

_____

2. Why do surgical clients have a reduced circulatory volume?

_____

_____

_____

Activity N *Answer the following questions focusing on nursing roles and responsibilities.*

1. A nurse is caring for a client who is to undergo surgery the following day.
   a. What potential risk factors increase the likelihood of perioperative complications?

   _____

   _____

   _____

2. A nurse in a health care facility is caring for a mid-life adult client scheduled for an incisional cholecystectomy.
   a. What general preoperative information should the nurse provide for this client?

   _____

   _____

   _____

b. What preoperative physical preparations is the nurse likely to perform for the client?

_____

_____

_____

Activity O *Consider the following questions. Discuss them with your instructor or peers.*

A nurse is caring for a client who has received preoperative spinal anesthesia.

1. What postoperative nursing care will be appropriate for this client?

_____

_____

_____

2. How does client care differ for general anesthesia versus regional anesthesia?

_____

_____

_____

SECTION VI: GETTING READY FOR NCLEX

Activity P *Answer the following questions.*

1. A nurse is providing preoperative information to a client scheduled to undergo surgery. What explanation will the nurse give to the client regarding the benefits of deep breathing?
   a. Reduces postoperative risk for respiratory complications
   b. Eases postoperative pain and discomfort
   c. Decreases the risk for circulatory complications

2. A senior client is scheduled to undergo surgery. What assessments should a nurse perform before fluid restriction? Select all that apply.
   a. Fluid intake and output
   b. Vital signs
   c. Level of consciousness
   d. Weight
   e. Skin turgor

CHAPTER 28

Wound Care

Learning Objectives

- Define wound.
- Name phases of wound repair.
- Identify signs and symptoms classically associated with the inflammatory response.
- Discuss the purpose of phagocytosis, including the types of cells involved.
- Name ways in which the integrity of a wound is restored.
- Explain first-, second-, and third-intention healing.
- Name types of wound complications.
- State purposes for using a dressing.
- Explain the rationale for keeping wounds moist.
- Describe types of drains, including the purpose of each.
- Name the major methods for securing surgical wounds together until they heal.
- Explain reasons for using a bandage or binder.
- Discuss the purpose for using one type of binder.
- Give examples of methods used to remove nonliving tissue from a wound.
- List commonly irrigated structures.
- State uses for applying heat and for applying cold.
- Identify methods for applying heat and cold.
- List risk factors for developing pressure ulcers.
- Discuss techniques for preventing pressure ulcers.

SECTION I: ASSESSING YOUR UNDERSTANDING

Activity A   FILL IN THE BLANKS

1. A _____ is damaged skin or soft tissue that results from trauma.

2. _____ is the physiologic defense immediately after tissue injury that lasts for approximately 2 to 5 days.

3. _____ is a process by which the white blood cells consume pathogens, coagulated blood, and cellular debris.

4. _____ is the period during which new cells fill and seal a wound, and it occurs from 2 days to 3 weeks after the inflammatory phase.

5. _____ (a period during which the wound undergoes changes and maturation) follows the proliferative phase and may last 6 months to 2 years.

6. _____ debridement is appropriate for uninfected wounds or for clients who cannot tolerate sharp debridement.

7. One of the chief advantages of _____ dressings is that they allow a nurse to assess a wound without removing the dressing.

8. _____ are tubes that provide a means for removing blood and drainage from a wound.

9. _____ are knotted ties, generally constructed from silk or synthetic materials such as nylon, which hold an incision together.

10. A _____ is a type of bandage generally applied to a particular body part such as the abdomen or breast.

Activity B   *Consider the following figure.*

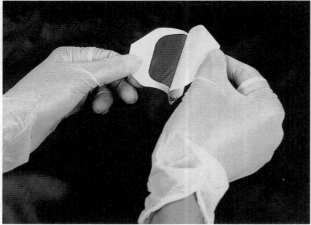

1. Identify the type of dressing.

   _____

   _____

   _____

2. What is the chief advantage of using this type of dressing?

   _____

   _____

   _____

Activity C   *Match the terms related to wounds in Column A with their descriptions in Column B.*

Column A	Column B
____ **1.** Open wound	**a.** Occurs more often from blunt trauma or pressure
____ **2.** Closed wound	
____ **3.** Granulation tissue	**b.** Wound caused by prolonged capillary compression
____ **4.** First-intention healing	**c.** Surface of the skin or mucous membrane is no longer intact
____ **5.** Pressure ulcer	**d.** A combination of new blood vessels, fibro-blasts, and epithelial cells
	e. A reparative process during which the wound edges are di-rectly next to each other

Activity D   *Presented here, in random order, are descriptions of the stages of a pressure ulcer. Place them in the correct sequence in the boxes provided.*

1. Ulcer is red and accompanied by blistering or skin tear.

2. Tissue is deeply ulcerated, exposing muscle and bone.

3. Characterized by intact but reddened skin.

4. Ulcer has a shallow skin crater that extends to the subcutaneous tissue.

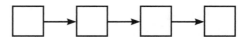

Activity E   *Briefly answer the following questions.*

1. What is the purpose of inflammation during the process of wound repair?

   _____

   _____

   _____

2. How is the integrity of skin and damaged tissue restored?

   _____

   _____

   _____

3. What are the factors that affect wound healing?

   _____

   _____

   _____

4. What are the factors that affect blood flow to the injured tissue?

   _____

   _____

   _____

5. What are the possible causes of surgical wound complication?

   _____

   _____

   _____

6. What purpose does the dressing of a wound serve?

_____

_____

_____

SECTION II: APPLYING YOUR KNOWLEDGE

Activity F *Heat and cold have various therapeutic uses and each can be used in several ways. Examples include an ice bag, collar, chemical pack, compress, and aquathermia pad. Answer the following questions involving a nurse's role in the application of a compress.*

A nurse is caring for a 2-year-old client who is being treated for viral fever at a health care facility. The nurse uses a cold compress for the child.

1. What is the purpose of a cold compress?

_____

_____

_____

2. How should the nurse apply the compress to the client?

_____

_____

_____

SECTION III: PRACTICING FOR NCLEX

Activity G *Answer the following questions.*

1. A nurse is caring for a client with an open wound at a health care facility. The wound is a clean separation of skin and tissue with smooth, even edges. How should the nurse document this wound?
   a. Incision
   b. Abrasion
   c. Laceration
   d. Ulceration

2. A nurse is caring for a diabetic client with pressure ulcers on the sole of their feet.

What is the best description of this type of ulceration?
   a. A clean separation of skin and tissue with smooth, even edges
   b. A separation of skin and tissue in which the edges are torn and irregular
   c. A wound in which the surface layers of the skin are scraped away
   d. A shallow crater in which skin or mucous membrane is missing

3. A nurse is caring for a client who has an open wound on their leg caused by a cut from a piece of glass. How would the nurse describe the inflammation stage of this wound repair?
   a. Physiologic defense immediately after tissue injury
   b. The period during which new cells fill and seal the wound
   c. Process by which damaged cells recover and reestablish normal functioning
   d. The period during which the wound undergoes changes and maturation

4. A nurse is caring for a client who accidentally injured themselves when using a knife. What action would the nurse describe as occurring during the first stage of inflammation?
   a. Leukocytes and macrophages migrate to the injury site
   b. The body keeps producing white blood cells
   c. Increased neutrophils and monocytes
   d. Blood vessels constrict to control blood loss

5. A nurse is caring for a client with an open wound. What characteristic is indicative of a wound that heals by second intention?
   a. Wound edges are directly next to each other
   b. Wound edges are widely separated, leading to complex reparative process
   c. Wound edges are widely separated and brought together with closure material
   d. Wound edges are close to each other but require closure material

6. A nurse is caring for a client who has been confined to bed for a long time. During an assessment of the client's skin, the nurse observes redness accompanied by blistering or tearing of skin. How should the nurse document this pressure ulcer?
   a. Stage I
   b. Stage II
   c. Stage III
   d. Stage IV

7. Which factor that might affect nutrition , and consequently impair wound healing, should a nurse assess for when caring for a senior client?
   a. Cognitive impairment
   b. Diminished collagen
   c. Decreased subcutaneous tissue
   d. Decreased blood supply

8. A nurse is treating an 11-year-old client who scraped their knee when they tripped and fell during a soccer match. The wound is bleeding and has some drainage. What type of dressing would be appropriate for this wound?
   a. Gauze
   b. Transparent
   c. Hydrocolloid
   d. Bandage

9. A nurse is caring for a client on intravenous therapy and uses a transparent dressing for the intravenous site. What is the benefit of using a transparent dressing?
   a. Occludes air and water from the wound
   b. Allows assessment of the wound without removing the dressing
   c. Allows treatment of wounds that are likely to bleed
   d. Keeps the wound moist, which promotes quick healing

10. A client who was severely injured with stab wounds has a closed suction drain. How should a nurse manage a closed drain site?
    a. Clean the insertion site in a circular manner
    b. Attach a safety pin or long clip
    c. Pull the drain for specified length
    d. Reposition a safety pin or long clip

11. A nurse is caring for a client with a superficial incision. What should the nurse use to manage the client's wound in this case?
    a. Hydrocolloid dressing
    b. Bandage
    c. Steri-Strip
    d. Gauze dressing

12. A nurse needs to bandage the arm of a client with a sprain resulting from a horse-riding accident. What techniques of wrapping the roller bandage should the nurse use in this case?
    a. Spiral turn
    b. Figure-of-eight turn
    c. Spica turn
    d. Recurrent turn

13. A nurse uses the spica turn technique to bandage a client at a health care facility. Where on the body is the nurse most likely using this technique?
    a. Elbow
    b. Legs
    c. Chest
    d. Knee

14. In which case would a nurse use the sharp debridement technique to promote healing?
    a. To treat clients with extensive necrotic tissue
    b. To treat clients with uninfected wounds
    c. To treat clients with small wounds
    d. To treat clients whose wounds are free of infection

15. A nurse is treating a 4-year-old with a solid object lodged in their ear. Before performing ear irrigation, the nurse performs a gross inspection of the client's ear. Why is this nursing intervention justified?
    a. The tapped object may swell and get more tightly fixed
    b. The pressure of the trapped solution could rupture the eardrum
    c. Drainage should be absorbed but should not obstruct its flow
    d. The tympanic membrane may become perforated

16. A nurse at a health care facility is caring for an 80-year-old client whose tests show reduced T-lymphocyte cells. The nurse should be aware that diminished immune response from reduced T-lymphocyte cells predisposes senior adults to:
    a. Pressure ulcers
    b. Shear-type injuries
    c. Delayed healing
    d. Wound infection

SECTION IV: REVIEWING WHAT YOU HAVE LEARNED

Activity H   *Fill in the blanks by choosing the correct word from the options given in parentheses.*

1. _____ is confirmed and monitored by counting the number and type of white blood cells in a sample of a client's blood. (Leukocytosis, Phagocytosis, Pinocytosis)

2. _____ dressings are self-adhesive, opaque, air- and water-occlusive wound coverings. (Gauze, Hydrocolloid, Transparent)

Activity I *Mark each statement as either T (True) or F (False). Correct any false statements.*

1. **T F** A wound is damaged skin or soft tissue that results from trauma.

2. **T F** Inflammation, the immediate physiologic response to tissue injury, lasts about 10 days.

Activity J *Write the correct term for each description below.*

1. The period from 2 days to 3 weeks after the inflammatory phase during which new cells fill and seal a wound _____

2. A process by which damaged cells recover and reestablish their normal function _____

3. The procedure of cleansing the vaginal canal to treat an infection _____

Activity K *Match the terms related to wounds and wound care in Column A with their description in Column B.*

Column A
____ 1. Collagen
____ 2. Remodeling
____ 3. Dehiscence
____ 4. Debridement
____ 5. Capillary action

Column B
a. Removal of dead tissue
b. Tough and inelastic protein
c. Movement of a liquid at the point of contact with a solid
d. Separation of wound edges
e. The period during which the wound undergoes changes and maturation

Activity L *Answer the following question.*

1. What are the three types of wound healing?

_____
_____
_____

SECTION V: APPLYING YOUR KNOWLEDGE

Activity M *Give rationales for the following questions.*

1. Why are transparent dressings less bulky than gauze dressings?

_____
_____
_____

2. Why is it important to keep wounds moist?

_____
_____
_____

Activity N *Answer the following questions focusing on nursing roles and responsibilities.*

1. A nurse is to perform an ear irrigation on a client.
   a. What process will the nurse follow?

   _____
   _____

   b. What postirrigation technique should the nurse implement?

   _____
   _____
   _____

2. What six basic techniques should a nurse follow to wrap a roller bandage?

   _____
   _____
   _____

SECTION VI: GETTING READY FOR NCLEX

Activity O   *Answer the following question.*

A physician has ordered a cold application for a client with a bruised and painful ankle. What explanation will a nurse give to the client regarding the benefit of cold applications?

a. Speeds healing

b. Relieves muscle spasm

c. Promotes circulation

d. Numbs sensation

CHAPTER 29

Gastrointestinal Intubation

Learning Objectives

- Define intubation and list reasons for gastrointestinal intubation.
- Identify general types of gastrointestinal tubes.
- Name assessments that are necessary before inserting a tube nasally.
- Explain the purpose of and how to obtain a *n*ose-to-*e*arlobe-to-the-*x*iphoid (NEX) measurement.
- Describe methods for determining distal placement in the stomach.
- Discuss ways by which nasointestinal feeding tubes or their insertion differs from their gastric counterparts.
- Name schedules for administering tube feedings.
- Explain the purpose of assessing gastric residual.
- Name nursing activities involved in managing the care of clients who are being tube-fed.
- Name nursing responsibilities for assisting with the insertion of a tungsten-weighted intestinal decompression tube.

SECTION I: ASSESSING YOUR UNDERSTANDING

Activity A   FILL IN THE BLANKS

1. A(n) _____ is an artificial opening into the stomach.

2. Gastric _____ tubes are used exclusively to remove fluid and gas from the stomach.

3. Belching often indicates that the tip of the tube is still in the _____.

4. A(n) _____ decompression tube is inserted in the same manner as a nasogastric tube.

5. Intestinal tubes like the Maxter tube and the Andersen tube are weighted with _____.

6. A(n) _____ tube is used in an emergency to remove toxic substances that have been ingested.

7. Some nasogastric tubes have more than one _____ within the tube.

8. A gastrostomy tube is placed surgically or with the use of a(n) _____.

9. A(n) _____ feeding usually involves 250 to 400 mL formula per administration.

10. _____ generally means the placement of a tube into a body structure.

Activity B *Consider the following figure.*

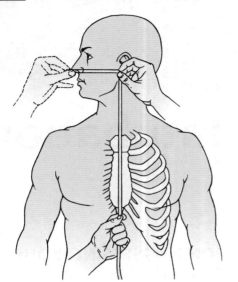

1. Identify the image.

_____

_____

_____

2. How is this procedure performed?

_____

_____

_____

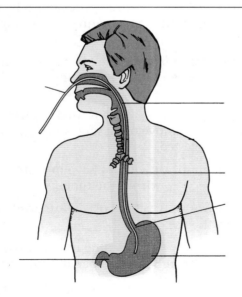

3. Identify and label the image.

_____

_____

_____

4. What are the disadvantages of this procedure?

_____

_____

_____

Activity C *Match the types of tube feeding formulas in Column A with their description in Column B.*

Column A

____ **1.** Balanced

____ **2.** High nitrogen

____ **3.** High fiber

____ **4.** Partially hydrolyzed

____ **5.** Isotonic balanced

Column B

a. Given to people with malabsorption syndromes

b. Meets total nutrition needs

c. Furnishes more protein than other formulas

d. Provides nutrition and decreases constipation or diarrhea

e. Supplements nutrition without altering water distribution

Activity D *Presented here, in random order, are steps that occur during the assessment of the pH of aspirated fluid. Write the correct sequence in the boxes provided.*

1. Aspirate a small volume of fluid with a clean syringe.

2. Perform an alcohol-based hand rub.

3. Compare the color on the test strip with color guide.

4. Drop a sample of gastric fluid onto an indicator strip.

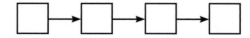

Activity E *Briefly answer the following questions.*

1. Why is intubation performed on clients?

_____

_____

_____

2. What are the problems faced with narrow-diameter feeding tubes?

_____

_____

_____

3. What are the nurse's functions regarding nasogastric tubes?

_____

_____

_____

4. When are tube feedings performed?

_____

_____

_____

5. What are the problems associated with bolus feedings?

_____

_____

_____

6. How can a dietitian help a tube-fed client in a home setting?

_____

_____

_____

SECTION II: APPLYING YOUR KNOWLEDGE

Activity F   _Nursing skills are activities that are unique to the practice of nursing. One of these skills is the counseling skill that the nurse implements during exchanges of information, offering pertinent health teaching and providing emotional support to the clients. Answer the following questions, which involve implementation of nursing skills._

A nurse is administering a tube-feeding formula to a senior client with severe abdominal pain. The client also experiences malabsorption syndromes.

1. What should the nurse do if the senior client develops hyperglycemia when tube-feeding?

_____

_____

_____

2. Which tube-feed formula should the nurse administer to the older client?

_____

_____

_____

SECTION III: PRACTICING FOR NCLEX

Activity G   _Answer the following questions._

1. A nurse has to administer liquid nourishment to a client over 30 to 60 minutes at the rate of 250 to 400 mL per administration with a feeding pump. What tube-feeding cycles should the nurse follow?
   a. Intermittent feeding
   b. Cyclic feeding
   c. Continuous feeding
   d. Bolus feeding

2. A nurse needs to insert a nasointestinal tube inside the nostril of a client. What action should the nurse ask the client to perform when assessing each nostril?
   a. Use a nebulizer for half an hour
   b. Perform presurgical skin preparation
   c. Avoid clearing nasal debris
   d. Ask the client to exhale

3. A nurse has to insert an intestinal decompression tube from the pyloric valve into the small intestine of a client. Which nursing action is appropriate?
   a. Observe the graduated marks on the tube
   b. Move the client into the Fowler position
   c. Ambulate the client if possible
   d. Request an X-ray confirmation

4. A nurse has to remove an intestinal decompression tube from a client. Which action should the nurse perform first when removing the tube?
   a. Remove the tube within 10 minutes
   b. Disconnect the tube from the suction source
   c. Secure the tube to the face with tape
   d. Verify the tube placement with a radiograph

5. A nurse is performing a preintubation assessment for a client who has been prescribed a nasogastric tube. What is the main goal of the assessment?
   a. Determine whether there is any nausea and vomiting
   b. Determine the client's ability to swallow, cough, and gag
   c. Detect the nostril best suited for tube insertion
   d. Check the client's level of consciousness

6. A nurse is inserting a gastric sump tube inside a client. A gastric sump tube is used exclusively to:
   a. Remove fluid and gas from the stomach
   b. Provide nourishment to the small intestine
   c. Remove liquid contents from the small intestine
   d. Reduce trauma to intestinal tissue

7. A nurse is caring for a client who is being provided with liquid nourishment on a cyclic feeding schedule. At what time of day would the nurse feed the client?
   a. Early morning
   b. Afternoon
   c. Late evening
   d. After lunch

8. A nurse is checking the gastric residual of a client who is being tube-fed. As a rule of thumb, how much should the volume of gastric residual be?
   a. Less than 250 mL
   b. Approximately 150 mL
   c. 1 mL/kcal, on a daily basis
   d. No more than 100 mL

9. A physician has ordered a nurse to provide enteral nutrition to a client. Which actions would the nurse perform? Select all that apply.
   a. Provide nourishment via the stomach
   b. Administer a liquid tube-feeding formula
   c. Provide nourishment via the intestine
   d. Use a tube that is short in length
   e. Use a tube that is small in diameter

10. A nurse is preparing a home care note for a tube-fed client who is being discharged from the health care facility. Which teaching point is most important when preparing clients for self-care at home?
    a. Demonstrate each procedure
    b. Provide detailed written instructions
    c. Make a referral to a home health agency
    d. Teach self-administration techniques

11. A nurse is inserting an intestinal decompression tube inside a client. Which action will help the nurse to monitor the tube's progression and approximate anatomic location?
    a. Observe graduated marks on the tube
    b. Reinsert the stylet when the tube is inside
    c. Ambulate the client if possible
    d. Mark the tube before inserting

12. A nurse is assessing a feeding tube smaller than 12 Fr, which is prone to obstruction. What actions should the nurse perform to maintain tube patency? Select all that apply.
    a. Wash the tube every 2 hours
    b. Give plenty of water to the client
    c. Flush the tube with 30 to 60 mL water
    d. Flush the tube with cranberry juice
    e. Flush the tube with carbonated beverages

13. A nurse has to tube-feed a client. Which tube-feeding schedule is least desirable because it distends the stomach rapidly, causes gastric discomfort, and increases risk of reflux?
    a. Continuous
    b. Bolus
    c. Intermittent
    d. Cyclic

14. A nurse is rectifying a gastrostomy leak that has occurred in a feeding tube inserted in a client. What causes a gastrostomy leak? Select all that apply.
    a. Infusion of the feed when the gastrointestinal tube is clamped
    b. Reduction in abdominal pressure
    c. Disconnection between the feeding tube and the gastrointestinal tube
    d. Instillation of highly concentrated nutritional formula
    e. Underinflation of the balloon beneath the skin

15. A client with a nasogastric tube complains of a vomiting sensation. The nurse assesses the client and notices that the client's bowel sounds are less than 5/minute. Which nursing diagnosis should the nurse document based on the data collected during client care?
    a. Imbalanced nutrition
    b. Self-care deficit
    c. Impaired swallowing
    d. Risk for aspiration

16. A nurse is administering a tube feeding to a client. The nurse pinches the feeding tube just as the last volume of water is administered. Why is this nursing action appropriate?
    a. To provide access to formula
    b. To prevent the tube from leaking
    c. To prevent air from entering the tube
    d. To purge air from the tube

17. A nurse is caring for a tube-fed client who has inflammation of the middle ear. Which nursing intervention will reduce the inflammation?
    a. Insert a small-diameter feeding tube
    b. Provide nasal and oral hygiene
    c. Keep the tubing filled with water
    d. Maintain the client's neck in a neutral position

SECTION IV: REVIEWING WHAT YOU HAVE LEARNED

Activity H *Fill in the blanks by choosing the correct word from the options given in parentheses.*

1. The use of gastrointestinal tubes to provide nourishment is called _____ feeding. (bolus, gavage, lavage)

2. _____ tubes are inserted through the nose for distal placement below the stomach. (Nasogastric, Nasointestinal, Orogastric)

Activity I *Mark each statement as either T (True) or F (False). Correct any false statements.*

1. **T F** Gastric reflux is the reverse flow of gastric contents.

2. **T F** Enteral nutrition is nourishment provided by the oral route.

Activity J *Write the correct term for the description below.*

1. Measuring the length from the nose-to-earlobe-to-the-xiphoid process

   _____

Activity K *Match the terms related to tube-feeding in Column A with their description in Column B.*

Column A	Column B
____ 1. Intermittent feeding	a. Instillation of liquid nutrition without interruption at a rate of approximately 1.5 mL/minute
____ 2. Continuous feeding	b. Instillation of liquid nourishment for 8 to 12 hours followed by a pause of 12 to 16 hours
____ 3. Cyclic feeding	c. Instillation of liquid nourishment four to six times a day

Activity L *Consider the following figure.*

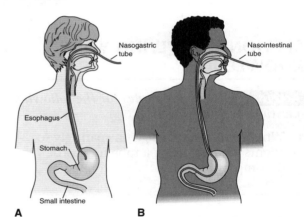

1. Label and identify what is shown in the figure.

   _____

   _____

   _____

2. What could be the adverse effects of this procedure?

_____

_____

_____

Activity M   _Answer the following questions._

1. What are the causes of gastrostomy leaks?

_____

_____

_____

2. What are the uses of gastric or intestinal tubes?

_____

_____

_____

SECTION V: APPLYING YOUR KNOWLEDGE

Activity N   _Give rationales for the following question._

1. Why should water be given sparingly to clients who are using a tube for gastric decompression?

_____

_____

_____

Activity O   _Answer the following questions focusing on nursing roles and responsibilities._

1. A nurse at an extended-care facility is caring for a client receiving tube feedings. The client has asked for self-care at home even if tube feeding is required.
   a. What written instructions should the nurse provide when preparing the client for home care?

_____

_____

_____

b. What are some nursing diagnoses that might be appropriate for this client?

_____

_____

_____

2. What are common nursing guidelines for clients with intestinal decompression tubes?

_____

_____

_____

Activity P   _Consider the following questions. Discuss them with your instructor or peers._

A client has been brought to the health care facility in a semiconscious state following a suicide attempt by drug overdose.

1. What immediate care should the nurse provide for this client?

_____

_____

_____

2. What assistance should the nurse provide during a lavage procedure for this client?

_____

_____

_____

SECTION VI: GETTING READY FOR NCLEX

Activity Q   _Answer the following questions._

1. How can the nurse clear a small-diameter orogastric feeding tube that is obstructed? Select all that apply.
   a. Aspirate as much as possible from the tube
   b. Instill 5 mL of an enzymatic solution
   c. Reinstill the aspirated fluid
   d. Measure the aspirated fluid and record
   e. Clamp the tube and wait for 15 minutes

2. A physician has ordered tube feedings for a hospitalized client. What conditions contribute to the development of diarrhea in a tube-fed client? Select all that apply.
   a. Highly concentrated formula
   b. Rapid administration
   c. Bacterial contamination
   d. Incorrect tube placement
   e. Inadequate calories

3. A nurse is caring for a senior adult client receiving tube feedings. What sign should the nurse closely monitor to identify hyperglycemia?
   a. Malabsorption syndrome
   b. Hydration status
   c. Change in skin turgor
   d. Elevated body temperature

CHAPTER 30

Urinary Elimination

Learning Objectives

- Identify the functions of the urinary system.
- Describe the physical characteristics of urine and factors that affect urination.
- Name types of urine specimens that nurses commonly collect.
- Identify alternative devices for urinary elimination.
- Define continence training.
- Name types of urinary catheters.
- Describe principles that apply to using a closed drainage system.
- Explain why catheter care is important in the nursing management of clients with retention catheters.
- Discuss the purpose of irrigating a catheter and methods for performing this skill.
- Define urinary diversion.
- Discuss factors that contribute to impaired skin integrity in clients with a urostomy.

SECTION I: ASSESSING YOUR UNDERSTANDING

Activity A   FILL IN THE BLANKS

1. A(n) _____ specimen is a sample of fresh urine collected in a clean container.

2. _____ means the absence of urine or a urinary volume of 100 mL or less in 24 hours.

3. In _____ the urine output is less than 400 mL per 24 hours, which indicates the inadequate elimination of urine.

4. _____ is difficult or uncomfortable voiding and a common symptom of trauma to the urethra or a bladder infection.

5. _____ refers to using a device inside the bladder or externally about the urinary meatus.

6. A(n) _____ catheter is a urine drainage tube inserted, but not left in place; it drains urine temporarily or provides a sterile urine specimen.

7. A(n) _____ irrigation instills irrigating solution into a catheter by gravity over a period of days.

8. Age-related changes, such as diminished bladder capacity and relaxation of the pelvic floor muscle tone, increase the risk of _____.

9. A(n) _____ catheter is not inserted within the bladder; instead, it surrounds the urinary meatus.

10. A(n) _____ is a seat-like container for elimination that is used to collect urine or stool.

Activity B *Consider the following figure.*

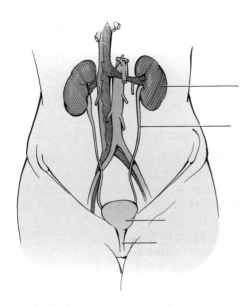

1. Identify and label the figure.

_____

_____

_____

2. What are the functions of the various parts in the figure?

_____

_____

_____

Activity C *Match the terms related to urinary elimination in Column A with their descriptions in Column B.*

Column A

_____ **1.** Urinary elimination

_____ **2.** Clean catch

_____ **3.** Polyuria

_____ **4.** Urinal

_____ **5.** Catheter irrigation

Column B

a. Voided sample of urine that is considered sterile

b. Cylindrical container for collecting urine

c. Technique for restoring or maintaining catheter patency

d. Process of releasing excess of fluid and metabolic waste

e. Greater-than-normal urinary volume and may accompany minor dietary variations

Activity D *Presented here, in random order, are steps that occur when providing a continuous irrigation. Write the correct sequence in the boxes provided.*

1. Connect the tubing to the catheter port for irrigation.

2. Monitor the appearance of the urine and volume of urinary drainage.

3. Purge the air from the tubing.

4. Regulate the rate of instillation according to the medical order.

5. Hang the sterile irrigating solution from an intravenous pole.

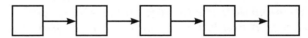

Activity E *Briefly answer the following questions.*

1. What are the common disorders associated with polyuria?

_____

_____

_____

2. What is a urinary catheter used for?

_____

_____

_____

3. What are the problems that may accompany the use of a condom catheter?

_____

_____

_____

4. What physiologic changes could lead older adults to experience urinary urgency and frequency?

_____

_____

_____

5. What are the resources available to assist older adults in evaluating and treating incontinence?

_____

_____

_____

6. What are the problems that a client with oliguria is likely to face?

_____

_____

_____

SECTION II: APPLYING YOUR KNOWLEDGE

Activity F   _A closed drainage system is a device used to collect urine from a catheter. It consists of a calibrated bag that can be opened at the bottom, tubing of sufficient length to accommodate the turning and positioning of clients, and a hanger from which to suspend the bag from the bed. Answer the following questions related to the use of a closed drainage system._

A nurse is caring for a client with a urinary catheter at a health care facility. The client has a distended bladder and is unable to void.

1. What care should the nurse take when a closed drainage system is used to collect urine from the catheter?

_____

_____

_____

2. How can the nurse prevent the drainage system from becoming a reservoir of pathogens?

_____

_____

_____

SECTION III: PRACTICING FOR NCLEX

Activity G   _Answer the following questions._

1. Order the following steps on how the need to urinate becomes apparent.
   a. Distention with urine causes increased fluid pressure
   b. This creates a desire to urinate
   c. The bladder distends with 150 to 300 mL urine
   d. This stimulates the stretch receptors in the bladder wall

2. When collecting a clean-catch urine specimen, what nursing action can prevent the urine sample from being contaminated by microorganisms or substances other than those in the urine?
   a. Collect the sample in a clean container
   b. Clean external structures through which the urine passes
   c. Collect the sample over a period of 24 hours
   d. Use a catheter to collect the sample

3. A nurse at a health care facility notes that the volume of the client's urine is more than 3,500 mL/day. What assessment might the nurse make that accounts for the increase in volume of the client's urine?
   a. Kidney dysfunction
   b. Gallbladder disease
   c. Diuretic medication
   d. Infection

4. A nurse at a health care facility needs to collect a sample of the client's urine. However, when collecting the sample, the nurse notes that the client's urine appears cloudy. What is a likely reason for the appearance of the urine?
   a. Stasis
   b. Blood
   c. Water-soluble dyes
   d. Dehydration

5. The laboratory test of a client's urine indicates the presence of plasma proteins in the urine. What term could a nurse use to document this type of urine?
   a. Hematuria
   b. Pyuria
   c. Proteinuria
   d. Albuminuria

6. An assessment of a client's urinary pattern indicates that the client has dysuria. What condition is indicative of dysuria?
   a. Absence of urine
   b. Inadequate elimination of urine
   c. Greater-than-normal urinary volume
   d. Difficult or uncomfortable voiding

7. The abnormal urinary elimination pattern in a client has been diagnosed as oliguria. Which problem is commonly seen in clients with oliguria?
   a. Urinary stones
   b. Diabetes mellitus
   c. Diabetes insipidus
   d. Enlarged prostate gland

8. At a health care facility, there are some clients who are men who require assistance with urinary elimination. To what type of clients should the nurse provide a urinal?
   a. Clients who can ambulate
   b. Clients who are weak
   c. Clients who are unable to walk
   d. Clients who are confined to bed

9. A nurse at a health care facility is caring for a client with urinary incontinence. The client has been provided with a catheter. For what reasons is a catheter used? Select all that apply.
   a. Restraining the client from urinating
   b. Keeping the incontinent client dry
   c. Measuring the residual urine
   d. Instilling medication within the bladder
   e. Preventing urinary tract infection

10. A nurse uses a urinary bag to collect a urine specimen from an infant boy at a health care facility. How would the nurse describe the urinary bag to the parents?
    a. A urine drainage tube inserted but not left in place
    b. A urine drainage tube that is left in place over a period of time
    c. A bag attached by adhesive backing to the skin around genitals
    d. A flexible sheath that is rolled around the penis

11. A nurse is caring for a female client who complains of the loss of a small amount of urine whenever she sneezes or laughs. What nursing intervention should the nurse suggest for this client?
    a. Clothing modification
    b. Weight reduction
    c. Absorbent undergarment
    d. Cutaneous triggering

12. A client with urge incontinence complains to a nurse that they perceive the need to void frequently and have a short-lived ability to sustain control of the flow. What is the possible cause of the client's condition?
    a. Loss of perineal and sphincter muscle tone
    b. Damage to the motor and sensory tracts in the lower spinal cord
    c. Altered consciousness related to head injury
    d. Bladder irritation secondary to infection

13. A nurse is caring for a client who has a retention catheter for urinary incontinence. When providing catheter care, why should the nurse clean the meatus and nearby section of the catheter at least once a day?
    a. To reduce the colonizing of microorganisms
    b. To remove gross secretions and transient microorganisms
    c. To protect the bed linen from becoming wet or soiled
    d. To reduce the potential for transmitting microorganisms

14. Order the following steps for irrigating a closed drainage system.
    a. Attach a needle to the syringe containing the sterile irrigation solution
    b. Clean the port with an alcohol swab
    c. Clamp the tubing beneath the port and instill the solution
    d. Pierce the port with an 18- or 19-guage 1.5-inch needle
    e. Release the tubing for drainage

15. Order the following steps with regard to providing continuous irrigation.
    a. Hang the sterile irrigating solution from an intravenous pole
    b. Regulate the rate of infusion according to the medical order
    c. Purge the air from the tubing
    d. Monitor the appearance of the urine and volume of urinary drainage
    e. Connect the tubing to the catheter port for irrigation

16. A nurse is caring for a senior client at a health care facility. What age-related condition should the nurse be observant of that could increase the risk for a urinary infection?
    a. Diminished bladder capacity
    b. Pelvic floor muscle tone relaxation
    c. Chronic residual urine
    d. Enlargement of the prostate

17. A nurse at a health care facility teaches double voiding to a client who is being treated for urinary tract infection resulting from residual urine. How would the nurse describe this procedure to the client?
    a. Clients void, then wait a few more minutes to allow any urine to be voided
    b. Clients void within 30 to 120 minutes after medication administration
    c. Clients plan toilet breaks every 60 to 90 minutes
    d. Clients have a routine toileting schedule every 90 to 120 minutes

18. A nurse provides a bedpan to a client who has been confined to the bed. Before using the pan, the nurse palpates the lower abdomen. Which statement justifies the nurse's action?
    a. Demonstrates concern for the client's comfort
    b. Prevents unnecessary exposure
    c. Promotes use of good body mechanics
    d. Checks for bladder fullness

19. When collecting a urine sample from the client for laboratory tests, the nurse notes that the client's urine appears dark amber in color. What is the possible cause for the appearance of the urine?
    a. Dehydration
    b. Liver disease
    c. Blood
    d. Water-soluble dyes

SECTION IV: REVIEWING WHAT YOU HAVE LEARNED

Activity H   *Fill in the blanks by choosing the correct word from the options given in parentheses.*

1. _____ means greater-than-normal urinary volume. (Anuria, Oliguria, Polyuria)

2. A _____ is a bedside seat-like container used for the elimination of body waste. (bedpan, commode, urinal)

Activity I   *Mark each statement as either T (True) or F (False). Correct any false statements.*

1. T F   Catheterization is the insertion of a hollow tube inside the bladder.

2. T F   The urinary meatus is the opening to the urethra.

3. T F   A straight catheter is an indwelling catheter left in place for a period of time.

Activity J   *Write the correct term for the description below.*

Urine containing blood _____

Activity K   *Consider the following figures.*

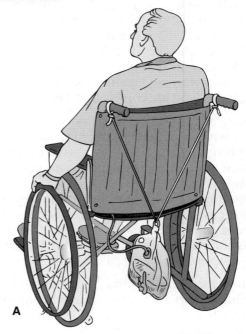

A

1. Identify what is shown in the figures.

   _____

   _____

   _____

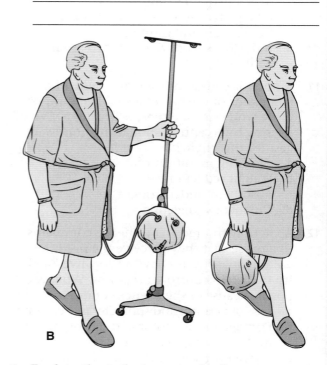

B

2. Explain the techniques in the figures.

   _____

   _____

   _____

Activity L   *A catheter is removed when it needs to be replaced or when its use can be discontinued. Write in the boxes provided below the correct sequence for removing a Foley catheter.*

1. Empty the balloon by aspirating the fluid with a syringe.

2. Measure the volume of each voiding for the next 8 to 10 hours.

3. Wash hands and put on clean gloves.

4. Inspect the catheter and discard it, if it appears to be intact.

5. Gently pull the catheter to the point where it exits from the meatus.

6. Clean the urinary meatus.

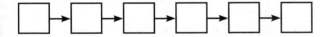

Activity M   *Answer the following questions.*

1. What are the four physical characteristics of urine?

_____

_____

_____

2. What are the uses of a urinary catheter?

_____

_____

_____

3. What are the potential problems of using condom catheters?

_____

_____

_____

SECTION V: APPLYING YOUR KNOWLEDGE

Activity N   *Give rationales for the following questions.*

1. Why is the first-voided specimen of the day preferred as a urine sample?

_____

_____

_____

2. Why is urination during the night considered unusual?

_____

_____

_____

Activity O   *Answer the following questions focusing on nursing roles and responsibilities.*

1. A nurse is caring for a client with urinary incontinence. What nursing diagnoses might be applicable in this situation?

_____

_____

_____

2. A middle-aged client has an indwelling retention catheter. What nursing care is appropriate for this client?

_____

_____

_____

Activity P   *Consider the following questions. Discuss them with your instructor or peers.*

A nurse is caring for a senior client with urinary incontinence who has an indwelling catheter.

1. What possible problems could occur in this client?

   _____

   _____

   _____

2. Describe the appropriate nursing care for this client.

   _____

   _____

   _____

SECTION VI: GETTING READY FOR NCLEX

Activity Q   *Answer the following questions.*

1. A client who is paralyzed from the waist down is experiencing spontaneous loss of urine. How should a nurse document this client's condition?
   a. Reflex incontinence
   b. Stress incontinence
   c. Functional incontinence
   d. Urge incontinence

2. A nurse is teaching a client to perform a Credé maneuver as part of urinary continence training. What instruction should the nurse teach the client regarding this maneuver?
   a. Massage or tap the skin lightly above the pubic area.
   b. Bend forward and apply hand pressure over the bladder.
   c. Relax the urinary sphincter in response to physical stimulation.
   d. Contract and relax the muscles alternately for 10 seconds.

3. A senior client with a musculoskeletal disorder cannot elevate the hips. The nurse is using a fracture pan to collect the client's urine and stool. What interventions should the nurse follow when using a nonmetallic fracture pan? Select all that apply.
   a. Warm the bedpan with warm running water.
   b. Palpate the client's lower abdomen.
   c. Place soiled tissue in the fracture pan.
   d. Slip the fracture pan just beneath the buttocks.
   e. Raise the head of the client's bed.

CHAPTER 31

Bowel Elimination

Learning Objectives

- Describe the process of defecation.
- Name components of a bowel elimination assessment.
- List common alterations in bowel elimination.
- Name types of constipation.
- Identify measures within the scope of nursing practice for treating constipation.
- Identify interventions that promote bowel elimination when it does not occur naturally.
- Name categories of enema administration.
- List common solutions used in a cleansing enema.
- Explain the purpose of an oil retention enema.
- Describe nursing activities involved in ostomy care.

SECTION I: ASSESSING YOUR UNDERSTANDING

Activity A   FILL IN THE BLANKS

1. _____ is the rhythmic contractions of intestinal smooth muscle that facilitate defecation.

2. _____ is eventually released when the anal sphincters relax.

3. _____ is an elimination problem characterized by dry, hard stool that is difficult to pass.

4. The incidence of constipation tends to be high among those whose dietary habits lack adequate _____.

5. Prolonged use of narcotic analgesia tends to cause _____ constipation.

6. Clients with a fecal _____ usually report a frequent desire to defecate but an inability to do so.

7. _____ results from swallowing air while eating or sluggish peristalsis.

8. A(n) _____ enema holds a solution within the large intestine for a specified period, usually at least 30 minutes.

9. _____ constipation is a consequence of a pathologic disorder such as a partial bowel obstruction.

10. Dietary fiber that becomes undigested cellulose attracts _____ within the bowel.

Activity B *Consider the following figure.*

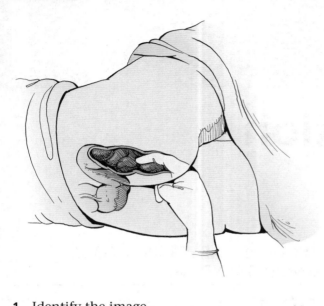

1. Identify the image.

   _____

   _____

   _____

2. When is the procedure required?

   _____

   _____

   _____

Activity C *Match the factors affecting bowel elimination in Column A with their effects in Column B.*

Column A

_____ **1.** Types of food consumed

_____ **2.** Fluid intake

_____ **3.** Neuromuscular function

_____ **4.** Abdominal muscle tone

_____ **5.** Opportunity for defecation

Column B

a. Inhibits or facilitates elimination

b. Influence color, odor, and volume

c. Influences moisture content of stool

d. Ability to control rectal muscles

e. Ability to increase intra-abdominal pressure

Activity D *Presented here, in random order, are steps that occur during the procedure of testing stool for occult blood. Write the correct sequence in the boxes provided.*

1. Take the sample from the center of the stool.

2. Place two drops of chemical reagent onto the test space.

3. Collect stool within a toilet liner or bedpan.

4. Apply a thin smear of stool onto the test area.

5. Wait for 60 seconds and observe for a blue color.

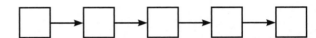

Activity E *Briefly answer the following questions.*

1. What problems with elimination do clients with musculoskeletal disorders face?

   _____

   _____

   _____

2. What is defecation?

   _____

   _____

   _____

3. What is involved in a comprehensive assessment of bowel elimination?

   _____

   _____

   _____

4. What are the common problems faced by clients related to bowel elimination?

   _____

   _____

   _____

5. How does a client develop pseudoconstipation?

   _____

   _____

   _____

6. What is diarrhea?

_____

_____

_____

SECTION II: APPLYING YOUR KNOWLEDGE

Activity F _Infrequent elimination of stool does not necessarily indicate that a person is constipated. Some people may be constipated, even though they have a daily bowel movement, whereas others who defecate irregularly may have normal bowel function. Answer the following questions, which involve the nurse's role when caring for a client with constipation._

A nurse is caring for a client who is complaining of constipation. During the initial assessment, the nurse finds out that the client has a sedentary job and eats convenience store food for lunch and dinner.

1. What kind of diet should the nurse recommend to the client to promote quick and easy elimination?

_____

_____

_____

2. What are the various signs and symptoms that accompany constipation?

_____

_____

_____

SECTION III: PRACTICING FOR NCLEX

Activity G _Answer the following questions._

1. A nurse is caring for a client with abnormal stool. The nurse knows that abnormal stool can appear in what colors? Select all that apply.
a. Black
b. Green
c. Brown
d. Yellow
e. Dark brown

2. A nurse is caring for a client with severe pain in the abdomen and constipation resulting from fecal impaction. Which intervention should the nurse perform to facilitate easy insertion into the rectum when removing the fecal impaction?
a. Lubricate the forefinger
b. Place the client in the Sims position
c. Lubricate the rectal tube
d. Warm the cleansing solution

3. A nurse is caring for a client with fecal impaction accompanied by rectal pain. The nurse knows that the rectal pain is the result of which factor?
a. Contractions in higher bowel areas
b. Unsuccessful efforts to empty the lower bowel
c. Insufficient intake of liquids
d. Retained barium from a radiographic procedure

4. A nurse is caring for a client who is extremely uncomfortable because of flatulence. Which nursing intervention can provide immediate relief to the client?
a. Insertion of a rectal suppository
b. Administration of a cleansing enema
c. Insertion of a rectal tube
d. Offering a glass of prune juice

5. A nurse is caring for a client with an intestinal disorder. Which intervention should the nurse perform to get accurate findings when testing the stool for occult blood?
a. Avoid placing reagent onto the test space
b. Cover the entire test space with the sample
c. Apply a thin smear of stool onto test area
d. Avoid taking the sample from the center of the stool

6. A physician has asked the nurse to include a power pudding recipe in a senior client's diet. Which ingredients should the nurse incorporate in the power pudding recipe? Select all that apply.
a. One cup prune juice
b. One cup applesauce
c. One cup of milk
d. One cup wheat bran
e. One cup water

7. A physician has ordered the nurse to increase the fluid intake in a client's diet. What will be the effect of increased liquid intake on the client's bowel elimination?
   a. Influence the odor and volume of stool
   b. Alter the bowel motility
   c. Influence the moisture content of stool
   d. Influence the fecal velocity

8. A nurse is removing the fecal impaction of a client. Which action is most appropriate for facilitating digital manipulation of the stool?
   a. Move the finger slowly and carefully
   b. Place the client in the Sims position
   c. Lubricate and insert the finger periodically
   d. Insert the finger to the level of the hardened mass

9. A nurse is administering a water-and-soap-solution enema to a client. Which step should the nurse perform to purge air from the tubing?
   a. Open the clamp and fill the tube with solution
   b. Hold the solution container 20 inches above the client's anus
   c. Lubricate the tip of the tube generously
   d. Instill the solution gradually over 5 to 10 minutes

10. A nurse is caring for a client with constipation related to inadequate dietary habits. Which food items should the nurse encourage the client to eat to promote hydration and avoid dry stool? Select all that apply.
    a. Prune juice
    b. Apple juice
    c. Oral fluids
    d. Banana pulp
    e. Cottage cheese

11. A nurse is administering a prescribed cleansing enema to a client with colitis. What condition may occur if the nurse administers a large-volume cleansing enema to a client?
    a. Increase the fecal velocity
    b. Rupture the bowel
    c. Irritate the local tissue
    d. Draw fluid from body tissue

12. A physician has ordered the nurse to administer an oil retention enema to a client for easier expulsion. For how long should the nurse ask the client to retain the cleansing solution within the large intestine?
    a. At least 1 hour
    b. At least 10 minutes
    c. At least 5 minutes
    d. At least half an hour

13. A nurse is assessing an older client who is self-conscious of her poor bowel elimination habits. Which habit would the nurse recommend to instill healthy elimination habits in older adults?
    a. Avoid high-fiber products like polycarbophil
    b. Increase dosage of laxatives gradually
    c. Use bulk-forming products with psyllium
    d. Use mineral oil retention enemas regularly

14. A nurse is assessing a client for fecal impaction. Which assessment aptly indicates that the client has fecal impaction?
    a. The client passes liquid stool frequently
    b. The client has foul breath
    c. The client has lost weight drastically
    d. The client has poor physical reflexes

15. A nurse is administering prescribed medicine to a client with diarrhea. The nurse points out that which factors can lead to diarrhea? Select all that apply.
    a. Poor fluid intake
    b. Laxative abuse
    c. Physical inactivity
    d. Bowel disorder
    e. Emotional stress

16. A nurse is digitally removing the hardened mass of stool from the rectum of a client. Why is it important for the nurse to remove the impaction gently?
    a. To prevent bleeding and tissue trauma
    b. To preserve the client's dignity and self-esteem
    c. To develop healthy bowel elimination
    d. To provide privacy and prevent soiling

SECTION IV: REVIEWING WHAT YOU HAVE LEARNED

Activity H *Fill in the blanks by choosing the correct word/value from the options given in parentheses.*

1. Hypertonic enema solutions are available in commercially prepared disposable containers that hold approximately _____ mL of solution. (60, 120, 180)

2. _____ constipation results from medical treatment. (Iatrogenic, Pseudo, Secondary)

Activity I *Mark the statement as either T (True) or F (False). Correct a false statement.*

1. **T F**   Vegetables such as cabbage and cucumbers are known to prevent intestinal gas.

Activity J *Write the correct term for each description below.*

1. Skin around the stoma _____

2. The rhythmic contraction of intestinal smooth muscle that facilitates defecation _____

3. Chemical injury to the skin resulting from enzymes present in stool _____

Activity K *Match the terms in Column A with their descriptions in Column B.*

Column A

___ **1.** Gastrocolic reflex

___ **2.** Anal sphincter

___ **3.** Stoma

___ **4.** Valsalva maneuver

Column B

a. Entrance to a surgically created opening to an organ of elimination

b. Closing the glottis and contracting the pelvic and abdominal muscles to increase abdominal pressure

c. Accelerated intestinal peristalsis that usually occurs during or after eating

d. Ring-shaped band of muscles

Activity L *Differentiate between fecal impaction and fecal incontinence in relation to the following.*

1. Definition

2. Causes

3. Symptoms

Activity M *Answer the following questions.*

1. What are the two components of a bowel elimination assessment?

_____

_____

_____

2. What are the various signs and symptoms of constipation?

_____

_____

_____

SECTION V: APPLYING YOUR KNOWLEDGE

Activity N *Give rationales for the following questions.*

1. Why is it important for the nurse to be cautious when administering large-volume enemas to clients?

_____

_____

_____

2. Why is tap water used when administering an enema?

_____

_____

_____

Activity O *Answer the following questions focusing on nursing roles and responsibilities.*

1. A nurse is caring for a client with a colostomy. What are the steps in performing a colostomy irrigation?

_____

_____

_____

2. A nurse is caring for a client with constipation.
    a. What are two interventions used to promote bowel elimination for this client?

_____

_____

_____

b. How should the nurse administer a commercially prepared disposable container of hypertonic enema solution?

_____

_____

_____

Activity P   *Consider the following questions. Discuss them with your instructor or peers.*

A midlife client who is scheduled to undergo a colostomy is concerned about how the surgery and its outcomes will affect their everyday life.

1. How can the nurse prepare the client physically and emotionally for managing the ostomy independently?

_____

_____

_____

2. How can the nurse prepare the family who may need to assist with the care of the client with an ostomy after discharge?

_____

_____

_____

SECTION VI: GETTING READY FOR NCLEX

Activity Q   *Answer the following questions.*

1. A client at a health care facility reports a frequent desire to defecate but has been passing liquid stool in small quantities for 2 days. What interventions should the nurse follow when removing a fecal impaction? Select all that apply.
   a. Ask the client to contract the gluteal muscles
   b. Instruct the client to breathe slowly and deeply
   c. Place the client in the Sims position
   d. Use a lubricated gloved forefinger to break up the mass of stool
   e. Provide periods of rest until the mass is removed

2. Which statement accurately describes a nursing action involved in draining accumulated urine or stool from a continent ileostomy?
   a. Keep the external end of the catheter at the level of the stoma
   b. Leave the stoma uncovered at all times
   c. Clean the removed catheter with cold soapy water
   d. Expect resistance after inserting the tube approximately 2 inches

CHAPTER 32

Oral Medications

Learning Objectives

- Define medication.
- Name components of a drug order.
- Explain the difference between trade and generic drug names.
- Name common routes for medication administration.
- Describe the oral route and general forms of medication administered this way.
- Explain the purpose of a medication record.
- Name ways drugs are supplied.
- Give the formula for calculating a drug dose.
- Discuss nursing responsibilities that apply to the administration of opioids.
- Name the five "rights" of medication administration.
- Discuss guidelines that apply to the safe administration of medications.
- Discuss points to stress when teaching clients about taking medications.
- Explain the circumstances involved in giving oral medications by an enteral tube and commonly associated problem.
- Describe appropriate actions in the event of a medication error.

SECTION I: ASSESSING YOUR UNDERSTANDING

Activity A FILL IN THE BLANKS

1. Medications are _____ substances that change body function.

2. A(n) _____ tablet is convenient when only part of a tablet is needed.

3. _____ orders are instructions for client care that are given during face-to-face conversations.

4. Decreased blood albumin levels reduce _____ binding of medications.

5. Older people taking more than one medication are more likely to develop _____ changes as an early and common sign of adverse effects.

6. _____ therapists are helpful in evaluating dysphagia and recommending safe and effective methods of administering oral medications.

7. _____ name is the chemical name not protected by a company's trademark.

8. The oral route facilitates drug absorption through the _____ tract.

9. A(n) _____ supply remains on the nursing unit for use in an emergency so that a nurse can give a drug without delay.

10. The nurse accesses the computerized system by using a(n) _____ and then selects the appropriate choice from a computerized menu.

Activity B   *Consider the following figure.*

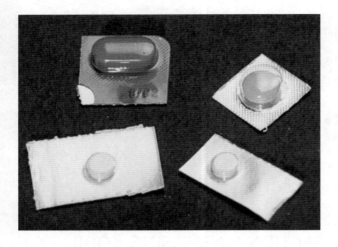

1. Identify the figure shown here.

_____

_____

_____

2. What is the purpose of this method of supplying medications?

_____

_____

_____

Activity C   *Match the terms related with oral medication in Column A with their description in Column B.*

Column A

_____ **1.** Trade name

_____ **2.** Oral route

_____ **3.** Enteric-coated tablets

_____ **4.** Medication administration record

_____ **5.** Pill organizer

Column B

a. Administration of drugs by swallowing or instillation through an enteral tube

b. A simple-to-use medication management system

c. Agency form used to document drug administration

d. The name by which a pharmaceutical company identifies its drug

e. Solid drug covered with a substance that dissolves beyond the stomach

Activity D   *Briefly answer the following questions.*

1. What is meant by frequency of drug administration?

_____

_____

_____

2. What are the components of a medical order?

_____

_____

_____

3. What is the importance of health teaching with regard to the administration of medication?

_____

_____

_____

4. Why is the client's medication not added to the formula during tube feeding?

_____

_____

_____

5. How does the computerized documentation of medication help at the health care agency?

_____

_____

_____

6. What should the nurse do when a medication error occurs?

_____

_____

_____

SECTION II: APPLYING YOUR KNOWLEDGE

Activity E   *One of the nurse's most important responsibilities is the administration of medications. Providing health teaching helps to ensure that clients administer their own medications safely and remain compliant.*

Answer the following questions related to health teaching regarding the administration of medication.

A nurse is providing health teaching with regard to the administration of medication for a senior client who is being discharged from the health care facility.

1. What should the nurse do if the senior client is having difficulty comprehending information about the medication routines?

   _____

   _____

   _____

2. What should the nurse include in the health teaching for this client?

   _____

   _____

   _____

SECTION III: PRACTICING FOR NCLEX

Activity F *Answer the following questions.*

1. A client has been admitted to the health care facility with complaints of abdominal pain. Under what condition would the nurse be permitted to write a medication order?
   a. If the nurse is a registered nurse
   b. If it is permitted by the health care facility
   c. If the nurse has a baccalaureate degree
   d. If it is legally permitted by the state's statutes

2. A physician prepares a medication order for a client who is being treated for chickenpox. The nurse should be aware that which components form a part of a valid medication order? Select all that apply.
   a. Name of the client
   b. Age of the client
   c. Dose to be administered
   d. Route of administration
   e. Name of the primary nurse

3. A nurse administers medication to the client per the medication order prepared by the physician. The medication order contains the trade name of the drug. The nurse knows that the chemical name of the drug that is

not protected by the company's trademark is known as:
   a. Trade name
   b. Proprietary name
   c. Generic name
   d. Brand name

4. A nurse needs to administer medication to a client with influenza via the oral route. What method would be appropriate?
   a. Administration of the drug by swallowing
   b. Administration of the drug by application on the skin
   c. Administration of the drug through an aerosol
   d. Administration of the drug by injections

5. Per the physician's medication order, a client needs to be administered half a tablet three times a day. What type of solid medication would allow this type of administration?
   a. Enteric-coated tablets
   b. Scored tablets
   c. Sustained-release capsules
   d. Pellets

6. Per the physician's medication orders, the nurse needs to administer a particular drug four times a day. What standard abbreviation would the physician use in this case?
   a. q4h
   b. b.i.d.
   c. t.i.d.
   d. q.i.d.

7. A physician at the health care facility orders a "qh" administration of medication to a client who is critically ill. What is the frequency of administration of the medication?
   a. Immediately
   b. Every day
   c. Hourly
   d. Twice a day

8. A physician dictates the medication order to a nurse over the telephone. What should the nurse do to ensure the accuracy of the medication order? Select all that apply.
   a. Repeat the dosage of drugs
   b. Spell the drug name for confirmation
   c. Write "VO" at the end of the order
   d. Write down the order on a notepad
   e. Have a second nurse listen simultaneously

9. A nurse at the health care facility requests the drugs from the pharmacy once the medication order has been transcribed to the MAR.

The nurse uses the individual supply method to dispense medication. An individual supply of medications:

a. Contains enough prescribed drugs for several days
b. Holds one tablet or capsule for individual clients
c. Remains on the nursing unit for use in emergency
d. Contains frequently used medication for that unit

10. A physician at the health care facility prescribes an opioid for a client. What are the responsibilities of the nurse with regard to the administration of these controlled substances? Select all that apply.
a. Have an accurate account of their use
b. Keep them on the nursing unit for emergency
c. Record each controlled substance used from stock supply
d. Place it in the container with prescribed drugs
e. Count each controlled substance at the change of each shift

11. A nurse at the health care facility needs to administer prescribed drugs to a client at the health care facility. What precaution should the nurse take before, during, and after every administration to avoid potential medication errors?
a. Calculate the drug dosage accurately per the medication order
b. Request a second nurse to confirm the drug dosage calculation
c. Ask the physician to mention the dosage in the medication order
d. Count the number of drugs that have been supplied

12. Per the physician's medication order, the nurse needs to administer 250 mg of the drug to the client orally, three times a day. However, the drug is available in 500 mg/5 mL. What quantity of the drug should the nurse administer to the client?
a. 5.5 mL
b. 2.5 mL
c. 1.5 mL
d. 7.5 mL

13. A nurse at the health care facility prepares the drug dosage to be administered to the client. Before administering the drugs to the client, why should the nurse compare the MAR with the written medical order?
a. Avoids potential complication
b. Ensures appropriate administration
c. Demonstrates compliance with the medical order
d. Prevents medication errors

14. The nurse needs to administer medication through an enteral tube for a client who has difficulty swallowing medication through the mouth. When administering the medication, the nurse interrupts the tube feeding for 15 to 30 minutes before and after administration of the drug, which should be given on an empty stomach. What is the rationale for the nurse's actions?
a. Facilitates the drug's therapeutic action
b. Facilitates access to the medication
c. Facilitates mixing into the liquid form
d. Facilitates instillation in the enteral tube

15. A nurse at the health care facility is providing the discharge instructions for a senior client. What teaching points should the nurse include in the client education regarding administration of drugs? Select all that apply.
a. Visual description of the drug and action, dose, and time of administration
b. List of health care facilities where the client can receive treatment
c. Instruction regarding whether food or liquid should accompany administration
d. Telephone number for the health care provider to contact should side effects occur
e. Client's insurance number should the client require emergency treatment

SECTION IV: REVIEWING WHAT YOU HAVE LEARNED

Activity G   *Fill in the blanks by choosing the correct word from the options given in parentheses.*

1. Drugs have a _____ name, which is the chemical name and is not protected by a company's trademark. (brand, generic, proprietary)

Activity H *Mark each statement as either T (True) or F (False). Correct any false statements.*

1. **T F** Drugs that dissolve at timed intervals are called sustained-release medications.

2. **T F** A scored tablet is a solid drug manufactured with a groove in the center.

3. **T F** The nurse asks the client to swallow the drug during sublingual or buccal administration.

Activity I *Write the correct term for each description below.*

1. Chemical substances that change body function _____

2. The term given to drugs covered with a substance that dissolves beyond the stomach _____

Activity J *Answer the following questions.*

1. What are the seven components of a medication order?

   _____

   _____

   _____

2. What is the purpose of a medication administration record?

   _____

   _____

   _____

SECTION V: APPLYING YOUR KNOWLEDGE

Activity K *Give rationales for the following questions.*

1. Why are enteric-coated tablets never cut, crushed, or chewed?

   _____

   _____

   _____

2. When are metric doses converted to household measurements?

   _____

   _____

   _____

Activity L *Answer the following questions focusing on nursing roles and responsibilities.*

1. A physician has listed drug names and directions for administering them in a client's medication order. The nurse, while transcribing the medication order, observes that the drug order is incomplete.

   a. What immediate actions should the nurse perform in this situation?

      _____

      _____

      _____

   b. What are the five rights of medication administration?

      _____

      _____

      _____

2. A nurse is caring for an adult client recovering from an appendectomy who is experiencing postoperative pain and discomfort. The physician provides telephone instructions for follow-up care to the nurse. What steps should the nurse take when receiving telephone orders from the physician?

   _____

   _____

   _____

Activity M *Consider the following question. Discuss it with your instructor or peers.*

A nurse is caring for a teenager who has been prescribed antibiotics.

1. What actions can the nurse take if the client cannot swallow the drugs?

   _____

   _____

   _____

SECTION VI: GETTING READY FOR NCLEX

Activity N   *Answer the following questions.*

1. A nurse is caring for a client whose medication administration record reads amoxicillin t.i.d. How often should the nurse administer this drug?
   a. Three times a day
   b. Every 3 hours
   c. Every 3rd day
   d. For 3 days

2. What intervention should the nurse perform when administering liquid oral medications?
   a. Pour liquids with the drug label toward the palm of the hand
   b. Leave the medication cup on a side table if the client is absent
   c. Offer a cup of water along with the medication
   d. Ask the client to hyperextend the neck when taking the drug

Topical and Inhalant Medications

Learning Objectives

- Explain how topical medications are administered and commonly applied.
- Identify forms of drugs applied by the transdermal route and principles to follow when applying a skin patch.
- Describe where eye medications are applied.
- Explain how the administration of ear medications differs for adults and children.
- Explain the rebound effect that accompanies the administration of nasal decongestants.
- Describe the difference between sublingual and buccal administration.
- Name a common reason for vaginal applications.
- Give the form of medication used most often for rectal administration.
- Explain why inhalation is a good route for medication administration.
- Name types of inhalers and alternatives for administering inhaled medications.

SECTION I: ASSESSING YOUR UNDERSTANDING

Activity A FILL IN THE BLANKS

1. A(n) _____ is a medication incorporated into an agent that is administered by rubbing it into the skin.

2. Drugs incorporated into patches or pastes are administered as _____ applications.

3. A(n) _____ contains a drug within a thick base and is applied not rubbed, into the skin.

4. Monitoring heart rate and blood pressure of older adults who use inhaled _____ is important because these medications commonly cause tachycardia and hypertension.

5. A(n) _____ application is a drug instilled in the outer ear.

6. A tablet given by _____ application is placed under the tongue to dissolve slowly and become absorbed by the rich blood supply in the area.

7. Symptoms of a(n) _____ infection include intense vaginal itching and a white vaginal discharge.

8. The _____ route administers drugs to the lower airways.

9. A(n) _____ results after a liquid drug is forced through a narrow channel using pressurized air or an inert gas.

10. Drugs administered rectally are usually in the form of _____; however, creams and ointments also may be prescribed.

Activity B   *Consider the following figure.*

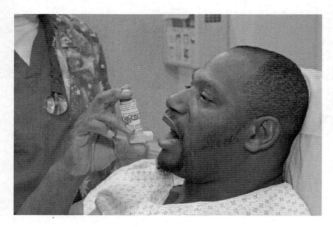

1. Identify the figure.

   _____

   _____

   _____

2. What does the device consist of?

   _____

   _____

   _____

Activity C   *Match the terms related to topical and inhalant medications in Column A with their descriptions in Column B.*

Column A

____ **1.** Topical route

____ **2.** Cutaneous applications

____ **3.** Skin patches

____ **4.** Rebound effect

____ **5.** Buccal application

Column B

a. Drugs rubbed into or placed in contact with the skin

b. Swelling of the nasal mucosa within a short time of drug administration

c. Drugs placed against the mucous membranes of the inner cheek

d. Drugs bonded to an adhesive bandage and applied to the skin

e. Administration of the medication to the skin and mucous membrane

Activity D   *Presented here, in random order, are steps that occur during instillation of ear medication. Write the correct sequence in the boxes provided.*

1. Place a small cotton ball loosely in the ear to absorb excess medication.

2. Tilt the client's head away from the ear into which the medication will be instilled.

3. Press and release the tragus, the projection of skin-covered cartilage at the opening of the external ear, to facilitate moving the medication toward the eardrum.

4. Manipulate the client's ear by straightening the auditory canal.

5. Compress the container and instill the prescribed number of drops on the side of the ear canal rather than directly onto the tympanic membrane.

6. If a bilateral administration is prescribed, wait at least 5 minutes before instilling medication in the opposite ear.

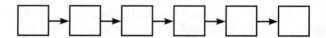

Activity E   *Briefly answer the following questions.*

1. What are skin patches?

   _____

   _____

   _____

2. What are otic applications?

   _____

   _____

   _____

3. What warning should a nurse give to a client who uses over-the-counter decongestant nasal sprays frequently?

   _____

   _____

   _____

4. What nursing instruction should a nurse give during the administration of sublingual or buccal application?

_____

_____

_____

5. What are the advantages of administering drugs through the inhalant route?

_____

_____

_____

6. What are the types of inhalers available to administer medication?

_____

_____

_____

SECTION II: APPLYING YOUR KNOWLEDGE

Activity F *Ophthalmic application is a method of applying drugs to the mucous membrane of one or both eyes. Answer the following question related to the nurse's role when administering ophthalmic drugs.*

A nurse is caring for a client with conjunctivitis at the health care facility.

1. What care should the nurse take when administering ophthalmic medication to this client?

_____

_____

_____

SECTION III: PRACTICING FOR NCLEX

Activity G *Answer the following questions.*

1. A client has been ordered hydrocortisone. What nursing intervention would the nurse perform for this client when applying this inunction?
   a. Clean the area with soap and water
   b. Apply the inunction with the palm
   c. Cool the inunction before application
   d. Lightly spread the inunction over the area

2. A client has been prescribed a vaginal application for yeast infection. What point should the nurse include in the teaching plan regarding administration of the vaginal application?
   a. Instill the medication in the morning after a bath
   b. Avoid emptying the bladder after application
   c. Lubricate the applicator tip with water-soluble jelly
   d. Remain recumbent for 5 minutes after application

3. A client at the health care facility has been prescribed nitroglycerin cream to dilate the coronary arteries. Which route would the nurse select to administer this medication to the client?
   a. Cutaneous
   b. Sublingual
   c. Otic
   d. Buccal

4. A client with pulmonary edema has been prescribed nitroglycerin. Which statement describes the application of nitroglycerin paste?
   a. It is bonded to an adhesive and applied to the skin
   b. It is placed against the mucous membrane of the inner cheek
   c. It is applied not rubbed, into the skin
   d. It is placed under the tongue and left to dissolve slowly

5. A physician prescribes the use of a contraceptive patch to a female client at the health care facility. How would the nurse describe the use of the patch to the client?
   a. A patch is mostly applied to the upper part of the body
   b. The drug in the patch becomes inactive immediately when the patch is removed
   c. A new patch is placed in exactly the same location as the previous one
   d. The drug in the patch takes 15 minutes to reach the therapeutic level after application

6. A nurse applies nitroglycerin paste to a client per the direction of the physician. What care should the nurse take to avoid irritating the client's skin?
   a. Avoid using the bare fingers to apply the paste
   b. Tape all edges of the application paper to the skin
   c. Remove one application before applying another
   d. Rotate the application site of the medicine

7. A nurse is caring for a client who has developed a sty in the left eye. When administering the eye medication, what action should the nurse take to prevent the drug from passing into the nasolacrimal duct?
   a. Position the sleeping client with the head tilted back
   b. Instruct the client to look toward the ceiling
   c. Make a pouch in the lower lid by pulling the skin downward
   d. Instruct the client to close the eyelids gently

8. A nurse needs to monitor the heart rate and blood pressure in a client who has been prescribed the use of bronchodilators. The nurse should monitor the client for what adverse effect?
   a. Bradycardia
   b. Hypertension
   c. Bronchitis
   d. Asthma

9. A client visits the health care facility with complaints of an earache resulting from an infection. The nurse needs to perform an otic application for this client. For what conditions are otic drugs used? Select all that apply.
   a. Moistening impacted cerumen
   b. The removal of a foreign body
   c. Treating local bacterial infection
   d. Clearing the auditory canal
   e. Treating local fungal infection

10. A nurse at the health care facility is caring for a client who complains of nasal congestion resulting from swelling of the nasal mucosa. The nurse further learns that the client has been using more than the recommended dosage of nasal medication. What should the nurse suggest to avoid this condition?
    a. Use a nasal spray that contains normal saline solution
    b. Use a nasal spray that contains a decreased dose of the medication

c. Use a nasal spray that contains antiinflammatory medication
d. Use a nasal spray that contains antiallergy medication

11. A client has been prescribed nasal drops for difficulty in breathing resulting from severe nasal congestion. What nursing action would help to distribute the medication?
    a. Place a rolled towel or pillow behind the client's neck
    b. Instruct the client to breathe as the container is squeezed
    c. Aim the tip of the dropper toward the nasal passage
    d. Instruct the client to breathe through the mouth

12. The physician has prescribed sublingual application of medication for a client with hypertension. What direction would the nurse give the client when administering the drug?
    a. Place the drug against the mucous membrane of the inner cheek
    b. Administer the drug by rubbing it into the skin
    c. Place the drug under the tongue and allow it to dissolve slowly
    d. Place the adhesive bandage, which is bonded to the drug, onto the skin

13. A nurse at the health care facility needs to administer nasal medication to a client with complaints of breathing difficulty. Before administering the medication, what should the nurse do to ensure that the right drug is given at the right time by the right route?
    a. Administer the medication 30 to 60 minutes within the scheduled time
    b. Read and compare the labels on the drug with the MAR
    c. Compare the MAR with the written medical record
    d. Review the client's drug, allergy, and medical histories

14. A client visits the health care facility for a routine physical assessment. During the assessment, the client complains to the nurse that recently she has been experiencing intense itching around the vaginal area and has noticed a white discharge. The nurse is aware that these are symptoms of a yeast infection. What medication would the nurse anticipate administering to the client?
    a. Suppository cream
    b. Scopolamine
    c. Nitroglycerin cream
    d. Estrogen

15. An asthmatic client has been prescribed the use of a dry powder inhaler. How would the nurse explain how the device works to the client?
    a. A device that forces a liquid drug through a narrow channel using pressurized air
    b. A device that consists of a canister that releases a dose of medication when compressed
    c. A device that delivers aerosolized medication, which is a liquid drug, forced through a narrow channel via a chemical propellant
    d. A device that holds a reservoir of pulverized drug and a carrier substance and depends on the client's inspiratory effort for medication delivery

SECTION IV: REVIEWING WHAT YOU HAVE LEARNED

Activity H   *Fill in the blanks by choosing the correct word from the options given in parentheses.*

1. The application of a drug to the skin or mucous membrane is an example of the _____ route of drug administration. (inhalant, parental, topical)

2. _____ application is the method of applying a drug on the skin and allowing it to be passively absorbed. (Cutaneous, Inunction, Transdermal)

3. _____ is a drug used to dilate the coronary arteries. (Estrogen, Nitroglycerin, Scopolamine)

Activity I   *Mark the statement as either T (True) or F (False). Correct a false statement.*

1. T F   The nurse asks the client to swallow the drug during sublingual or buccal administration.

Activity J   *Write the correct term for each description below.*

1. Swelling of the nasal mucosa that accompanies the overuse of nasal decongestants
   _____

2. The chamber attached to an inhaler
   _____

Activity K   *Differentiate between dry powder and metered-dose inhalers based on the categories given below.*

1. Description
2. Method of Medication Delivery
3. Ease of Use

Activity L   *When administering topical drugs, the nurse takes steps to maintain the integrity of the skin and mucous membranes. Write in the boxes provided below the correct sequence for topical vaginal administration.*

1. Depress the plunger once it reaches the proper distance within the vagina.

2. Insert the applicator into the vagina to the length recommended in the package directions.

3. Apply a sanitary pad and ask the client to remain recumbent for at least 10 to 30 minutes.

4. Place the drug in the applicator and apply lubricant to the tip.

5. Remove the applicator and place it on a clean tissue.

6. Have the client empty the bladder before inserting the medication.

□ → □ → □ → □ → □ → □

Activity M   *Answer the following question.*

1. What are ophthalmic applications?
   _____
   _____
   _____

SECTION V: APPLYING YOUR KNOWLEDGE

Activity N   *Give rationales for the following questions.*

1. Why are certain drugs administered by application to the skin?
   _____
   _____
   _____

2. Why should extremely hairy areas be clipped before applying skin patches?

_____

_____

_____

Activity O   *Answer the following questions focusing on nursing roles and responsibilities.*

1. A client undergoing nicotine withdrawal therapy has been ordered medication in the form of skin patches. How should these skin patches be applied?

_____

_____

_____

2. A physician has prescribed otic application of neomycin for a client with severe itching in his ear.
   a. How will the nurse instill this application?

   _____

   _____

   _____

   b. How does administration of otic drugs differ for adults and children?

   _____

   _____

   _____

Activity P   *Consider the following questions. Discuss them with your instructor or peers.*

A physician has prescribed timolol (Timoptic) for a client with glaucoma.

1. What care should the nurse take when administering an ophthalmic application?

_____

_____

_____

2. What should the nurse do if the applicator tip becomes contaminated?

_____

_____

_____

SECTION VI: GETTING READY FOR NCLEX

Activity Q   *Answer the following questions.*

1. What instructions should the nurse provide when teaching a client to use a metered-dose inhaler? Select all that apply.
   a. Shake the canister prior to use
   b. Exhale quickly through open lips
   c. Float the canister in a water bowl
   d. Inhale while depressing the canister
   e. Ask the client to hold their breath for 20 seconds

2. What is the most accurate instruction the nurse can provide when teaching a client how to use prescribed nasal medication?
   a. Place a rolled towel or pillow beneath the neck before administration
   b. Place the tip of the container in front of the nostril
   c. Ensure that both the nostrils are open during administration
   d. Remain in position for 1 full minute after administration

Parenteral Medications

Learning Objectives

- Name the parts of a syringe.
- List factors to consider when selecting a syringe and needle.
- Explain the rationale for redesigning conventional syringes and needles.
- Name ways that pharmaceutical companies prepare parenteral drugs.
- Discuss an appropriate action before combining two drugs in a single syringe.
- List injection routes.
- Identify common sites for intradermal, subcutaneous, and intramuscular injections.
- Name types of syringes commonly used to administer an intradermal, subcutaneous, and intramuscular injection.
- Describe the angles of entry for intradermal, subcutaneous, and intramuscular injections.
- Discuss why most insulin combinations must be administered within 15 minutes of being mixed.
- Describe techniques for preventing bruising when administering heparin subcutaneously.

SECTION I: ASSESSING YOUR UNDERSTANDING

Activity A   FILL IN THE BLANKS

1. Nurses draw an imaginary line at the _____ when administering an injection in the deltoid site.

2. A(n) _____ syringe holds 1 mL fluid and is calibrated in 0.01-mL increments.

3. When administering _____ injections, nurses use a 90-degree angle for piercing the skin.

4. _____ is unnecessary when injecting insulin with an insulin pen because the needle is only 5-mm long and unlikely to enter a muscle.

5. There is a risk of damaging the _____ nerve and artery if the deltoid site is not identified properly.

6. Conventional syringes and needles are being redesigned to avoid _____ injuries.

7. _____ is the process of adding a diluent to a powdered substance before administering the drug parenterally.

8. _____ needles contain a membrane that acts as a barrier blocking the entrance of glass shards when withdrawing medication from a glass ampule.

9. _____ is a hormone required by some clients with diabetes.

Activity B   *Consider the following figure.*

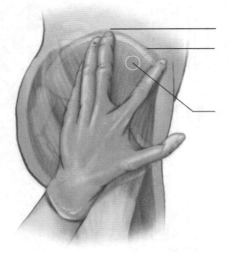

1. Identify and label the image.

_____

_____

_____

2. What are the names of the muscles used in this injection site?

_____

_____

_____

3. How is this site located to perform injections?

_____

_____

_____

Activity C   *Match the type of injection in Column A with the size of syringe used in Column B.*

Column A

_____ **1.** Intradermal

_____ **2.** Subcutaneous

_____ **3.** Insulin

_____ **4.** Intramuscular

Column B

a. 3 or 5 mL calibrated in 0.2-mL increments

b. 1 mL calibrated in units

c. 2, 2.5, or 3 mL calibrated in 0.1-mL increments

d. 1 mL calibrated in 0.01 mL in minims

Activity D   *Presented here, in random order, are steps that occur during the withdrawal of medication from an ampule. Write the correct sequence in the boxes provided.*

1. Tap the top of the ampule.

2. Tap the barrel of the syringe near the hub.

3. Insert the filter needle attached to a syringe into the ampule.

4. Snap the neck of the ampule away from your body.

5. Remove the filter needle and attach a sterile needle.

☐ → ☐ → ☐ → ☐ → ☐

Activity E   *Briefly answer the following questions.*

1. What is the meaning of parenteral route?

_____

_____

2. What are the components of a syringe?

_____

_____

_____

3. Why is a lower drug dose indicated in senior clients?

_____

_____

_____

4. Why is it important to pinch tissue for an intramuscular injection?

_____

_____

_____

5. Why are conventional syringes and needles being redesigned?

_____

_____

_____

6. Why is it important to rotate insulin injection sites?

_____

_____

_____

SECTION II: APPLYING YOUR KNOWLEDGE

Activity F   *The most common route for administering insulin is through a subcutaneous or intravenous injection. Answer the following questions, which involve the nurse's role in caring for a diabetic client.*

A nurse is caring for a client who is obese and has diabetes. The physician has ordered the nurse to administer a combined low dose of insulin to the client per the prescription.

1. What type of syringe should the nurse use to administer the insulin?

_____

_____

_____

2. When should the nurse administer the combined low dose of insulin to the client?

_____

_____

_____

SECTION III: PRACTICING FOR NCLEX

Activity G   *Answer the following questions.*

1. A nurse has reconstituted a prescribed vial drug for administering to a client. Which action should the nurse perform if the medication needs to be reused for more than one administration?
   a. Write the client's name on the vial label
   b. Write the date, time, and initials on the vial label
   c. Write the client's illness on the vial label
   d. Write the syringe details on the vial label

2. A nurse needs to administer an intramuscular injection to a client in the rectus femoris site. What are appropriate actions in this procedure? Select all that apply.
   a. Palpate the posterior iliac spine and greater trochanter
   b. Place the injection in the middle third of the thigh
   c. Ask the client to lie in a supine position on the bed
   d. Ask the client to sit on the edge of the bed
   e. Place one hand on the knee and below the trochanter

3. A nurse is administering a heparin injection subcutaneously to a client. The normal gauge of a needle when administering medications subcutaneously is:
   a. 25 gauge
   b. 27 gauge
   c. 20 gauge
   d. 21 gauge

4. A nurse has administered a prescribed injection to a client in the ventrogluteal site. What intervention should the nurse make to help reduce injection discomfort?
   a. Massage the injection with local anesthetic
   b. Have the client take deep breaths before receiving the injection
   c. Have the client lie in a prone position and point the toes outward
   d. Ask the client to avoid ambulating for 10 minutes after receiving the injection

5. A nurse is withdrawing medication from an ampule. Which technique should the nurse follow to prevent injecting glass particles into the client?
   a. Insert the filter needle into the ampule
   b. Tap the barrel of the syringe near the hub
   c. Use a needle with a small diameter
   d. Attach a sterile needle for administering the injection

6. Per the physician's order, a nurse is combining two prescribed drugs into a single syringe. Which action should the nurse perform before combining the two drugs?
   a. Use a larger gauge needle for combining drugs
   b. Withdraw an equal amount of drug from their containers
   c. Consult a drug reference chart before withdrawing
   d. Fix a filter needle on the syringe before withdrawing

7. A nurse is withdrawing a prescribed narcotic drug from a vial to administer it to a client with chronic back pain. What measure should the nurse take to prevent illegal drug use of the excess medication?
   a. Avoid discarding the excess medication in the trash
   b. Label the vial container with a secret code
   c. Aspirate and dispose of the excess medication in the presence of a witness
   d. Dilute the excess medication with saline solution

8. A nurse needs to administer an intramuscular injection to a client. How can the nurse reduce injection discomfort?
   a. Avoid changing needles when there is tissue irritation
   b. Apply an ice pack to numb the skin before the injection
   c. Avoid applying pressure to the site when removing the needle
   d. Instill the medication quickly and steadily

9. A nurse needs to flush all the medication from the syringe at the time of injection. Which action is appropriate?
   a. Use a needle with a smaller gauge
   b. Attach a long shaft needle to the syringe
   c. Avoid using filter needles when withdrawing
   d. Add 0.1 to 0.2 mL air to the syringe

10. A nurse is assessing the stock of safety injection devices in the health care facility. Which are modified safety injection devices? Select all that apply.
    a. Injections with plastic shields that cover the needle after use
    b. Injections with reusable needles that are immersed in an alcohol solution
    c. Injections with disposable needles that are cleaned with cotton swabs
    d. Injections with needles that retract into the syringe
    e. Gas-pressured devices that inject medications without needles

11. A nurse has placed one hand above the knee and one hand below the greater trochanter before administering a prescribed intramuscular injection to an infant. In which of the following sites is the nurse administering the injection?
    a. Deltoid site
    b. Vastus lateralis site
    c. Rectus femoris site
    d. Ventrogluteal site

12. A nurse has administered a prescribed dosage of heparin injection to a client subcutaneously. Which nursing action is appropriate?
    a. Administer the dosages of heparin in small volumes
    b. Use the same needle for withdrawing and administering heparin
    c. Avoid rotating injection sites when administering heparin
    d. Massage the injection site after administering injection

13. A nurse is bunching the tissue of a client between the thumb and fingers before administering an injection subcutaneously. For which clients is this technique most appropriate? Select all that apply.
    a. Diabetic clients
    b. Infants
    c. Children
    d. Thin clients
    e. Obese clients

14. A nurse needs to administer an irritating medication to a client. Which type of injection is most suitable?
    a. Intravenous
    b. Subcutaneous
    c. Intradermal
    d. Intramuscular

15. A nurse is administering an intramuscular injection to a client in the ventrogluteal site. What is an advantage offered by this site over the dorsogluteal site?
    a. It has large nerves and blood vessels
    b. It is less fatty and fecal contamination is rare
    c. It can hold a large amount of injected medication
    d. It can be massaged immediately after injection

16. A nurse is mixing insulins before administering them to a client with diabetes. Which action would the nurse perform to mix the insulins without damaging the protein molecules?
    a. Administer it within 15 minutes of mixing
    b. Insert the needle in the insulin itself
    c. Roll the medication in the palms
    d. Withdraw specific units of insulin from the vial with an additive

SECTION IV: REVIEWING WHAT YOU HAVE LEARNED

Activity H *Fill in the blanks by choosing the correct word from the options given in parentheses.*

1. The part of the syringe that holds the medication is called the _____. (barrel, plunger, tip)

2. With a(n) _____ injection, a drug is administered parenterally between the layers of the skin. (intradermal, intravenous, subcutaneous)

Activity I *Mark each statement as either T (True) or F (False). Correct any false statements.*

1. **T F** Needle lengths vary from approximately 2.5 to 3.5 inches.

2. **T F** Lipoatrophy is an accumulation of subcutaneous fat at the site of repeated insulin injections.

Activity J *Match the terms related to intramuscular injection sites in Column A with their explanations in Column B.*

Column A	Column B
a. Muscles in the quadriceps group of the outer thigh	_____ **1.** Ventrogluteal site
b. Lateral aspect of the upper arm	_____ **2.** Vastus lateralis site
c. Anterior aspect of the thigh	_____ **3.** Rectus femoris site
d. Medius and minimus muscles in the hip	_____ **4.** Deltoid site

Activity K *Consider the following figure.*

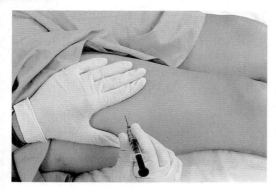

1. Identify what is shown in the figure.

   _____

   _____

   _____

2. Explain the technique being used.

   _____

   _____

   _____

Activity L *Answer the following questions.*

1. What are five factors to consider when selecting a syringe and needle?

   _____

   _____

2. What are prefilled cartridges?

   _____

   _____

   _____

SECTION V: APPLYING YOUR KNOWLEDGE

Activity M *Give rationales for the following questions.*

1. Why is an 18-gauge needle wider than a 27-gauge needle?

   _____

   _____

   _____

2. Why are conventional syringes and needles being redesigned?

   _____

   _____

   _____

Activity N *Answer the following questions focusing on nursing roles and responsibilities.*

1. A client with diabetes has been prescribed a combination of regular and intermediate-acting insulin. What

interventions should the nurse follow when mixing insulins?

_____

_____

_____

2. What actions should the nurse take if a needlestick injury occurs?

_____

_____

_____

SECTION VI: GETTING READY FOR NCLEX

Activity O   *Answer the following question.*

1. What important considerations should the nurse keep in mind when using the Z-track technique to inject medications? Select all that apply.
   a. Use the Z-track technique only in the deltoid muscles
   b. Massage the injection site after Z-track administration
   c. Insert the needle, aspirate, and inject the medication
   d. Select a large muscular site for injection
   e. Withdraw the needle and immediately release the taut skin

2. A nurse is preparing to perform a subcutaneous injection. What important measure should the nurse take when drawing up this medication from an ampule?
   a. Hold the ampule at an angle of 45 degrees from the body
   b. Avoid tapping the top of the ampule
   c. Insert the filter needle along the rim of the ampule
   d. Snap off the ampule's neck away from the body

Intravenous Medications

Learning Objectives

- Name the types of veins into which intravenous medications are administered.
- Describe appropriate situations for administering intravenous medications.
- Describe one method for giving bolus administrations of intravenous medications.
- Name ways by which intravenous medications are administered.
- Describe methods for administering medicated solutions intermittently.
- Explain the technique for administering a piggyback infusion.
- Discuss purposes for using a volume-control set.
- Describe a central venous catheter.
- Name types of central venous catheters.
- Discuss techniques for protecting oneself when administering antineoplastic drugs.

SECTION I: ASSESSING YOUR UNDERSTANDING

Activity A FILL IN THE BLANKS

1. The _____ route of drug administration is the most dangerous.

2. Senior clients with _____ often experience more confusion and disorientation with an acute illness.

3. A nontunneled _____ catheter is inserted through the skin in a peripheral vein such as the basilic, cephalic, jugular, or subclavian vein.

4. A(n) _____ administration is also described as a drug given by intravenous push.

5. The _____ attaches a special label to a container of antineoplastic drugs to warn nurses.

6. The end of the tunnel catheter exits from the skin lateral to the _____ process.

7. A(n) _____ lock is also called a *saline* or *heparin lock*, or an *intermittent infusion device*.

8. _____ drugs are commonly also referred to as *chemotherapy* or just *chemo*.

9. _____ catheters have a self-sealing port pierced through the skin with a special noncoring needle.

Activity B   *Consider the following figures.*

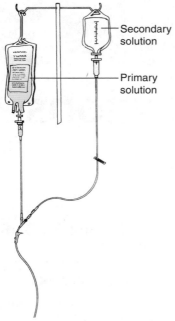

1. Identify the image.

   _____

   _____

   _____

2. What is the advantage of this arrangement?

   _____

   _____

   _____

3. Identify the image.

   _____

   _____

   _____

4. What is the advantage of this arrangement?

   _____

   _____

   _____

Activity C *Match the types of intravenous administration in Column A with their features in Column B.*

Column A

_____ **1.** Bolus administration

_____ **2.** Continuous administration

_____ **3.** Secondary infusion

_____ **4.** Volume-control set

Column B

a. Parenteral drug that is instilled over several hours

b. IV tubing chamber that holds a portion of the solution from a larger container

c. Undiluted or diluted medication given into a vein in 1 or more minutes

d. Parenteral drug that has been diluted in a small volume of intravenous solution

Activity D *Presented here, in random order, are steps that occur during administration of medication through an intravenous port. Write the correct sequence in the boxes provided.*

1. Pull back on the plunger of the syringe.

2. Gently instill a few tenths of a milliliter of medication.

3. Locate the port nearest to the intravenous insertion site.

4. Pierce the port with needle and pinch the tubing.

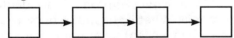

Activity E *Briefly answer the following questions.*

1. When is it appropriate to seek another drug route for senior clients?

_____

_____

_____

2. How is a bolus administration given to a client?

_____

_____

_____

3. What is a medication lock?

_____

_____

_____

4. What is the purpose of antineoplastic drugs?

_____

_____

_____

5. What is a central venous catheter?

_____

_____

_____

6. What information should the nurse provide to clients about intravenous route drugs?

_____

_____

_____

_____

SECTION II: APPLYING YOUR KNOWLEDGE

Activity F *Senior clients comprise the largest age group of clients cared for in acute and long-term health care facilities. Administration of intravenous medications is quite common in senior clients. Answer the following questions, which involve the nurse's role in caring for clients on intravenous therapy.*

A nurse is preparing the discharge sheet of a senior client with an intravenous drug administered to them through a tunneled catheter.

1. What should the nurse do if the client needs continued intravenous therapy?

_____

_____

_____

2. What should a nurse teach to a senior client when there is emphasis on an early discharge?

_____

_____

_____

SECTION III: PRACTICING FOR NCLEX

Activity G   *Answer the following questions.*

1. When administering an intermittent secondary infusion, a nurse removes a refrigerated secondary solution 30 minutes before administering it to the client. What is the rationale for the nurse's action?
   a. Ensures medication accuracy
   b. Promotes comfort
   c. Prevents medication errors
   d. Ensures client safety

2. A nurse is administering antineoplastic drugs to a client with cancer. Which are the possible ways through which nurses or caregivers can absorb antineoplastic drugs? Select all that apply.
   a. Through skin contact
   b. Through inhalation of fluid droplets
   c. Through oral intake of drug residue
   d. Through radiation of heat
   e. Through chemical vapors

3. A nurse is administering intravenous medication to a client with the aid of a medication lock. What is the most popular feature of a medication lock?
   a. It eliminates the need for a continuous administration of intravenous fluid
   b. It can be flushed with saline and heparin
   c. It can withstand approximately 2,000 punctures
   d. It can maintain patency without obtaining a blood return

4. A nurse is administering a prescribed dosage of intravenous drug to a senior client. Why are seniors predisposed to toxic effects from intravenous drugs?
   a. Senior clients have decreased visual acuity and manual dexterity
   b. Senior clients face confusion and disorientation with an acute illness
   c. Senior clients have a slower metabolism and excretion process
   d. Senior clients have diminished protein components in their blood

5. A nurse needs to use a central venous catheter to administer 150 mL medication to a client. What step should the nurse perform to prevent complications such as air embolism?
   a. Regulate the flow of infusion
   b. Reclamp the catheter
   c. Remove the needle from the port
   d. Instill 5 mL normal saline in tubing

6. A nurse is caring for a senior client who is being administered an intravenous drug intermittently. Which drugs' adverse effects should the nurse be on the lookout for in senior clients? Select all that apply.
   a. Anticoagulants
   b. Opiates
   c. Insulin
   d. Sulfonamides
   e. Normal saline

7. A nurse is assessing the condition of a client with an implanted catheter. The client complains of skin discomfort to the nurse. What nursing action would reduce the skin discomfort?
   a. Replace the special needle
   b. Apply anesthetic topically
   c. Change the self-sealing port
   d. Cease the intravenous solution

8. A nurse needs to dilute a parenteral drug in a secondary infusion before delivering the prescribed dosage to the client. What is the volume of intravenous solution that is usually used to dilute during a second infusion?
   a. 100 to 250 mL over 5 to 60 minutes
   b. 500 to 1,000 mL over 5 to 6 hours
   c. 100 to 500 mL over 30 to 60 minutes
   d. 50 to 100 mL over 30 to 60 minutes

9. A nurse is assessing the health of a client who has a prescribed dosage of bolus administration after a cesarean operation. The client is showing symptoms of accidental hypothermia. What is the initial nursing action taken when a client's condition changes for any reason during a bolus administration?
   a. Call for the lead physician
   b. Stop the administration of intravenous fluid
   c. Reduce the prescribed rate of intravenous fluid
   d. Call the emergency service for help

10. When preparing a prescribed dosage of an antineoplastic drug, the nurse covers the drug preparation area with a disposable paper pad. What is the rationale for the nurse's action?
    a. To reduce the potential of skin contact
    b. To inactivate the prescribed drug
    c. To avoid inhalation of the drug spill
    d. To absorb a small drug spill

11. A nurse needs to administer an intravenous medication to a client through an intermittent infusion device. What solution is used to fill the intravenous tubing before administration?
    a. Sterile bacteriostatic water
    b. Sterile normal saline
    c. Sterile isopropyl alcohol
    d. Sterile hydrogen peroxide

12. A nurse is administering intravenous medications and fluid to a senior client. The client complains to the nurse about a bloated abdomen and frequent urination. The nurse stops the intravenous administration and fixes the volume-control set to administer the intravenous medications and fluids. What nursing diagnosis should the nurse identify?
    a. Risk for injury
    b. Risk for infection
    c. Excess fluid volume
    d. Acute pain

13. A nurse is administering an intermittent secondary infusion to a client. Which actions are appropriate for this procedure? Select all that apply.
    a. Hang the secondary solution higher than the primary solution
    b. Avoid inserting the modified adapter within the port
    c. Avoid clamping the tubing when the solution has instilled
    d. Release the roller clamp on the secondary solution
    e. Regulate the rate of flow by counting the drip rate

SECTION IV: REVIEWING WHAT YOU HAVE LEARNED

Activity H   *Fill in the blanks by choosing the correct word from the options given in parentheses.*

1. An undiluted medication given quickly into a vein is called a _____ administration. (bolus, piggyback, soluset)

2. _____ catheters are inserted into a central vein, with part of the catheter secured in the subcutaneous tissue. (Implanted, Percutaneous, Tunneled)

Activity I   *Mark each statement as either T (True) or F (False). Correct any false statements.*

1. T F   Volume-control set infusions require connecting a second bag of intravenous solution to a primary infusing solution.

2. T F   Hickman and Broviac catheters are examples of implanted catheters.

Activity J   *Write the correct term for the description below.*

1. Medications used to destroy or slow the growth of malignant cells _____

Activity K   *Match the terms related to intravenous medications in Column A with their explanations in Column B.*

Column A

____ 1. Central venous catheter

____ 2. Intravenous route

____ 3. Continuous administration

____ 4. Intermittent administration

Column B

a. Instillation of parenteral drug over several hours

b. Instillation of parenteral drug in the short term (several minutes up to 1 hour)

c. A device that extends to the superior vena cava

d. Drug administration via peripheral veins

Activity L   *Differentiate between tunneled and percutaneous catheters based on the categories given below.*

1. Method of Insertion

2. Uses

Activity M   *Answer the following questions.*

1. When are intravenous administrations appropriate for clients?

_____

_____

_____

2. What are the advantages of using a medication lock?

_____

_____

_____

SECTION V: APPLYING YOUR KNOWLEDGE

Activity N *Give rationales for the following questions.*

1. Why is the intravenous route of drug administration considered the most dangerous?

_____

_____

_____

2. Why do some central venous catheters have multiple lumens?

_____

_____

_____

Activity O *Answer the following question focusing on nursing roles and responsibilities.*

A physician has prescribed a bolus drug administration for a client. What interventions should the nurse perform when using a medication lock?

_____

_____

_____

Activity P *Consider the following question. Discuss it with your instructor or peers*

A nurse is caring for a client with severe burns for whom the physician has prescribed pain medication by the intravenous route. What is a possible rationale for administering pain medication by this route?

_____

_____

_____

SECTION VI: GETTING READY FOR NCLEX

Activity Q *Answer the following questions.*

1. A nurse is caring for a client with a malignant tumor who has been prescribed antineoplastic drugs. What measure should the nurse take to avoid self-contamination with antineoplastic drugs?
   a. Wear one or two pairs of nonpowdered surgical gloves
   b. Pour 10% alcohol over every drug spill
   c. Wear a short-sleeved gown with a closed front
   d. Clean the spilled drug area with water

2. A nurse is caring for a client receiving a piggyback infusion along with a primary intravenous solution. What action should the nurse perform when administering the secondary infusion?
   a. Remove a refrigerated secondary solution 10 minutes before the infusion
   b. Administer the secondary infusion at the same rate as that of the primary infusion
   c. Set the height of the secondary solution 10 inches below the primary solution
   d. Wipe the uppermost port of the primary tubing with an alcohol swab

CHAPTER 36

Airway Management

Learning Objectives

- Define airway management.
- Identify the structural components of the airway.
- Discuss natural mechanisms that protect the airway.
- Explain the methods used by nurses to help maintain the natural airway.
- Name techniques for liquefying respiratory secretions.
- Explain techniques of chest physiotherapy.
- Describe suctioning techniques used to clear secretions from the airway.
- Name examples of artificial airways.
- Discuss indications for inserting an artificial airway.
- Identify components of tracheostomy care.

SECTION I: ASSESSING YOUR UNDERSTANDING

Activity A FILL IN THE BLANKS

1. The _____ is a protrusion of flexible cartilage above the larynx.

2. Hairlike projections called _____ beat debris that collects upward in the lower airway.

3. The volume of water in mucus affects its _____, or thickness.

4. _____ therapy improves breathing, encourages spontaneous coughing, and helps clients to raise sputum for diagnostic purposes.

5. Evaluation of _____ is important for implementing appropriate interventions to prevent aspiration.

6. _____ relies on negative (vacuum) pressure to remove liquid secretions with a catheter.

7. Nurses perform _____ suctioning with a suctioning device called a Yankauer-tip or tonsil-tip catheter.

8. _____ suctioning means removing secretions from the upper portion of the lower airway through a nasally inserted catheter.

9. A nasopharyngeal airway, sometimes called a(n) _____, can be used to protect the nostril if frequent suctioning is necessary.

10. Respiratory cilia become less efficient with age, predisposing older adults to a high incidence of _____.

Activity B *Consider the following figures.*

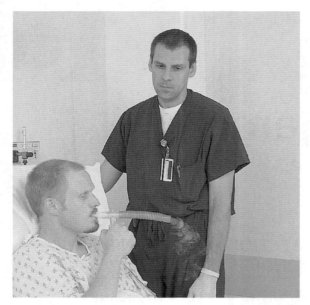

1. Identify the type of therapy being performed here.

   _____

   _____

   _____

2. How does this therapy help the client?

   _____

   _____

   _____

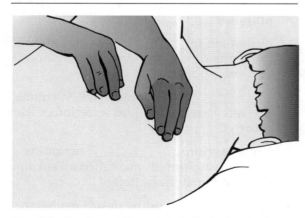

3. Identify the type of postural drainage technique used here.

   _____

   _____

   _____

4. What is the purpose of this technique?

   _____

   _____

   _____

Activity C *Match each term related to airway management in Column A with its description in Column B.*

Column A

____ 1. Ventilation

____ 2. Inhalation therapy

____ 3. Chest physiotherapy

____ 4. Postural drainage

____ 5. Oropharyngeal suctioning

Column B

a. Respiratory treatments that provide a mixture of oxygen, humidification, and aerosolized medications directly to the lungs

b. Positioning technique that promotes gravity drainage of secretions from various lobes or segments of the lungs

c. Removing secretions from the throat through an orally inserted catheter

d. Indicated for clients with chronic respiratory diseases who have difficulty coughing or raising thick mucus

e. Movement of air in and out of the lung

Activity D *Presented here, in random order, are the steps that occur when the nurse performs percussion on a client. Write the correct sequence in the boxes provided.*

1. Keep the fingers and thumb together.

2. Percuss for 3 to 5 minutes in each postural drainage position.

3. Cup the hands.

4. Apply the cupped hands to the client's chest.

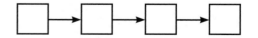

Activity E *Briefly answer the following questions.*

1. What are the factors that can jeopardize airway patency?

_____

_____

_____

2. What are the structures that protect the airway from a wide variety of inhaled substances?

_____

_____

_____

3. What are the most common methods of maintaining the natural airway?

_____

_____

_____

4. What are the two common types of artificial airway management?

_____

_____

_____

5. What is the purpose of an oral airway?

_____

_____

_____

6. What are the common causes of pathologic pulmonary changes in older adults?

_____

_____

_____

SECTION II: APPLYING YOUR KNOWLEDGE

Activity F *Clients at risk for airway obstruction or requiring long-term mechanical ventilation are candidates for an artificial airway. Answer the following question related to the nursing care for a client with a tracheostomy tube.*

A nurse is caring for a client who requires prolonged mechanical ventilation and oxygenation.

1. What intervention should the nurse perform for the client who is unable to talk because of the tracheostomy tube?

_____

_____

_____

SECTION III: PRACTICING FOR NCLEX

Activity G *Answer the following questions.*

1. The nurse is caring for an asthmatic client at the health care facility. The nurse is aware of which of the following structures forming part of the lower airway? Select all that apply.
   a. Trachea
   b. Nose
   c. Bronchi
   d. Alveoli
   e. Pharynx

2. A client at the health care facility is being treated for an injury to the tracheal cartilages. How would the nurse explain the function of the tracheal cartilages to the client?
   a. Act as a lid that closes during swallowing and helps direct food
   b. Ensure a portion of the airway beneath the larynx remains open
   c. Type of tissue that lines the respiratory passage to trap particulate matter
   d. Hairlike projections that beat debris collected in lower airways

3. A nurse uses aerosol therapy for a client with complaints of chest congestion. The nurse is aware that aerosol therapy:
   a. Helps in raising sputum for diagnostic purposes
   b. Helps in dislodging respiratory secretions
   c. Helps in loosening retained secretions
   d. Helps in draining secretions from various lobes of the lungs

4. A nurse at the health care facility needs to send a client's sputum specimen to the laboratory for diagnostic purposes. What is the best time to collect this specimen?
   a. Just before the client goes to sleep
   b. Just after the client undergoes physiotherapy
   c. Just after the client awakens
   d. Just after percussion is performed on the client

5. A client with a chronic respiratory disorder has been prescribed a postural drainage technique. The nurse understands that the outcome of postural drainage is to:
   a. Promote gravity drainage of secretion
   b. Encourage spontaneous coughing
   c. Help loosen retained secretions
   d. Help dislodge respiratory secretions

6. A physician directs the nurse to perform percussion on a client who is having difficulty coughing. During therapy, how long should the nurse perform percussion on each postural drainage position?
   a. For 3 to 5 minutes
   b. For 10 minutes
   c. For 10 to 15 minutes
   d. For 15 minutes

7. A nurse is caring for an infant client with chest congestion. The doctor has ordered the nurse to use suctioning to relieve the client's condition. What negative pressure should be applied for the infant if the nurse uses a wall suctioning machine?
   a. 100 to 140 mm Hg
   b. 50 to 95 mm Hg
   c. 95 to 100 mm Hg
   d. 45 to 50 mm Hg

8. A nurse has been directed to use suction to relieve a client with chest congestion. When performing the suctioning, what should the nurse do to break up mucus and raise secretions?
   a. Occlude the air vent of the suction
   b. Rotate the catheter, as it is withdrawn
   c. Encourage the client to cough
   d. Wait until the client takes a breath

9. A physician directs the nurse to use nasopharyngeal suctioning for a client with chest congestion. How would the nurse describe this process to the client?
   a. Removing secretions from the throat through a nasally inserted catheter
   b. Removing secretions from the upper portion of the lower airway through a nasally inserted catheter
   c. Removing secretions from the throat through an orally inserted catheter
   d. Removing secretions from the mouth using a Yankauer-tip or tonsil-tip catheter

10. A nurse caring for clients who require an artificial airway should understand which clients are candidates for a tracheostomy? Select all that apply.
    a. A client recovering from general anesthesia
    b. A client who has an upper airway obstruction
    c. A client recovering from a seizure
    d. A client who requires prolonged mechanical ventilation
    e. A client who is less stable and requires oxygenation

11. A nurse is caring for a client who is recovering from surgery for removal of a brain tumor. The nurse uses an oral airway to manage the client's airway. What should the nurse do to prevent aspiration in the client?
    a. Perform oral suctioning if necessary
    b. Position the client supine with the neck hyperextended
    c. Hold the airway so that the curved tip points upward
    d. Rotate the airway over the top of the tongue

12. A client at the health care facility is receiving mechanical ventilation through a tracheostomy tube. The nurse needs to perform suctioning because of the presence of copious secretions. The nurse inserts the catheter tube a shorter distance—that is, until resistance is felt. The nurse should understand that the cause of resistance may be due to:
    a. Contact between the catheter tip and the main bronchi
    b. Contact between the carina and the main bronchi
    c. Contact between the catheter tip and the carina
    d. Contact between the catheter tip and the end of the tube

13. A nurse needs to perform tracheostomy care for a client on mechanical ventilation. Which interventions should the nurse perform? Select all that apply.
    a. Cleaning the skin around the stoma
    b. Changing the outer cannula
    c. Changing the inner dressing
    d. Clearing the outer airway
    e. Cleaning the inner cannula

14. A nurse is caring for an older client with pneumonia. The nurse should be aware of which of the following age-related changes predisposing older clients to a higher incidence of pneumonia?
    a. Retention of secretions
    b. Diminished efficiency of cilia
    c. Decreased air exchange
    d. Compromised ventilation

15. The nurse is caring for an older client who complains of difficulty in coughing. What interventions should the nurse perform for this client? Select all that apply.
    a. Inquire about the client's current history of cough
    b. Determine how long the cough has been present
    c. Inquire whether the physician has been informed
    d. Observe and describe sputum if present
    e. Check the client's medication against the medical order

16. The nurse at the health care facility is caring for a client with difficulty swallowing (or dysphagia). For what related condition would the nurse assess this client?
    a. Cardiac dysrhythmias
    b. Hypoxemia
    c. Aspiration pneumonia
    d. Chronic pulmonary diseases

SECTION IV: REVIEWING WHAT YOU HAVE LEARNED

Activity H *Fill in the blanks by choosing the correct word from the options given in parentheses.*

1. The lower airway contains the _____. (alveoli, laryngopharynx, oropharynx)

2. Removing secretions from the upper portion of the lower airway through a nasally inserted catheter is called _____ suctioning. (nasopharyngeal, nasotracheal, oropharyngeal)

Activity I *Mark each statement as either T (True) or F (False). Correct any false statements.*

1. T F Nurses perform nasotracheal suctioning with a device called the Yankauer tip.

2. T F Tracheal cartilage is a protrusion of flexible cartilage above the larynx.

Activity J *Write the correct term for each description below.*

1. The collective system of tubes in the upper and lower respiratory tracts _____

2. A surgically created opening in the trachea _____

Activity K *Consider the following figure.*

1. Identify and label the figure.

   _____

   _____

   _____

2. What is the function of these structures?

   _____

   _____

   _____

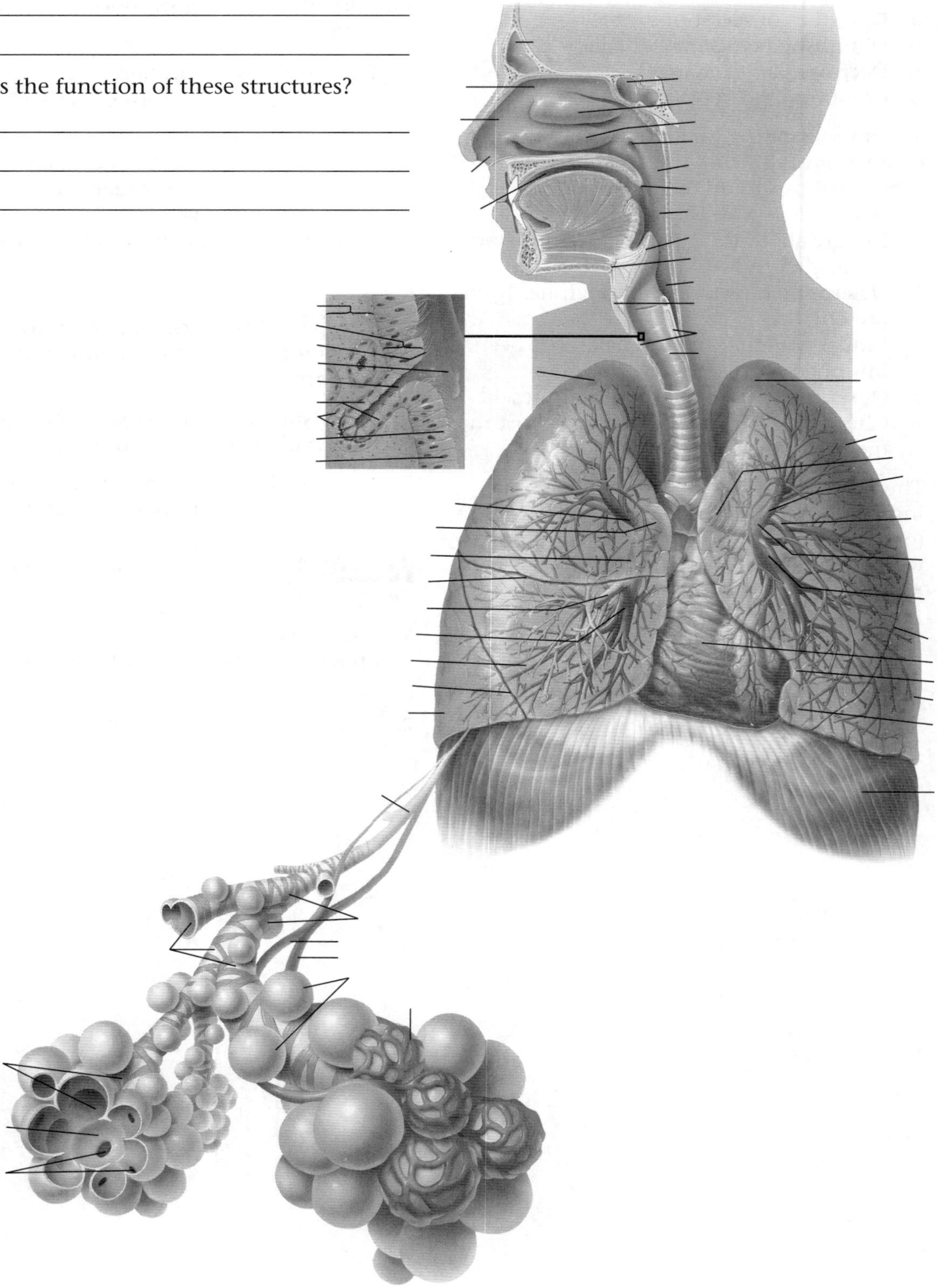

Activity L *Answer the following questions.*

1. What four natural mechanisms protect the airway?

_____

_____

_____

2. What conditions may result in the need to insert an artificial airway?

_____

_____

_____

SECTION V: APPLYING YOUR KNOWLEDGE

Activity M *Give rationales for the following questions.*

1. Why is it important for the nurse to frequently assess clients who have a tracheostomy?

_____

_____

_____

2. Why should nurses ensure adequate hydration in clients with a severe cough?

_____

_____

_____

Activity N *Answer the following questions focusing on nursing roles and responsibilities.*

1. A physician has asked a nurse to perform chest physiotherapy using percussion and vibration techniques for a client with a chronic respiratory disorder.
   a. What interventions should the nurse perform during the percussion technique?

   _____

   _____

   _____

   b. What interventions should the nurse perform during the vibration technique?

   _____

   _____

   _____

2. Describe instructions that a nurse should provide when teaching postural drainage to a client with thick mucus and their family.

_____

_____

_____

SECTION VI: GETTING READY FOR NCLEX

Activity O *Answer the following questions.*

1. A nurse is to obtain a sputum specimen from a client who has been receiving aerosol treatments for a respiratory disease. What action should the nurse perform when collecting the sputum specimen?
   a. Tell the client to avoid rinsing the mouth before the specimen collection
   b. Instruct the client to attempt a forceful cough and expectorate
   c. Obtain the sputum specimen before an aerosol treatment
   d. Obtain saliva from within the mouth

2. A nurse is caring for a client with a weak and persistent cough. Which intervention should the nurse follow when caring for this client?
   a. Maintain 2,000 to 3,000 mL fluid intake for 24 hours
   b. Instruct the client to breathe through the mouth
   c. Ensure that the client is supine at all times
   d. Provide the client with warm milk three or four times a day

3. A client has undergone a tracheotomy for an upper airway obstruction. Which intervention should the nurse perform when providing tracheostomy care for this client?
   a. Remove the inner cannula and place it in a saline solution
   b. Clean the area around the stoma with diluted peroxide
   c. Blow-dry the cannula after cleaning it with a saline solution
   d. Remove the used ties before applying new ties

CHAPTER 37

Resuscitation

Learning Objectives

- Identify signs of an airway obstruction and explain why an airway obstruction is life-threatening.
- Describe appropriate actions if a client has a partial airway obstruction.
- Explain the purpose of the Heimlich maneuver and describe the circumstances for using subdiaphragmatic and chest thrusts.
- Identify the recommended action for relieving an airway obstruction in an infant and in an unconscious person.
- List the five steps in the chain of survival.
- Explain cardiopulmonary resuscitation and the associated steps in circulation, airway, and breathing (CAB).
- Describe the purpose of chest compression.
- Name techniques for opening the airway and list ways a trained rescuer administers rescue breathing.
- Discuss the appropriate use of an automated external defibrillator.
- Describe criteria used in the decision to discontinue resuscitation efforts.

SECTION I: ASSESSING YOUR UNDERSTANDING

Activity A FILL IN THE BLANKS

1. To open the airway of a person with cardiac arrest, nurses position the client _____ on a firm surface.

2. Nurses place a breathing client in the _____ position to maintain an open airway and prevent aspiration of fluid.

3. Giving a breath that lasts a full second reduces the potential for distending the _____ and stomach.

4. Squeezing the heart between the _____ and vertebrae increases pressure in the ventricles.

5. A(n) _____ of food or some other foreign object may cause mechanical airway obstruction.

6. When performing CPR, senior clients are at a greater risk for fractured _____.

7. Nurses perform _____ breathing through the victim's mouth, nose, or stoma.

8. Correct placement of the _____ and the body is essential during chest compressions.

9. Unrelieved airway obstruction will lead to loss of _____ and eventually death.

10. A _____ team comprises a group of people trained and certified in advanced cardiac life support.

Activity B *Consider the following figures.*

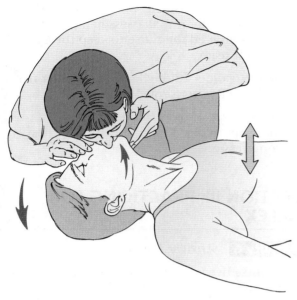

1. Identify the image.

_____

_____

_____

2. How is the action shown in the figure performed?

_____

_____

_____

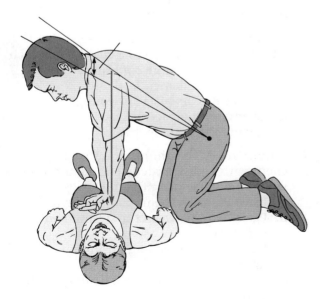

3. Identify and label the image.

_____

_____

_____

4. How do nurses assess whether this procedure is required?

_____

_____

_____

Activity C *Match the different resuscitation techniques in Column A with their specific features in Column B.*

Column A	Column B
____ **1.** Mouth-to-mouth breathing	**a.** Rescuer closes the infant or child's mouth
____ **2.** Mouth-to-nose breathing	**b.** Promotes circulation and increases pressure in the ventricles
____ **3.** Mouth-to-stoma breathing	**c.** Reduces the potential for distending the esophagus
____ **4.** Chest compression	**d.** Rescuers use a tube with the mouth or a one-way valve mask

Activity D *Presented here, in random order, are the steps that occur during chest thrusts performed on infants. Write the correct sequence in the boxes provided.*

1. Give five chest thrusts of one per second to the middle of the breastbone just below the nipple line.

2. Use the heel of the hand to give five back slaps between the shoulder blades.

3. Turn the infant supine and with two fingers give five chest thrusts.

4. Support the infant over the forearm and hold the infant prone with the head downward.

5. Repeatedly give five back blows and chest thrusts until the object is dislodged.

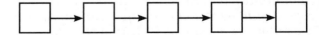

Activity E   *Briefly answer the following questions.*

1. What is partial airway obstruction?

_____

_____

_____

2. What is rescue breathing?

_____

_____

_____

3. What do CAB and CPR stand for?

_____

_____

_____

4. When is mouth-to-nose breathing performed?

_____

_____

_____

5. What is an automated external defibrillator (AED)?

_____

_____

_____

6. Why should a one-way mask be used when performing rescue breathing?

_____

_____

_____

SECTION II: APPLYING YOUR KNOWLEDGE

Activity F   *Older adults need to be informed that they may change their minds about advance directives and instructions for resuscitation at any time. All changes must be communicated to the physician, and a written copy should be stored in a safe location. Answer the following questions, which involve the nurse's role in caring for senior clients.*

A nurse is taking care of an older adult client who has been complaining of mild pain in the chest. The client has had two cardiac arrests in the past, and after initial assessment, the physician has ordered the nurse to keep the CPR equipment ready.

1. Why are older adult clients at a greater risk when CPR is performed on them?

2. Which type of older adult clients are more apt to bleed internally during chest compressions?

SECTION III: PRACTICING FOR NCLEX

Activity G   *Answer the following questions.*

1. A nurse needs to perform the chin-lift technique on an adult client who has a partial airway obstruction. In what position would the nurse place the client?
   a. Lateral position
   b. Fowler position
   c. Supine position
   d. Sims position

2. A nurse is attending to a client with an airway obstruction. What evidence should the nurse observe before performing a Heimlich maneuver on the client?
   a. Insufficient chewing
   b. Compromised swallowing
   c. Inability to speak
   d. Aspiration of vomitus

3. A nurse is preparing to administer a shock with the aid of an AED to a client. For which client is this procedure contraindicated?
   a. Clients with dementia
   b. Clients 8 years of age or younger
   c. Clients with a pacemaker
   d. Clients with osteoporosis

4. A nurse needs to administer a shock to a client with an implanted defibrillator. Where would the nurse place the AED pads?
   a. Place them on the implanted device itself
   b. Place them between the sternum and vertebrae
   c. Place them 1 inch away from the implanted device
   d. Place them on the brachial artery in the upper arm

5. A nurse is performing CPR on a client without defibrillation. The nurse knows they should assess the client's condition after how many cycles of compression and ventilations?
   a. 5 cycles
   b. 10 cycles
   c. 15 cycles
   d. 20 cycles

6. A nurse who is part of emergency services is caring for a client who had cardiac arrest. Which steps should the nurse take to initiate the chain of survival? Select all that apply.
   a. Provide the client with early CPR
   b. Arrange for the cardiac defibrillator
   c. Place the client in a recovery position
   d. Keep the advanced life support services ready
   e. Assess the client's pulse rate and circulation

7. A person accidentally swallows a large piece of food that causes partial airway obstruction. Which is the initial color on a person's face when there is partial or complete obstruction?
   a. Red
   b. Pink
   c. Blue
   d. White

8. A nurse is attaching an AED to a middle-age client who had cardiac arrest. Which institutions/areas generally have accessibility to an AED? Select all that apply.
   a. Schools
   b. Airports
   c. Police stations
   d. Amusement parks
   e. Subways

9. A nurse needs to perform rescue breathing on a client with a laryngectomy. What is an appropriate nursing action?
   a. Seal the client's nose with the fingers
   b. Use a one-way valve mask
   c. Cover the client's mouth with a hand
   d. Seal the client's stoma with the mouth

10. A nurse needs to perform the Heimlich maneuver on an infant who has partial obstruction resulting from aspiration of vomitus. The nurse is holding the infant prone with the head downward. What is the nurse's next action?
    a. Use two fingers to give back thrusts
    b. Use the heel of the hand to give five back blows

    c. Alternate the client between supine and prone positions
    d. Use finger sweeps to remove the obstruction from the throat

11. After opening the partial airway obstruction of a client, a nurse needs to assess the spontaneous breathing pattern of the client. What would be the appropriate observation?
    a. Observe for the rising and falling of the chest
    b. Check the pulse rate at the wrist
    c. Observe the mouth and nose for movement
    d. Observe the change in skin color

12. A physician has ordered a nurse to discontinue resuscitation attached to a client with cardiac arrest. What factors contribute toward the discontinuing of resuscitation? Select all that apply.
    a. Data obtained from blood gas results and electrolyte studies
    b. The client's condition deteriorates despite resuscitation efforts
    c. Rescuers and emergency service nurses are exhausted
    d. The client's family is against the use of resuscitation
    e. The age of the client and the diagnosis given to the client

13. A nurse is performing chest compression on a middle-age adult client with cardiac arrest. How would the nurse deliver a straight-down motion with each compression?
    a. Use two fingers to thrust the chest
    b. Avoid interlocking the fingers
    c. Rock back and forth over the client
    d. Position the body over the hands

14. A nurse is assisting a client who has symptoms of cardiac arrest within the health care facility premises. Which action should the nurse perform to provide early emergency services to the client?
    a. Alert the lead physician of emergency service
    b. Notify the switchboard operator for assistance
    c. Assess the client and then dial 911
    d. Describe the client's age and physical appearance

SECTION IV: REVIEWING WHAT YOU HAVE LEARNED

Activity H   *Fill in the blanks by choosing the correct word from the options given in parentheses.*

1. The CAB of cardiopulmonary resuscitation are _____, airway, and breathing. (circulation, congestion, cyanosis)

2. The rate for compressions for infants receiving CPR is _____/minute. (100, 125, 150)

Activity I   *Mark the statement as either T (True) or F (False). Correct a false statement.*

1. T F   The jaw-thrust maneuver helps to remove any foreign material within the client's mouth.

Activity J   *Write the correct term for each description below.*

1. In a hospital, the summoning of personnel trained in advanced life support techniques _____

2. A side-lying position in resuscitation that helps a breathing person maintain an open airway and prevent aspiration of fluid _____

Activity K   *Match the terms related to resuscitation in Column A with their explanations in Column B.*

Column A

____ 1. Heimlich maneuver

____ 2. Subdiaphragmatic thrusts

____ 3. Cardiopulmonary resuscitation

____ 4. Head-tilt/chin-lift technique

____ 5. Rescue breathing

Column B

a. Using techniques to restore breathing and circulation

b. Ventilating the lungs

c. The preferred method for opening the airway

d. Relieving a mechanical airway obstruction

e. Applying pressure to the abdomen

Activity L   *Differentiate between mouth-to-mouth breathing and mouth-to-stoma breathing based on the categories given below.*

1. Technique

2. Sealing of the client's nose

Activity M   *Cardiac arrest may lead to unresponsiveness. Rescuers implement a five-step survival process known as the Chain of Survival. Write in the boxes provided below the correct sequence of the chain of survival.*

1. Effective advanced life support

2. Integrated postcardiac arrest care

3. Early cardiopulmonary resuscitation with a focus on compressions

4. Immediate recognition and access to emergency services

5. Rapid defibrillation

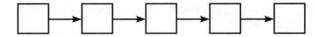

Activity N   *Answer the following questions.*

1. What are various signs of a partial and complete airway obstruction?

_____

_____

_____

2. For how long and for what reasons can basic cardiopulmonary resuscitation be interrupted?

_____

_____

_____

SECTION V: APPLYING YOUR KNOWLEDGE

Activity O   *Give rationales for the following questions.*

1. Why is a one-way valve mask used for rescue breathing?

_____

_____

_____

2. In what cases would a monitor display an error message during the attachment of an AED's electrode pad?

_____

_____

_____

Activity P *Answer the following questions focusing on nursing roles and responsibilities.*
An 8-year-old client develops an obstructed airway.

1. What immediate steps should the nurse take to relieve the client's obstruction?

_____

_____

_____

2. What should the nurse do if the child is unconscious?

_____

_____

_____

Activity Q *Consider the following questions. Discuss them with your instructor or peers.*

A 9-month-old infant accidentally inhales a button used for an eye on a toy.

1. How is clearing the airway for an infant different from clearing the airway of an adult?

_____

_____

_____

2. What suggestions should the nurse impart to the client's family to prevent such a situation?

_____

_____

_____

SECTION VI: GETTING READY FOR NCLEX

Activity R *Answer the following questions.*

1. A triage nurse is examining an unresponsive 6-year-old child. When performing CPR, what should the nurse do?
   a. Apply compression in the midline one finger width below the nipples
   b. Compress using two thumbs with the hands encircling the chest
   c. Place the heel of the hand at the center of the chest between the nipples
   d. Provide one breath every 5 seconds at the rate of 10 breaths/minute

2. A nurse is caring for a client with impaired ventilation. Which intervention should the nurse perform for this client?
   a. Administer oxygen at 20% using a Venturi mask
   b. Ensure that the client is supine at all times
   c. Replace the Venturi mask with a non-rebreather mask if SpO_2 is 90%
   d. Continually monitor the client's SpO_2 with a pulse oximeter

CHAPTER 38

End-of-Life Care

Learning Objectives

- Define terminal illness.
- Name the stages of dying.
- Describe methods by which nurses can promote acceptance of death in dying clients.
- Define respite care.
- Discuss the philosophy of hospice care.
- List aspects of terminal care.
- Name signs of multiple organ failure.
- Explain why a discussion of organ donation must take place as expeditiously as possible after a client's death.
- Explain the difference between a clinical autopsy and a forensic autopsy and the manner in which postmortem care is implemented.
- Name components of postmortem care.
- Discuss the benefit of grieving and signs that grief is being resolved.

SECTION I: ASSESSING YOUR UNDERSTANDING

Activity A   FILL IN THE BLANKS

1. A(n) _____ illness means a condition from which recovery is beyond reasonable expectation.

2. The term _____ is the concept of caring for terminally ill clients.

3. _____ involves the maintenance of an adequate fluid volume.

4. _____ is determined on the basis that breathing and circulation have ceased.

5. _____ is one of the last reflexes to disappear as death approaches.

6. A(n) _____ is an examination of the organs and tissues of a human body after death.

7. A(n) _____ is a person legally designated to investigate deaths that may not be the result of natural causes.

8. The _____ is a person who prepares the body for burial or cremation.

9. A person who cannot accept someone's death is in a state of pathologic or _____ grief.

10. Some survivors have _____ experiences such as seeing, hearing, or feeling the continued presence of the deceased.

Activity B   Consider the following figure.

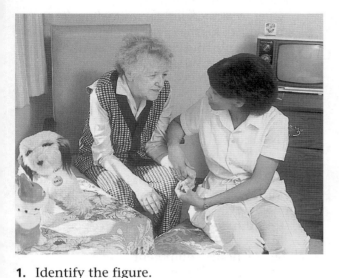

1. Identify the figure.

_____

_____

_____

2. What are the responsibilities of the nurse in this kind of setup?

_____

_____

_____

Activity C   Match the five stages of dying in Column A with their descriptions in Column B.

Column A

____ **1.** Denial

____ **2.** Anger

____ **3.** Bargaining

____ **4.** Depression

____ **5.** Acceptance

Column B

a. Clients confront potential losses

b. Clients have dealt with their losses and have completed unfinished business

c. Clients retaliate against fate

d. Clients refuse to believe that the diagnosis is accurate

e. Clients are willing to accept death but want to extend their life temporarily

Activity D   Presented here, in random order, are the stages of grief. Write the correct sequence in the boxes provided.

1. Developing awareness

2. Idealization

3. Shock and disbelief

4. Restitution period

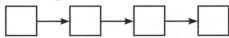

Activity E   Briefly answer the following questions.

1. What does "dying with dignity" mean?

_____

_____

_____

2. What is brain death?

_____

_____

_____

3. What is a death certificate?

_____

_____

_____

4. What is postmortem care?

_____

_____

_____

5. What is multiple organ failure?

_____

_____

_____

SECTION II: APPLYING YOUR KNOWLEDGE

Activity F   Nurses are more involved than any other group with people who experience impending death. Answer the following

questions, which relate to a nurse's role in caring for a dying client.

A nurse is caring for a young client with leukemia. The client asks the nurse to confirm if the laboratory reports are correct and to have them double-checked. The client is sure that there is a mistake, because all this happened while they were very healthy and active without any sign of illness.

1. What stage of dying is this client experiencing?

   _____

   _____

   _____

2. How should the nurse help dying clients to cope?

   _____

   _____

   _____

SECTION III: PRACTICING FOR NCLEX

Activity G   *Answer the following questions.*

1. A nurse is caring for a young client who has been severely injured in a motor vehicle accident. The client has multiple organ failure and is dying. Which statement by the client indicates that the client is in the depression stage of dying?
   a. "How can it be? No, I'm not dying."
   b. "What have I done wrong? Why me?"
   c. "I have just finished college."
   d. "Yes, I'm dying."

2. A nurse is caring for a senior client with a terminal illness. Which intervention by the nurse indicates respect for the rights of the dying client?
   a. Asking the client to avoid talking about death
   b. Informing the client about preparing an advance directive
   c. Avoiding any reference to spirituality when talking to the client
   d. Telling the client that the results of the diagnostic test look good

3. A nurse is caring for a senior client with acute renal failure who is dying. How might the

nurse cater to the basic needs of the client and their family members?
   a. Offer to secure spiritual counseling, if requested, for the client and family members
   b. Provide nursing care to the client without regard to the nurse's own feelings
   c. Discourage the client from talking to family members about their death
   d. Try to convince the client and family members to agree to organ or tissue donation

4. A nurse is caring for a client with a terminal illness in their home. What interventions can the nurse offer to this client? Select all that apply.
   a. Coordinate community services
   b. Arrange for home nursing visits
   c. Secure home equipment
   d. Provide round-the-clock nursing care
   e. Suggest transferring the client to residential care

5. A nurse is caring for a senior client with impaired swallowing. What care should the nurse take to prevent choking and aspiration in the client?
   a. Assist the client to a lateral position
   b. Ask the client to sleep without a pillow
   c. Assist the client to assume a semi-Fowler position
   d. Ensure that the client is supine at all times

6. A client is admitted to the health care facility for a major surgery. The client has prepared an advance directive expressing their wish to donate their eyes in case of death. The client died before the surgery. What should the nurse keep in mind when caring for the client's body?
   a. Harvest the eyes as soon as possible based on the client's directive
   b. Avoid placing hot or cold compresses over the client's eyes
   c. Avoid discussing the organ donation with the client's family members
   d. Discuss the possibility of harvesting the eyes after death with the client's next of kin

7. A nurse is caring for a terminally ill client who has been referred for hospice care. Which client is eligible for hospice care?
   a. Clients with less than 6 months to live
   b. Clients with difficult behavior
   c. Clients requiring high-tech palliative care
   d. Clients who cannot live independently

8. A client with carcinoma of the lung is receiving hospice care at their home. What service is offered by hospice care?
   a. The client receives subacute or intermediate care
   b. The client is provided with labor-intensive treatment
   c. Round-the-clock nursing care is provided to the client
   d. Care is provided by a multidisciplinary team of professionals

9. A nurse is caring for a senior client with impaired swallowing. What care should the nurse take to maintain adequate fluid volume in the client?
   a. Offer frequent small sips of water
   b. Offer small amounts of beverages
   c. Provide wrapped ice cubes to be sucked
   d. Inform the physician of the need for intravenous fluids

10. A nurse is caring for a client with bone cancer. The nurse identifies the risk of inadequate consumption of food. What is a possible cause for this diagnosis?
    a. Pressure sores
    b. Nausea
    c. Weakness
    d. Infection

11. A nurse is caring for a client who is terminally ill and prescribed oxygen therapy. Which intervention is important for the client on oxygen therapy?
    a. Need for intravenous fluids
    b. Need for total parenteral nutrition
    c. Need for lubrication of the lips
    d. Need for frequent mouth care

12. A client with acute renal failure is administered non-narcotic analgesics. The nurse caring for this client is aware that the goal of non-narcotic analgesics is
    a. To dull the consciousness
    b. To suppress respirations
    c. To inhibit the ability to communicate
    d. To provide relief from pain

13. A nurse is caring for an older client who has slipped into a coma. The client is showing signs of multiple organ failure. What care should the nurse take when summoning the family of the dying client? Select all that apply.
    a. Identify themselves by name, title, and location
    b. Ask the family to rush to the facility without explaining
    c. Ask for the family member by name and speak calmly
    d. Explain that the client's condition is deteriorating
    e. Tell the family all answers to queries will be given at the facility

14. A nurse is caring for a dying client who is in coma. Which conditions indicate brain death in the client? Select all that apply.
    a. Absence of brain stem reflexes
    b. Unreceptiveness or unresponsiveness to moderately painful stimuli
    c. $Paco_2$ less than 60 mm Hg after preoxygenation with 100% oxygen
    d. Complete absence of central and deep tendon reflexes
    e. No spontaneous respiration after being disconnected from a ventilator

15. A client at the health care facility has died after a prolonged illness. A nurse is assigned to perform postmortem care for the client. What one intervention should the nurse perform?
    a. Clean secretions from the skin
    b. Remove dentures from the mouth
    c. Keep all hairpins and clips
    d. Place a rolled towel under the head

SECTION IV: REVIEWING WHAT YOU HAVE LEARNED

Activity H *Fill in the blanks by choosing the correct word from the options given in parentheses.*

1. _____ involves a process of negotiation, usually with God or some higher power, in an attempt to delay the inevitability of death. (Bargaining, Denial, Depression)

2. _____ care provides round-the-clock nursing care for clients who cannot live independently. (Hospice, Residential, Respite)

3. The ability to _____ is one of the last reflexes to disappear as death approaches. (hear, smell, suck)

Activity I *Mark each statement as either T (True) or F (False). Correct any false statements.*

1. **T F** Diarrhea may be a common consequence of continuous narcotic analgesia.

2. **T F** An autopsy is the examination of human organs and tissues to treat a disease.

Activity J *Write the correct term for each description below.*

1. A person legally designated to investigate an unnatural death _____

2. A legal document attesting that the person named on the form is deceased _____

3. A condition in which two or more organ systems gradually cease to function _____

Activity K *Match the terms related to grieving in Column A with their explanations in Column B.*

Column A

_____ **1.** Anticipatory grief

_____ **2.** Pathologic grief

_____ **3.** Grief work

_____ **4.** Grief response

Column B

a. Activities involved in grieving

b. Psychological and physical experiences while grieving

c. Inability to accept someone's death

d. Feeling sad before someone's death

Activity L *Differentiate between home care and residential care based on the categories given below.*

1. Role of nurses

2. Delivery of care

Activity M *Dr. Elisabeth Kübler-Ross described stages through which terminally ill clients progress. Write in the boxes provided below the usual sequence of typical comments during the stages of dying.*

1. "Why me?"

2. "Yes, me."

3. "Yes, me, but if only ...."

4. "I am ready."

5. "No, not me."

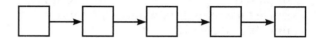

Activity N *Answer the following questions.*

1. What classifies an illness as terminal?

    _____

    _____

    _____

2. When can hospice care be terminated?

    _____

    _____

    _____

SECTION V: APPLYING YOUR KNOWLEDGE

Activity O *Give rationales for the following questions.*

1. Why is skin care important for terminally ill, incontinent clients?

    _____

    _____

    _____

2. Why do the lips of terminally ill clients need periodic lubrication?

    _____

    _____

    _____

3. Why are death certificates sent to the local health department?

_____

_____

_____

Activity P *Answer the following questions focusing on nursing roles and responsibilities.*

1. What are two methods that nurses can use to promote an acceptance of death in dying clients? What interventions can nurses use to provide emotional support to these clients?

_____

_____

_____

2. A nurse is caring for a client in the last stages of terminal brain cancer. What nursing diagnoses might apply for this client and their family members?

_____

_____

_____

3. A nurse is caring for a dying client.
   a. What nursing actions are appropriate related to the client's hygiene and nourishment?

_____

_____

_____

   b. How can the nurse ensure that the client receives adequate fluids?

_____

_____

_____

Activity Q *Consider the following questions. Discuss them with your instructor or peers.*

1. A nurse is providing postmortem care for a senior client who has died of cancer. How can the nurse demonstrate dignity and respect for the client's body?

2. A nurse is caring for a client who is unresponsive to even painful stimuli, cannot breathe independently, and has completely absent central and deep tendon reflexes. The physician has confirmed that the client is brain dead.
   a. What should the nurse do if the family asks to discontinue life support systems for the client?
   b. What information should the nurse provide to the family about the legal implications of their request?

SECTION VI: GETTING READY FOR NCLEX

Activity R *Answer the following questions.*

1. A nurse at an extended care facility is caring for a client with cancer and a limited prognosis for long-term survival. Which intervention is most appropriate?
   a. Share information, such as trends in vital signs, with the client
   b. Ask the client to identify goals that could be accomplished in 24 months
   c. Encourage the client to seek alternative forms of treatment
   d. Ask the client not to dwell on old memories and goals previously established

2. A nurse is caring for a client who had medical equipment attached to them at the time of death. What measures will the nurse implement when providing postmortem care of the client's body? Select all that apply.
   a. Obtain supplies for cleaning and wrapping the body
   b. Keep all the medical equipment attached to the body
   c. Contact individuals involved in organ procurement
   d. Ask for the approximate arrival time of the mortuary personnel
   e. Remove the disposable pads from between the legs

3. When caring for a dying client, which measures are appropriate for procuring organ or tissue donations? Select all that apply.
   a. Determine the dying client's wishes concerning organ and tissue donation
   b. Obtain permission from the next of kin as the client nears death
   c. Inform the mortician to remove specific organs when preparing the body
   d. Contact the pathologist in charge of performing autopsies
   e. Enlist the assistance of an organ procurement coordinator

4. A nurse is caring for a cold and stuporous client who has developed mottled skin. This condition may have been caused by failure of the:
   a. Brain and heart
   b. Liver and kidney
   c. Pancreas and stomach
   d. Intestine and bladder

Answers

CHAPTER 1

SECTION I: ASSESSING YOUR UNDERSTANDING

Activity A
1. Saint Thomas
2. Practical
3. Evidence-based practice
4. Art
5. Theory
6. Dorothea Orem
7. Practical nurses
8. Practical nurse
9. Baccalaureate
10. Counselor

Activity B
1. There are two basic educational options available for a nursing career: practical or vocational nursing and registered nursing. Several types of programs prepare graduates in registered nursing. Each educational track provides the knowledge and skills for a particular entry level of practice.
2. The factors that affect the choice of a nursing program are as follows:
   - Career goals
   - Geographic location of schools
   - Costs involved
   - Length of programs
   - Reputation and success of graduates
   - Flexibility in course scheduling
   - Opportunity for part-time versus full-time enrollment
   - Ease of movement into the next level of education

Activity C
1. b   2. c   3. d   4. a

Activity D
Question 1.

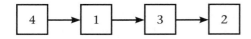

Question 2.

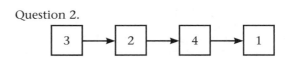

Activity E
1. In 1862, Dorothea Lynde Dix established the following selection criteria for nurses. Applicants were to be:
   - 35 to 50 years old
   - Matronly and plain looking
   - Educated
   - Neat, orderly, sober, and industrious, with a serious disposition
2. According to Virginia Henderson, "the unique function of the nurse is to assist the individual, sick or well, in the performance of those activities contributing to health or its recovery (or to a peaceful death) that he could perform unaided if he had the necessary strength, will, or knowledge; and to do this in such a way as to help him gain independence as rapidly as possible."
3. According to the ANA, the six essential features that characterize nursing are the following:
   - Provision of a caring relationship that facilitates health and healing
   - Attention to the range of human experiences and responses to health and illness within the physical and social environments
   - Integration of objective data with knowledge gained from an appreciation of the client's or group's subjective experience
   - Application of scientific knowledge to the processes of diagnosis and treatment through the use of judgment and critical thinking
   - Advancement of professional nursing knowledge through scholarly inquiry
   - Influence on social and public policy to promote social justice
4. The factors that influence the choice of a nursing program are career goals, geographic location of schools, costs involved, length of programs, reputation and success of graduates, flexibility in course scheduling, opportunity for part-time versus full-time enrollment, and ease of movement into the next level of education.

5. The guidelines to be kept in mind while delegating nursing tasks to staff members are right task, right circumstance, right person, right directions and communication, and right supervision and evaluation.

SECTION II: APPLYING YOUR KNOWLEDGE

Activity F

1. The nurse should use counseling skills to provide effective nursing care to this client. The nurse should try to understand the client's concerns by implementing active listening skills, thereby encouraging the client to express their problems. The nurse may then provide the client with required health teaching and education.

2. Active listening is the skill of demonstrating full attention to what is being said, hearing both the content being communicated and the unspoken message. The most important advantage of active listening is that it facilitates therapeutic interactions. Giving clients the opportunity to be heard helps them to organize their thoughts and to evaluate their situation more realistically.

SECTION III: PRACTICING FOR NCLEX

Activity G

1. Answer: a
   RATIONALE: During the Crimean War, the most important contribution of Florence Nightingale and her team of nurses was that the death rate of soldiers decreased from 60% to 1%. This was the result of improvement in ventilation, nutrition, sanitation, and the control of infection and gangrene in the soldiers.

2. Answer: b
   RATIONALE: Palpating the abdomen for liver enlargement is a technique for physical examination, which is an important assessment skill. In contrast, telling the client to exercise daily and educating the client about a hepatitis B vaccination program is a counseling skill. Ensuring that the client is taking their medications regularly is a caring skill.

3. Answer: d
   RATIONALE: The nurse should use counseling skills while dealing with the mother. These would include communicating with the client, actively listening during exchanges of information, and providing emotional support. Assessment and using comforting and caring skills may be required for her son, but are not applicable while dealing with the mother to help her cope with the situation. The mother needs emotional support to deal with the fact that her son has been diagnosed with a terminal illness.

4. Answer: b
   RATIONALE: The client would be emotionally disturbed as a result of loss of limb, so the nurse uses empathy to deal with the client. Empathy is the intuitive awareness of what the client is experiencing. The nurse uses empathy in clinical care to perceive the client's emotional state and need for support. This helps the nurse to provide effective nursing care without getting emotionally distraught by the client's condition. Empathy helps the nurse remain compassionately detached. A nurse who understands the client's condition would avoid hurting the client's emotions and feelings. Providing emotional support to the emotionally unstable client and counseling the client are basic caring activities and may not involve empathy.

5. Answer: d
   RATIONALE: The nurse uses assessment skills to interview the client's spouse to collect more information about the incidence of unconsciousness. Assessment skills include interviewing, examining, and observing. Counseling skills, however, are applicable if the nurse provides health education and discusses the condition. Caring skills are demonstrated when providing direct nursing care to the client. Comforting skills would be used if the client feels apprehensive and insecure.

6. Answer: a
   RATIONALE: While delegating a nursing task to the nursing staff, the nurse should follow the guidelines of right task, right circumstances, right person, right direction and communication, and right supervision and evaluation. Right person refers to knowing the unique competencies of the caregiver. The nurse should decide, based on the caregiver's competency, whether they will be able to perform the task, thereby ensuring the best possible nursing care for the client. Right person does not mean that care is given to the right client, nor does it have to do with the sincerity of the caregiver. Also, the delegation of work is not based on client criteria, but the competency of the caregiver.

7. Answer: a
   RATIONALE: The nurse should perform the procedure with the LPN. Even if the LPN does know the procedure, the nurse is responsible for the overall care provided to the client. Only the task is delegated, not the accountability. Requesting that the LPN refer to the manual and perform the procedure is risky because the LPN may make mistakes. The LPN is not confident about the procedure and therefore should not be asked to do the task alone. Requesting that the LPN observe another LPN perform the procedure does not ensure that the task would be done correctly.

8. Answer: d
   RATIONALE: The communication should be precise and clear when delegating the task. The nurse should mention clearly the client, their identification, and the task to be done. If not, it may lead to confusion and misinterpretation. The statement that says to complete the task and report back does not specify the client and their identification. The

other statements give clear instructions about the client but not the task.

9. Answer: b
RATIONALE: Asking the client to rate the pain on the pain scale is an example of assessment. This would give the details about the nature and intensity of the pain. Giving medicines for pain is a caring skill. Telling the client not to worry because the pain would subside indicates comforting skills. The statement that advises the client to support the incision site during movements is a counseling skill.

10. Answer: a
RATIONALE: The nurse should alleviate the client's anxiety by increasing their confidence in the health care team; the nurse may inform them about the general outcomes of the surgery. The nurse should not show an attitude of indifference by telling them that there is "always a first time." The nurse should not get personally involved by telling the client about the nurse's own experience. Everyone has their own concerns, so it is not appropriate to generalize about the anxiety the client is having.

11. Answers: a, c, e
RATIONALE: The factors that affect the choice of nursing programs include career goals, length of programs, and the cost involved. Career goals decide the direction and the type of course that would help to reach those goals. The program chosen also depends upon the affordability, the cost involved, and the length of the program. Types of training are more or less the same; hence, it does not have much of an impact on the choices made.

12. Answers: a, b, d
RATIONALE: Active listening encourages the client to express their concerns and evaluate them realistically. In an interaction with a client, the nurse demonstrates active listening by nodding their head, asking counterquestions, and repeating the matter to get the exact meaning. The nurse also observes the nonverbal communication of the client. The nurse never brings in their own emotions and concerns into the interaction because it may shift the focus from the client to the nurse.

13. Answer: a
RATIONALE: By asking the client to describe the incident, the nurse is using assessment skills to collect more information. The nurse is using the technique of interviewing to collect client-related data. It is not an example of comforting skills because the nurse is not providing any emotional support. Also, counseling skill is not used because no health education is provided. Caring skills include providing assistance in activities of daily living and are therefore not applicable in this scenario.

14. Answers: a, c, d
RATIONALE: Factors that have contributed to the shortage of nurses are an increased aging population requiring health care, heavier workloads and sicker clients, and the likelihood of mandatory overtime. As more and more people are aging, the population requiring health care is also increasing, putting heavier workloads on the nursing staff. Also, clients are sicker and require more intensive care than was the case in the past. People interested in joining nursing may become disinterested when they consider the working hours. Educational growth in nursing is not limited to one specific area, as nursing has multiple options for various types of growth and learning.

15. Answer: c
RATIONALE: Associate degree programs represent the shortest courses in registered nursing. Graduates from this type of program acquire an associate degree in nursing, which results in their being referred to as a *technical nurse*. Graduate nursing programs provide specialized courses that are available at the masters and doctoral levels. Baccalaureate programs are the longest and most expensive. A hospital-based diploma program generally lasts 3 years.

SECTION IV: REVIEWING WHAT YOU HAVE LEARNED

Activity H
1. Science
2. Nightingale

Activity I
1. True

Activity J
1. d   2. a   3. b   4. c

Activity K
1. Nightingale selected only people with upstanding characters to become potential nurses, trained people for their future work, improved sanitary conditions for the sick and injured, significantly reduced the death rate of British soldiers, provided classroom education and clinical teaching, and advocated lifelong nursing education.
2. Henderson's definition, later adopted by the International Council of Nurses, broadened nursing to include health promotion, not just illness care. She stated that "The unique function of the nurse is to assist the individual, sick or well, in the performance of those activities contributing to health or its recovery (or to a peaceful death) that he could perform unaided if he had the necessary strength, will, or knowledge. And to do this in such a way as to help him gain independence as rapidly as possible."

Activity L
1. Empathy, or intuitive awareness of what another person is experiencing, helps nurses to perceive the client's emotional state and need for support. Not

all clients are comfortable communicating their feelings to strangers.

Activity M

1. The nurse must first determine the client's needs and problems.
2. The nurse requires the assessment skills of interviewing, observing, and examining the client and, potentially, the client's family. The nurse also should review the client's medical record and talk with other health care workers to gather more information.

Activity N

There is no definite answer to this activity. Students may choose to discuss their thoughts with peers or instructors.

SECTION V: GETTING READY FOR NCLEX

Activity O

1. **Answer: a**
   RATIONALE: The demise of nursing in England before the time of Florence Nightingale began when hospitals were managed by the English state, which recruited criminals, widows, and orphans as the labor force. Recruitment of lay people by monasteries to assist in physical care, engagement of religious groups in many of the roles of nursing, or lack of resources during periods of plague and pestilence did not lead to the demise of nursing in England before the time of Florence Nightingale.

2. **Answers: b, d, e**
   RATIONALE: A hospital-based diploma program, an associate degree nursing program, and a baccalaureate degree nursing program provide the qualifications for taking the NCLEX-RN. A practical nursing program is a nursing preparatory program after which graduates are qualified to take their licensing examination. Licensed graduates who pass a licensed practical nursing (LPN) program are a vital link between the registered nurse and unlicensed assistive personnel.

CHAPTER 2

SECTION I: ASSESSING YOUR UNDERSTANDING

Activity A

1. Nursing process
2. Assessment
3. Objective
4. Client
5. Implementation
6. Focus
7. Diagnosis
8. Subjective
9. Physiologic
10. Collaborative

Activity B

1. The five steps of the nursing process are:
   - Assessment
   - Diagnosis
   - Planning
   - Implementation
   - Evaluation

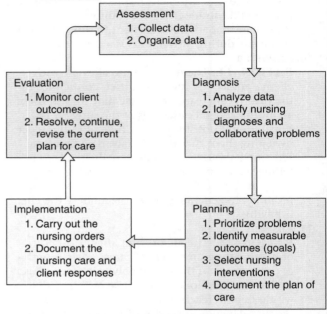

2. The types of data collected during assessment are:
   - Subjective data
   - Objective data
3. Collaborative problems are those potential complications from a disorder, test, or treatment that the nurse cannot treat independently, for example, hemorrhage. They represent an interdependent domain of nursing practice.
4. The role of the nurse is to monitor to detect the complication(s) and, if detected, manage the complication cooperatively with nurse- and physician-prescribed interventions. The nurse is specifically responsible and accountable for the following:
   - Correlating medical diagnoses or medical treatment measures with the risk for unique complications
   - Documenting complications for which clients are at risk
   - Making pertinent assessments to detect complications
   - Reporting trends that suggest development of complications
   - Managing the emerging problem with nurse- and physician-prescribed measures
   - Evaluating the outcomes

Activity C

1. c **2.** d **3.** b **4.** a

Activity D

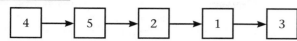

4 → 5 → 2 → 1 → 3

Activity E

1. The nursing process is an organized sequence of problem-solving steps used to identify and manage the health problems of clients. The nursing process is the very infrastructure of nursing practice in all health care settings. When nursing practice follows the nursing process, clients receive quality care in minimal time with maximal efficiency. In addition, the nursing process serves as a framework for nursing documentation in medical records, and when medical records are subpoenaed for court cases, the steps in the nursing process are the basis for determining whether standards of care have been met.

2. The nursing process has seven distinct characteristics:
   - Within the legal scope of nursing
   - Based on knowledge
   - Planned
   - Client centered
   - Goal directed
   - Prioritized
   - Dynamic

3. There are three types of assessments:
   - Database assessment: initial information about the client's physical, emotional, social, and spiritual health obtained during the admission interview and physical examination.
   - Focus assessment: the information that provides more details about specific problems and expands the original database.
   - Functional assessment: a comprehensive evaluation of a client's physical strengths and weaknesses in areas such as (1) the performance of activities of daily living, (2) cognitive abilities, and (3) social functioning.

4. Concept mapping is a method of organizing information in graphic or pictorial form. It is created by identifying a main subject with interconnected links to related components. This strategy promotes critical thinking while gathering data from the client and medical record or a written case study, selecting significant information, and organizing related concepts on a one- or two-page working document.

5. Short-term goals have the following characteristics:
   - Developed from the problem portion of the diagnostic statement
   - Client centered, reflecting what the client will accomplish, not the nurse
   - Measurable, identifying specific criteria that provide evidence of goal achievement
   - Realistic, to avoid setting unattainable goals, which can be self-defeating and frustrating
   - Accompanied by a target date for accomplishment, the predicted time when the goal will be met

SECTION II: APPLYING YOUR KNOWLEDGE

Activity F

1. The sources of data in this case would be the client themselves, their family members, their previous case files, and any other medical documents.

2. In the given case, the types of data obtained would be both subjective and objective. The subjective data would include pain, restlessness, anxiety, and palpitation. The objective data would include high blood pressure, increased heart rate, high temperature, and high respiratory rate.

SECTION III: PRACTICING FOR NCLEX

Activity G

1. **Answer: b**
   RATIONALE: Objective data are observable and measurable facts and are signs of a disorder. High blood pressure is considered objective data because it can be measured. Pain in the abdomen, a tingling sensation, and itching of the nose are all subjective data because none of these can be measured; they are all information that only the client can feel and describe.

2. **Answer: a**
   RATIONALE: The client with Cushing disease and with an open wound is at increased risk for infection as a result of excess hormone secretion and impaired immune function. The first priority should be risk for infection. The client may also have impaired mobility, disturbed body image, and risk for delayed surgical recovery, but none of these would be considered a high priority.

3. **Answer: c**
   RATIONALE: While caring for a stroke client, the first step is to perform a physical assessment to determine the needs of the client. Based on the identified needs, realistic goals are set and nursing actions are planned. Finally, the nursing actions are implemented. The nurse may evaluate the outcome of the nursing action to plan for further care.

4. **Answer: d**
   RATIONALE: According to Maslow's need hierarchy, risk for body image disturbance is of the lowest priority. An altered breathing pattern indicates a problem in the airway and is the most important nursing diagnosis. An altered elimination need is also a physiologic need, and therefore, it also has high priority. Ineffective coping is a social problem and, therefore, is more important than the body image disturbance.

5. **Answer: a**
   RATIONALE: Anticoagulants have an inhibitory effect on the body's coagulation mechanism. As a result, the client can bleed heavily from sustaining even a minor injury. The nursing action should include providing a safe environment to the client. Risk for infection, risk for imbalanced fluid volume, and ineffective health maintenance may or may not be present for the client.

6. **Answer: a**
RATIONALE: The short-term goal for the client should be to help the client ambulate to a bedside chair. The other goals, such as helping the client return to activities of daily life, to maintain a healthy and active lifestyle, and to prevent repeat surgery, are long-term goals.

7. **Answer: b**
RATIONALE: The client consumed foods that were restricted for them because they did not want to be considered different from others. The client is experiencing situational low self-esteem because they feel different from their peer group. The assessment data do not indicate risk for body image disturbance, ineffective health maintenance, or risk from impaired nutritional intake.

8. **Answer: b**
RATIONALE: Pain of grade 2 on a pain scale is a piece of objective data because it is measurable. The pricking pain, throbbing pain, and cramping pain are descriptive and cannot be measured; therefore, they are subjective data.

9. **Answer: c**
RATIONALE: The long-term goal for this client would be to prevent recurrence of disc prolapse by practicing body mechanics. To prevent infection at the surgical site, to avoid putting strain on the back during the immediate postoperative period, and to ambulate and perform activities of daily life are short-term goals that can be achieved in a week.

10. **Answer: b**
RATIONALE: The client is scared about the recurrence of pain and feels anxious anticipating the pain. The pain threatens the psychosocial integrity of the client, as evidenced by Maslow's Hierarchy of Human Needs. There is no evidence that there is urinary retention or an impaired coping mechanism.

11. **Answer: a**
RATIONALE: Risk for disuse syndrome is a risk diagnosis because it is not present in the client but may develop as a complication of the coma. An ineffective breathing pattern, impaired physical mobility, and total self-care deficit are problem-focused diagnoses because these are already present in the client.

12. **Answer: b**
RATIONALE: The client is concerned about the baby's safety and has fears of miscarriage. Fear is the most important diagnosis in this scenario. Spotting does not lead to a decrease in body fluid volume. The client may be advised bed rest, but the client's primary concern is her baby. There may or may not be a problem with impaired urinary elimination.

13. **Answer: c**
RATIONALE: Assessing the condition of the wound should be the first step performed by the nurse. The remaining steps would follow the findings obtained from the assessment of the wound. Assessment is followed by preparing articles for dressing, then dressing the wound, and finally documenting the findings.

14. **Answer: d**
RATIONALE: The client has an impaired gastrointestinal system and is on enteral feeding, which increases the risk of aspiration. Therefore, risk for aspiration is given highest priority in the nursing diagnosis. This nursing diagnosis directly addresses the problem in airway maintenance. Bowel elimination, imbalance in fluid volume, and risk for imbalanced nutrition are also possible problems, but are not as important as the problem of airway maintenance.

15. **Answers: a, c, d**
RATIONALE: Conducting postoperative surgical assessments, monitoring the client's level of pain before and after administering medications, and checking the neurologic status of a client with a head injury are focus assessments because they are done frequently or on a scheduled basis to know the client's progress. Conducting urine analysis on admission and inquiring about dietary habits of the client are database assessments.

16. **Answer: c**
RATIONALE: Ineffective coping is the appropriate diagnosis for the client. It is defined as the state in which an individual demonstrates impaired adaptive behaviors and problem-solving abilities in meeting life's demands and roles. Risk for disuse syndrome and deficient diversional activity are not related to the coping mechanism. Disturbed self-esteem may be related to it, but it does not have any effect on the displacement.

17. **Answer: a**
RATIONALE: Alopecia is the thinning or complete loss of hair; it is a complication of hormone therapy. Alopecia can cause body image disturbances, especially in females. It could be managed by the use of wigs, scarves, and hats. Teaching the client about use of cosmetics, shampoo, and washing of the hair and scalp may not help.

18. **Answers: b, c, d**
RATIONALE: Pain in the abdomen, tenesmus, and nausea are subjective data because none of them can be measured; they can only be described by the client. High temperature and high blood pressure are measurable and, therefore, are objective data.

SECTION IV: REVIEWING WHAT YOU HAVE LEARNED

Activity H

1. Diagnosis
2. Objective

Activity I

1. True.
2. False. The nurse assigned to the client refers to the plan of care, reviews it for appropriateness, and revises it according to changes in the client's condition.
3. True.

Activity J

1. Goal
2. Nursing process

Activity K

	Database Assessment	Focus Assessment
1. Definition	This lengthy and comprehensive method of assessment includes initial information about the client's physical, emotional, social, and spiritual health.	This method of assessment provides details about specific problems and expands the original database.
2. Purpose	Information obtained serves as a reference for comparing all future data and provides the evidence used to identify the client's initial problems.	Focus assessments are generally repeated frequently or according to a schedule to determine trends in a client's condition and responses to therapeutic interventions.
3. Example	• Health history • Family health history • Current health problem as perceived by the client • Social history (e.g., marital status, use of alcohol and tobacco) • Current prescription and nonprescription medications used	• Postoperative surgical assessments • Monitoring of the client's pain level before and after administering medications • Checking the neurologic status of a client with a head injury

Activity L

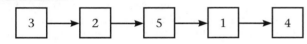

Activity M

1. Nursing diagnoses are categorized into four groups: problem-focused (formerly called actual), risk, syndrome, and health promotion.
2. Collaborative problems are those potential complications from a disorder, test, or treatment that the nurse cannot treat independently, for example, hemorrhage. They represent an interdependent domain of nursing practice. The role of the nurse is to monitor to detect the complication(s) and, if detected, manage the complication cooperatively with nurse- and physician-prescribed interventions.

SECTION V: APPLYING YOUR KNOWLEDGE

Activity N

1. Stays in acute care settings are usually less than 1 week. Because short-term goals are supposed to be achievable within 1 week, they are most appropriate for clients in acute care settings.
2. The nurse should document a nursing order so that all nursing team members understand exactly what to do for the client. The nurse should also sign the nursing order to indicate accountability.

Activity O

1.
   a. The nurse must first determine the client's needs and problems through assessment.
   b. The nurse requires the assessment skills of interviewing, observing, and examining the client and, potentially, the client's family. The nurse should also review the client's medical record and talk with other health care workers to gather more information.

2.
   a. The nurse first needs to assess the client and gather information to determine areas of abnormal function, risk factors that contribute to health problems, and client strengths. The nurse bases the nursing diagnosis on their analysis of these data and determines whether they suggest normal or abnormal findings.
   b.
      • Name of the health-related issue or problem as identified in the NANDA-I list
      • Etiology (its cause)
      • Signs and symptoms

3.
   a. Short-term goals should be achievable within 1 week. They should be developed from the problem portion of the diagnostic statement; client centered, reflecting what the client, not the nurse, will accomplish; measurable, identifying specific criteria that provide evidence that the goal has been reached; realistic, not unattainable, which can be self-defeating and frustrating; and accompanied by a target date for accomplishment (the predicted time when the goal will be met).
   b. Long-term goals are desirable outcomes that take weeks or months to accomplish. If a client achieves short-term goals in an acute setting, however, they are more likely to achieve long-term goals during home care or in other community settings.

c. One short-term goal for this client might be the ability to use a walking device and ambulate without assistance from another person. One long-term goal might be to be able to walk without any walking device or assistance.

Activity P

There are no definite answers to this activity. Students may choose to discuss their thoughts with peers or instructors.

SECTION VI: GETTING READY FOR NCLEX

Activity Q

1. **Answer: b**
   RATIONALE: Abdominal pain is information that only the client can feel and describe. The nurse should record temperature, pulse rate, and blood pressure as objective data, which are observable and measurable facts.

2. **Answer: a**
   RATIONALE: "Impaired Skin Integrity related to inactivity" is a problem-focused nursing diagnosis, meaning that signs or symptoms have been manifested. A risk nursing diagnosis indicates uncertainty because the problem does not yet exist. Syndrome and health promotion diagnoses are one-part statements and are not linked with an etiology or signs and symptoms.

CHAPTER 3

SECTION I: ASSESSING YOUR UNDERSTANDING

Activity A

1. Statutory
2. Veracity
3. Deontology
4. Liability
5. Defamation
6. Tort
7. Teleology
8. Felony
9. Common
10. Administrative

Activity B

1. The figure provided is an incident report.
2. The nurse has an important role in filling out the incident report. All witnesses are identified by name. Any pertinent statements made by the injured person, before or after the incident, are quoted. Accurate and detailed documentation often helps to prove that the nurse acted reasonably or appropriately in the circumstances.
3. The incident report should include five important pieces: when the incident occurred, where it happened, who was involved, what happened, and what actions were taken.

4. The figure is the format of a living will.
5. An advance directive is a written statement identifying a competent person's wishes concerning terminal care. The two types of advance directives are a living will and a durable power of attorney for health care.
6. The nurse and the health care workers cannot sign the living will of a client in their health care facility.

Activity C

1. b   2. c   3. d   4. a

Activity D

1. Allocation of scarce resources is the process of deciding how to distribute limited life-saving equipment or procedures among several people who could benefit. Such decisions are difficult. In effect, those who receive the resources have a greater chance to live, whereas those who do not may die prematurely. One strategy is that of first come, first served. Another is to project what would produce the most good for the most people, although predicting the future is impossible.
2. Code status refers to how health care personnel are required to manage care in case of cardiac or respiratory arrest. Without a written order from the physician to the contrary, the client is designated as a full code. A full code means that all measures to resuscitate the client are used. Some clients specify using drugs, but refuse cardiac defibrillation or endotracheal intubation for mechanical ventilation. For anything less than a full code, the physician must write an order to that effect in the client's medical record.
3. A living will is an instructive form of an advance directive, that is, it is a written document that identifies a person's preferences regarding medical interventions to use, or not to use, in a terminal condition, irreversible coma, or persistent vegetative state with no hope of recovery. Clients must share advance directives with health care providers to ensure that they are implemented.
4. Several ethical issues recur in nursing practice. Examples include telling the truth, maintaining confidentiality, withholding or withdrawing treatment, advocating for ethical allocation of scarce resources, and protecting vulnerable people from unsafe practices or practitioners.
5. Autonomy refers to a competent person's right to make their own choices without intimidation or influence. For a person to make a decision, they must have all relevant information, including treatment options, in a language they understand. The client always has the option of obtaining a second opinion from another practitioner. One outcome may be that the client declines all possible options for treatment—a decision that must be respected.

SECTION II: APPLYING YOUR KNOWLEDGE
Activity E

1. The health care team should conduct the surgery because it is lifesaving for the client. In an emergency, consent can be implied. In other words, it is assumed that in life-threatening circumstances, a client would give consent for treatment if they were able to understand the risks. However, another physician must concur that the emergency procedure is essential. Meanwhile, the nurse can track down the client's details and inform the family.
2. The act does not equate to battery because the surgery is done to save the life of the client, and consent in an emergency situation is implied.

SECTION III: PRACTICING FOR NCLEX
Activity F

1. **Answer: c**
   RATIONALE: The physician can be charged with slander for criticizing the nurse in the presence of the client. Battery (unauthorized physical contact) can include touching a person's body, clothing, chair, or bed. Assault is an act in which bodily harm is threatened or attempted. Such harm may be physical intimidation, remarks, or gestures. Libel is a damaging statement written and read by others. These are not applicable in this case.
2. **Answer: c**
   RATIONALE: Removal of the feeding tube from the comatose client carries legal implications. The nurse should check the client records for family authorization. The family members can make treatment decisions on behalf of the client if the client is unable to do so. Although a written order from the physician is necessary, the nurse should also check to determine whether the family members have given consent to it. The nurse should not carry out the orders without checking to see the orders in writing. The need for court orders may differ from one health care facility to another.
3. **Answer: a**
   RATIONALE: Taking monetary compensation from the client is unlawful. Whenever a problem such as this is identified, the first step is to report the situation to an immediate supervisor. The supervisor may take necessary action per the Nurses Act. Ignoring the incident and keeping silent is unethical and would encourage the colleague's behavior. It is not appropriate to call the police. Confronting the colleague may raise conflict and the colleague may become emotional or evasive. Moreover, the colleague may not cease the behavior after the confrontation.
4. **Answer: b**
   RATIONALE: The surgeons should operate upon the client, assuming that consent is implied. In an emergency, consent can be implied. It is assumed

that in life-threatening circumstances, a client would give consent for treatment if they were able to understand the risks. In most cases, another physician must concur that the emergency procedure is essential. The nurse should not wait for the family to come and give consent because it could prove fatal for the client. Neither the nurse nor the supervisor can sign the consent form; it is unlawful to do so.
5. **Answer: c**
   RATIONALE: Revealing confidential client-related information to someone without the client's permission is a violation of the client's right to privacy. Right to information is not applicable in this situation because the client's records are confidential. However, the scenario is not a breach of duty because there is no direct harm to the client. Defamation is also not applicable to this scenario because defamation is an act in which untrue information harms a person's reputation, which has not happened here.
6. **Answer: a**
   RATIONALE: Nurses are not supposed to carry out any verbal orders except in an emergency. The nurse should tell the physician to come back and write the orders. The nurse is not authorized to write orders on behalf of the physician. The nurse should not carry out any instructions if not in writing. It is the nurse's duty to inform the client about drug dosage change, but it does not imply that the nurse carries out verbal orders.
7. **Answer: b**
   RATIONALE: The nurse's action is an act of negligence. Negligence is the harm that results because a person did not act reasonably. The nurse did notice the sign of hypoglycemia but failed to act appropriately. Defamation, assault, and battery are not applicable in this case. Defamation is an act in which untrue information harms a person's reputation. Battery refers to unauthorized physical contact. Assault is an act in which bodily harm is threatened or attempted.
8. **Answer: c**
   RATIONALE: A living will is an instructive form of an advance directive—that is, it is a written document that identifies a person's preferences regarding medical interventions to use or not to use in a terminal condition, irreversible coma, or persistent vegetative state with no hope of recovery. The health care professionals of the same health care facility are not supposed to sign the will. Therefore, the nurse should not sign it and should politely indicate the reason to the client. Calling the physician or nurse supervisor is not an appropriate action.
9. **Answer: a**
   RATIONALE: In case of hazardous incidents, the nurse should inform the physician and the supervisor about the incident. The incident report is separate from a medical document and should not be

kept along with the client's records; neither should it be mentioned in the client's records. It is a legal document; therefore, a copy of the incident report should not be made. Incident reports determine how to prevent hazardous situations and serve as a reference in case of future litigation.

10. **Answer: b**
    RATIONALE: The nurse would get immunity from possible legal lawsuit through the provision of assumption of risk. The nurse had warned the client about walking without assistance, but the client ignored the nurse's warning and fell down. The nurse should document the whole incident, including the fact that warning was given to the client. Good Samaritan law, statute of limitations, and judicial law are not applicable here. Good Samaritan laws provide legal immunity to passersby who provide emergency first aid to victims of accidents. Statute of limitations is the designated time within which a person can file a lawsuit. Judicial laws are decisions based on prior similar cases.

11. **Answer: c**
    RATIONALE: A nurse threatening to turn off the signal system of communication is an appropriate example of assault. Assault is an act in which bodily harm is threatened or attempted. Such harm may be physical intimidation, remarks, or gestures. A nurse telling a client that they cannot leave the health care facility or restraining them from being discharged without the consent of the physician could amount to false imprisonment. A nurse discussing confidential client information with a friend is an example of invasion of privacy.

12. **Answer: b**
    RATIONALE: The determination of negligence is based on the fact that harm resulted because the nurse did not act reasonably. The client could not be taken for a barium ingestion test because of ingestion of food. The dietary department sending the wrong food tray is unrelated. The nurse insisting the client eat the food and not confirming the order with the physician only contributed to the situation.

13. **Answers: b, d**
    RATIONALE: Restraining a client against their will is not lawful. The nurse can be charged for battery and false imprisonment. Battery is unauthorized physical contact that can include touching a person's body, clothing, chair, or bed. False imprisonment is interference with a person's freedom to move about at will without legal authority to do so. It is applicable if a nurse detains a competent client from leaving the hospital or other health care agency. Assault is an act in which bodily harm is threatened or attempted. Such harm may be physical intimidation, remarks, or gestures. Slander and libel are not applicable because there is no harm done to the client's reputation in either oral or written form.

14. **Answers: b, c**
    RATIONALE: The nurse can be charged for invasion of privacy and libel. All information that the client renders to the nurse should be kept confidential. If any case reports have to be published, the names need to be changed to maintain privacy. By publishing the client's name in the research report, the nurse has caused invasion of privacy of the client. The nurse has written harmful statements about the client, which could be charged as libel. Libel is a damaging statement written and read by others. Felony, misdemeanor, and slander are not applicable here. A misdemeanor is a minor criminal offense, whereas a felony is a serious criminal offense, such as murder or falsifying medical records. Slander is a character attack uttered orally in the presence of others.

15. **Answers: b, c, e**
    RATIONALE: The nurse should inform the physician and take their orders for restraining the client. The nurse should also discuss it with the client's family and make them understand the reason for restraining the client. Mention of the type and duration of the restraint should also be made in the client's records. The nurse cannot make their own decision to restrain the client because this could lead to being charged with battery or false imprisonment. The nurse should not sedate the client or restrain them without a physician's orders.

SECTION IV: REVIEWING WHAT YOU HAVE LEARNED

Activity G

1. Libel
2. Veracity

Activity H

1. False. On the advice of an attorney, an anecdotal note can be used as evidence in court.
2. False. Negligence is harm that results from acting carelessly in a given circumstance; malpractice is professional negligence.

Activity I

	Teleologic Theory	Deontologic Theory
1. Definition	This theory of ethics is based on final outcomes.	This theory of ethics is based on duty or moral obligations.
2. Ideology	The ultimate ethical test for any decision is based on what is best for most people.	Decisions must be based on the ultimate morality of the act itself. The outcome is not an issue.
3. Example	A teleologist would argue that selective abortion is ethically correct because it is done to ensure the full-term birth of remaining healthy fetuses.	A deontologist would argue that destroying any fetus is wrong, whether it is done to save others or not because killing is always immoral.

Activity J

1. Laws are rules of conduct that governments establish and enforce to protect both the general public and each person. The six types of laws are constitutional, statutory, administrative, common, criminal, and civil.
2. A nurse practice act is a statutory law that legally defines the unique role of the nurse and differentiates it from that of other health care practitioners. Each state has its own nurse practice act that defines the scope of nursing practice, establishes the limits to that practice, identifies the titles that nurses may use, authorizes a board of nursing to oversee nursing practice, and determines what constitutes grounds for disciplinary action.

Activity K

1. The damages sought in malpractice lawsuits are so high that attorneys hired by health care facilities are sometimes more committed to defending the facility against liability and negative publicity than to defending the nurse employee whom they are also being paid to represent. By obtaining personal liability insurance, a nurse involved in a lawsuit will have a separate attorney working on their sole behalf.
2. Gross negligence indicates total disregard for another's safety. Nurses have training in safety beyond that of average people; hence, they are expected to provide a higher standard of care at all times.
3. Using untrained interpreters, volunteers, or family increases the risk for undermining the client's confidentiality and privacy. It may violate family roles and boundaries. It also may increase the potential for modifying, condensing, omitting, or adding information or projecting the interpreter's own values during communication between client and health care provider.
4. Derogatory remarks attack a person's character and good name and can lead to accusations of defamation.

Activity L

1. The nurse cannot detain a competent client from leaving the health care facility. The client can allege false imprisonment or interference with their freedom to move about at will without legal authority to do so.
2. If a client wants to leave without being medically discharged, the nurse should ask the client to sign a form indicating personal responsibility for leaving against medical advice (AMA). Even if the client refuses to sign the form, however, the nurse has no authority to prevent them from leaving the facility.

Activity M

There are no definite answers to this activity. Students may choose to discuss their thoughts with peers or instructors.

SECTION V: GETTING READY FOR NCLEX

Activity N

1. **Answer: b**
   RATIONALE: The nurse is at risk for being charged with a felony, a serious criminal offense. Examples include murder, falsifying medical records, insurance fraud, and stealing narcotics. A misdemeanor is a minor criminal offense such as shoplifting. Negligence is harm caused by an unreasonable act. Malpractice is professional negligence: professionals are required to maintain a higher standard of accountability.
2. **Answer: d**
   RATIONALE: The nurse should use a wanderer alarm to detect when the client leaves the bed. The nurse should not raise the side rails to restrain the client's movement because they could be accused of interfering with the client's freedom to move about without legal authority to do so. The nurse could be accused of assault if they verbally threaten to restrain the client. The nurse should obtain a medical order to use a restraint only if less restrictive alternatives are unsuccessful.

CHAPTER 4

SECTION I: ASSESSING YOUR UNDERSTANDING

Activity A

1. Hierarchy
2. Holism
3. Mortality
4. Hereditary
5. Primary
6. Infirmity
7. Morbidity
8. Secondary
9. Medicare
10. Team

Activity B

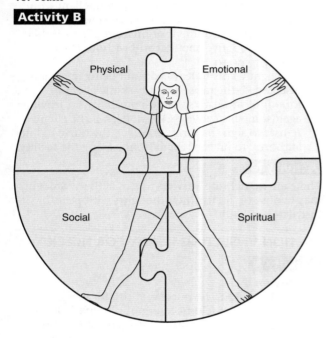

1. The figure represents holism as a concept that considers the sum of the physical, emotional, social, and spiritual health of a person.
2. The components of holism that determine how "whole" or well a person feels are physical, mental, social, and spiritual.
3. The components of holism are interrelated; if a person is physically ill, the affect can be seen in their social, mental, and spiritual well-being as well.

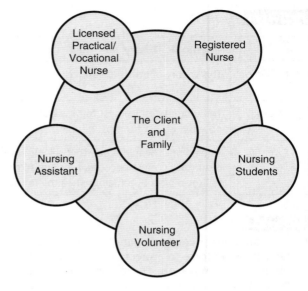

4. The nursing team.
5. The main purpose of the nursing team is to provide effective nursing care to the client and the client's family.

Activity C

1. b
2. c
3. d
4. a

Activity D

Question 1.

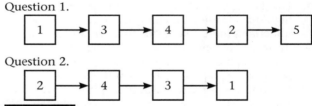

Question 2.

Activity E

1. According to Maslow, the first-level physiologic needs are the most important. They include activities necessary to sustain life. Maslow believed that until humans satisfied their physiologic needs, they could not or would not seek to fulfill other needs.
2. The types of illnesses based on their duration are acute illness, chronic illness, and terminal illness.
3. Managed care organizations are private insurers who carefully plan and closely supervise the distribution of their clients' health care services to control costs of health care. These organizations focus on prevention as the best way to manage costs.
4. Capitation is a payment system in which a preset fee per member is paid to a health care provider regardless of whether the member requires services. Capitation provides an incentive to providers to control tests and services as a means of making a profit. If members do not receive costly care, the provider makes money.

5. Nurse-managed care is a pattern in which a nurse manager plans the nursing care of clients based on their type of case or medical diagnosis. A clinical pathway is typically used in a managed care approach. In nurse-managed care, a professional nurse evaluates whether predictable outcomes are met on a daily basis. By meeting the outcomes in a timely manner, the client is ready for discharge by the time designated by prospective payment systems, if not before.

SECTION II: APPLYING YOUR KNOWLEDGE

Activity F

1. The nurse manager plans the nursing care of clients based on their type of case or medical diagnosis. They forecast outcomes and determine the best strategies for favorable outcomes, keeping in mind the cost factors. The nurse manager is responsible for the client's preoperative workup, hernioplasty, and postoperative care. The nurse manager evaluates whether predictable outcomes are met on a daily basis.

2. The nurse-managed care model ensures that standards of care are met with greater efficiency and cost savings. The recovery is fast, and the client is ready for discharge by the time designated by prospective payment systems. It also addresses the issues of nursing shortages and the need to balance the costs of medical care with limited reimbursement systems.

SECTION III: PRACTICING FOR NCLEX

Activity G

1. **Answer: d**
RATIONALE: The client would require extended care at a rehabilitation center to help them adapt to walking with the prosthesis. The client would have to undergo continuous assessments and evaluation of the prosthesis, followed by intense physiotherapy. The client does not require acute care provided in primary, secondary, or tertiary care centers.

2. **Answer: b**
RATIONALE: Depression is the first priority of nursing care. Wellness involves physical, emotional, social, and spiritual health. The client does not have any physical illness; rather, their emotional needs should be cared for. Dependability and low self-esteem are social and spiritual aspects of health and are dependent on physical and emotional health.

3. **Answer: a**
RATIONALE: Chronic illnesses have a gradual onset, usually with pain in the joints, and last for a long time. The incidence increases with age, and senior clients are more likely to suffer from chronic disorders like osteoarthritis. Osteoarthritis runs a long course and has an equally long treatment regimen. Chronic disorders are not hereditary and do not have a genetic predisposition; they are therefore not inherited from parents.

4. **Answer: c**
RATIONALE: Heart disease as a result of damaged lungs is a secondary disease. Lung disease resulting from smoking is a primary disorder, and smoking resulting from any cause is a causative factor. Heart disease resulting from fetal abnormality is not a *secondary disorder*. Any disease condition resulting from an underlying and preexisting disease condition is called a *secondary disorder*.

5. **Answer: a**
RATIONALE: Gout is a chronic disease with intermittent remissions and exacerbations. During the remission state, the client remains free of the symptoms, whereas during the exacerbated state, the symptoms of gout are aggravated. Heart attack, common cold, and varicose veins are not associated with a state of remission.

6. **Answer: d**
RATIONALE: Functional nursing is a pattern of nursing care in which each nurse on a client unit is assigned specific tasks. The approach is task-based, not client-based. The team leader in a team nursing care pattern heads a team of nursing staff who carry out the task together. A nurse manager is responsible for assessing and planning nursing care in a nurse-managed care pattern. Primary nursing care involves an admitting nurse, who is responsible for a client's care throughout their stay at a health care facility.

7. **Answer: c**
RATIONALE: The nurse manager is responsible for care and outcomes in a nurse-managed care pattern of nursing care. Team nursing has a team leader to supervise the members. In the functional nursing model, the nurse in charge ensures that all nursing tasks are carried out. The case manager is responsible for providing overall nursing care to a group of clients in case method nursing care.

8. **Answer: b**
RATIONALE: The diagnosis-related group is an important component of Medicare for reimbursement of health care costs. The disease conditions and procedures are classified into various groups. The reimbursement of cost is done according to the particular group in which the diagnosis is included, regardless of the actual cost incurred. Managed care organizations are private insurers with an objective to provide cost-effective health care. They carefully plan and closely supervise the distribution of their clients' health care services.

9. **Answer: c**
RATIONALE: Cystic fibrosis is a heredity disorder and is present at birth. The disorder can be genetically predicted and can be transferred from parents to children through genes. Atrial septal defect is a congenital disorder and is present at birth, but cannot be transferred from one generation to the other. Myositis and macular edema are acquired diseases.

10. **Answer: a**
    RATIONALE: Polydactyly is the result of faulty development of the embryo and not faulty gene transfer. Congenital disorders are present at birth but are not genetically predicted. This disorder cannot be transferred from one generation to the other. It may be the result of maternal exposure to toxins and infectious agents.

11. **Answer: c**
    RATIONALE: Mortality is a measure of death resulting from a particular disease or condition. In this case, neonatal mortality indicates the number of neonatal deaths per 1,000 live births of neonates. The other parameters are not standard for comparison.

12. **Answer: b**
    RATIONALE: Physiotherapy is an example of extended care. It does not involve acute care and is not compulsorily done on the hospital premises. The hospital providing surgical facilities is a tertiary care center. After being discharged from tertiary care, the client joins a physiotherapy unit for extended care.

13. **Answer: a**
    RATIONALE: The scenario is an example of team nursing. In team nursing, a team leader assigns the nursing task and supervises the care given. It is different from functional nursing during which a nurse is responsible only for the assigned task. It is also different from primary nursing because there are many nursing staff members responsible for client care. Nurse-managed care has a nurse manager responsible for assessing and planning client care according to the outcomes predicted.

14. **Answer: b**
    RATIONALE: The hospital makes the profit. The client is insured through a capitation scheme, which provides a preset fee per member to the health care provider regardless of whether the member requires services. If a client is discharged earlier, the hospital keeps the difference.

15. **Answer: c**
    RATIONALE: The client is referred to the medical specialist as a secondary level of health care. The family physician represents the primary care level; they are the first contact of the client with the health service. If, after the initial examination, the physician believes that the client requires specialist care, they can refer clients to specialized care facilities. These facilities are a secondary level of health care.

16. **Answer: b**
    RATIONALE: Mortality is a measure of deaths resulting from any disease or condition. Statistics note that 440,000 people die from cigarette smoking–attributable illness, which indicates death resulting from smoking-related illnesses; therefore, this is a measure of mortality. Lung cancer

accounting for 1% of all cigarette smoking–attributable illnesses indicates morbidity of illnesses as a result of cigarette smoking. The statement that cigarette smoking results in 5.6 million potential lives lost per year demonstrates the effect of smoking on health. A loss of $75 billion in direct medical costs results from smoking-attributable illnesses, representing a health care cost burden.

17. **Answers: b, c, d, a**
    RATIONALE: Pain in the wound is the first priority of nursing care. The first step should be alleviation of pain and closing the open wound to prevent infection. The second step should be to calm the client and alleviate their anxiety and apprehension related to the treatment. The client may avoid social interactions as a result of burns on the face; therefore, the client's social needs should be met. The need of self-esteem is also not met in the client because they feel dependent on others.

18. **Answers: b, c, e**
    RATIONALE: Influenza, measles, and conjunctivitis are acute disorders and have a short duration. Diabetes mellitus and hypertension are chronic diseases. The onset of these diseases is gradual, and the course of the disease runs longer, sometimes for one's whole life.

19. **Answer: c**
    RATIONALE: The team leader is responsible for overall care provided to clients in the nursing unit. The team leader assigns tasks, supervises the nursing staff, and evaluates the care provided by them. The team leader helps maintain a team spirit to provide efficient nursing care. The leader may assist other nursing staff in their assigned tasks, but the nurse is responsible for overall care.

20. **Answer: c**
    RATIONALE: The conference is the most important part of team nursing. Conferences may cover a variety of subjects, but are planned with certain goals in mind, such as determining the best approaches to each client's health problems, increasing team members' knowledge, and promoting a cooperative spirit among nursing personnel.

SECTION IV: REVIEWING WHAT YOU HAVE LEARNED

Activity H
1. Hereditary
2. Secondary

Activity I
1. True
2. True

Activity J
1. Holism
2. Sequela
3. Remission

Activity K

1. c   **2.** a   **3.** d   **4.** b

Activity L

1. The World Health Organization (WHO) defines health as "a state of complete physical, mental, and social well-being, not merely the absence of disease or infirmity."
2. The five common management patterns that nurses use to administer client care are functional nursing, case method, team nursing, primary nursing, and nurse-managed care.

SECTION V: APPLYING YOUR KNOWLEDGE

Activity M

1. In team nursing, nursing personnel with various levels of expertise divide clients into groups and complete their care together. Regular conferences cover various subjects but are planned with specific goals, such as determining the best approaches to each client's health problems, increasing team members' knowledge, and promoting a cooperative spirit among nursing personnel.
2. The team leader organizes and directs the team providing nursing care. They usually assign and supervise the care that other team members provide for the client; occasionally, the team leader may also assist with client care. All team members report the outcomes of care to the team leader, who evaluates if the goals of client care are met.

SECTION VI: GETTING READY FOR NCLEX

Activity N

1. **Answer: a**
   RATIONALE: The primary nursing pattern is being used in this case. With the functional nursing pattern, each nurse on a client unit is assigned specific tasks, such as giving medications or performing dressing changes, for all clients. With the case method, one nurse manages all care for a client or group of clients for a designated period. In nurse-managed care, a nurse manager plans the nursing care of clients based on their type of case or medical diagnosis.
2. **Answer: c**
   RATIONALE: Nurse-managed care is being used in this case. In primary nursing, the admitting nurse assumes responsibility for planning client care and evaluating the client's progress until discharge. With the functional nursing pattern, each nurse on a client unit is assigned specific tasks, such as giving medications or performing dressing changes, for all clients. With the case method, one nurse manages all care for a client or group of clients for a designated period.

CHAPTER 5

SECTION I: ASSESSING YOUR UNDERSTANDING

Activity A

1. Neurotransmitters
2. Postsynaptic
3. Neuropeptide
4. Serotonin
5. Norepinephrine
6. Spinal cord
7. Cortex
8. Subcortex
9. Hypothalamus
10. Pituitary

Activity B

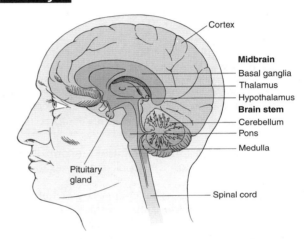

1. The figure shows the central nervous system.
2. The components of the central nervous system are the cortex, the subcortex, and the reticular activating system (RAS). The cortex is considered the higher functioning portion of the brain. It enables people to think abstractly, use and understand language, accumulate and store memories, and make decisions about information received. The cortex also influences other primitive areas of the brain located in the subcortex.

   The subcortical structures are primarily responsible for regulating and maintaining physiologic activities that promote survival. Examples include regulation of breathing, heart contraction, blood pressure, body temperature, sleep, appetite, and stimulation and inhibition of hormone production.

   The RAS, an area of the brain through which a network of nerves passes, is the communication link between the body and mind. Information about a person's internal and external environment is funneled through the RAS to the cortex on both conscious and unconscious levels. The cortex processes the information and generates behavioral and physiologic responses via activation by the hypothalamus.

Activity C
1. b   **2.** c   **3.** a

Activity D

Question 1.

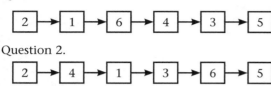

Question 2.

2 → 4 → 1 → 3 → 6 → 5

Activity E

1.

Sympathetic Nervous System	Parasympathetic Nervous System
The sympathetic nervous system prepares the body for fight or flight when a situation occurs that the mind perceives as dangerous.	The parasympathetic nervous system restores equilibrium after danger is no longer apparent.
It accelerates the physiologic functions that ensure survival through enhanced strength or rapid escape.	It inhibits the physiologic stimulation created by the sympathetic nervous system.
An example in which the sympathetic nervous system takes precedence is the increase of blood pressure and heartbeat when a person is faced with a dangerous situation.	An example in which the parasympathetic nervous system takes precedence is when animals being chased by predators simulate the appearance of death to save their lives.

2. A feedback loop is the mechanism for controlling hormone production. Feedback can be negative or positive.

3. When internal or external changes overwhelm homeostatic adaptation, stress results. Stress is the physiologic and behavioral responses to disequilibrium. It has physical, emotional, and cognitive effects.

4. The three stages of stress are the alarm stage, the stage of resistance, and, in some cases, stage of exhaustion. During the alarm stage, at the immediate onset of a stress response, storage vesicles within the sympathetic nervous system neurons rapidly release norepinephrine. Shortly thereafter, the adrenal glands secrete additional norepinephrine and epinephrine. These stimulating neurotransmitters and neurohormones prepare the person for a fight-or-flight response. Almost simultaneously, there is a hypothalamic–pituitary–adrenal cascade of hormones. The hypothalamus releases corticotropin-releasing factor (CRF), which triggers the pituitary gland to secrete adrenocorticotropic hormone (ACTH). The result is the release of cortisol, a stress hormone, from the adrenal cortex. Cortisol plays various important roles in responding to a stressor, such as raising blood glucose and inhibiting insulin to meet increased energy requirements.

5. Coping strategies are stress-reducing activities selected consciously that help people deal with stress-provoking events or situations. They can be therapeutic and nontherapeutic. Therapeutic coping strategies usually help the person acquire insight, gain confidence to confront reality, and develop emotional maturity. Examples of coping strategies include seeking professional assistance in a crisis, using problem-solving techniques, demonstrating assertive behavior, practicing progressive relaxation, and turning to a comforting other or higher power. Maladaptation results when people use nontherapeutic coping strategies such as mind- and mood-altering substances, hostility and aggression, excessive sleep, avoidance of conflict, and abandonment of social activities.

6. Stress-related illness can be prevented or minimized at three levels. Primary prevention involves eliminating the potential for illness before it occurs. An example is teaching principles of nutrition and methods to maintain normal weight and blood pressure to adolescents. Secondary prevention includes screening for risk factors and providing a means for early diagnosis of disease. An example is regularly measuring the blood pressure of a client with a family history of hypertension. Tertiary prevention minimizes the consequences of a disorder through aggressive rehabilitation or appropriate management of the disease. An example is frequently turning, positioning, and exercising a client who has had a stroke to help restore functional ability.

SECTION II: APPLYING YOUR KNOWLEDGE

Activity F

1. The nurse should implement stress-reduction and management techniques and promote the client's physiologic adaptive responses.

2. The nurse should ensure that the client understands all stress-related health problems. The nurse should take care when communicating with the client and explain the principles of nutrition and methods to maintain normal weight and blood pressure to the client. The nurse should also regularly measure the blood glucose of the client if they have a family history of hypertension.

SECTION III: PRACTICING FOR NCLEX

Activity G

1. Answer: b
   RATIONALE: The primary level of stress prevention involves eliminating the potential for illness before it occurs. The nurse, in this case, teaches the client the methods to maintain normal blood pressure to rule out the probability of disease. Monitoring the client's blood pressure and prescribing diet, exercise, and medicines are techniques for secondary and tertiary prevention.

2. Answer: a
   RATIONALE: Alternative thinking techniques facilitate a change in a person's perceptions from negative to positive thinking and help reframe a situation. Reframing helps a person to analyze a stressful situation from various perspectives and ultimately conclude that the situation is not as bad as it once seemed. Alternative behavior helps a person take actions to control a stressful situation. Alternative lifestyles and adaptive activities help a person adopt different lifestyles and take part in activities such as exercise to come out of a stressful situation.

3. Answer: a
   RATIONALE: The secondary level of stress prevention includes screening for risk factors and providing a means for early diagnosis of disease. The nurse, in this case, monitors the client's blood pressure regularly to diagnose the disease early. Teaching the client the methods to maintain normal blood pressure, to rule out the probability of disease, is primary prevention. Prescribing diet, exercise, and medicines is a technique for tertiary prevention.

4. Answer: a
   RATIONALE: The client is resorting to nontherapeutic coping strategies to deal with their stress. This has resulted in maladaptation, and the client's mood is altering. Therapeutic coping strategies usually help a person to acquire insight and maturity. Coping mechanisms are unconscious tactics to defend the ego.

5. Answer: b
   RATIONALE: Alternative behavior helps a person take actions to control a stressful situation. The nurse advises the client to adopt an alternative behavior by interacting with supportive people and taking control of the situation. Alternative lifestyles and adaptive activities help a person adopt different lifestyles and take part in activities such as exercise to come out of a stressful situation. Alternative thinking techniques facilitate a change in a person's perceptions, from negative to positive thinking, and helps reframe a situation.

6. Answer: b
   RATIONALE: Serotonin stabilizes mood, induces sleep, and regulates temperature. This would help the client with insomnia. Norepinephrine heightens arousal and increases energy, dopamine promotes coordinated movement, and endorphins help relieve pain.

7. Answer: a
   RATIONALE: Body massages trigger the release of endorphins, which help relieve pain and promote a sense of well-being. The release of acetylcholine promotes coordinated movement, whereas γ-aminobutyric acid inhibits the excitatory neurotransmitters. Substance P, when released, transmits the pain sensation in the body.

8. Answer: c
   RATIONALE: The nurse should advise the client to adopt alternative behavior and be more assertive at the workplace. Changing their job or accepting their current situation will not help them cope with stress. Only changing behavior will help cope with all problematic situations. The client could undergo therapy, but that would not reduce the stress immediately.

9. Answer: b
   RATIONALE: The boy is in a state of alarm after the death of his mother, which explains the high blood pressure and irregular heartbeat. The stages of resistance and exhaustion are the next stages of stress, during which the body tries to cope with stress and reach a stage of homeostasis. The boy has yet to reach homeostasis at this point.

10. Answer: a
   RATIONALE: The greatest stressor for a person is the death of a spouse. Therapeutic intervention would be most effective for this client because the client needs emotional support. In the other situations, the client can adapt to new surroundings and try to relieve stress by making changes in their living arrangements, getting a new job, and improving their financial situation.

11. Answer: c
   RATIONALE: Because the senior client is lonely after losing their spouse, they have gone into depression as a result of loneliness. By advising them to get a pet for company and listening to uplifting music, the nurse is advising the client to adopt an

alternative lifestyle. If the nurse needed to change the client's perception of the situation, they would have advised an alternative way of thinking. If they wanted the client to take control of their life, then they would have advised the client to alter behavior or perform adaptive activities.

12. Answer: d
RATIONALE: The first task that the nurse needs to do is to understand why the client is stressed. Only after analyzing the causes for stress should the nurse attempt to treat the client by administering medicines and implementing therapy.

13. Answer: a
RATIONALE: The client has been in a state of stress for a long time and has already gone through the alarm and resistance stages of stress. The client is now in the exhaustion stage of stress, during which the effects of stress-related neurohormones suppress the immune system. However, the client is not in a state of homeostasis or balance.

14. Answers: a, c, d
RATIONALE: Stress-reduction and management techniques include undergoing therapies, adopting alternative behavior and lifestyles, and stimulating the senses. All these help in reducing stress. Advising the client to accept their duties and situations and to take medication to counter stress would not help the client to reduce their stress levels.

15. Answers: c, b, e, a, d
RATIONALE: The first task that the nurse needs to perform is to identify the factors that are causing stress to the client. The nurse then needs to identify how the client responds to the stress and try to reduce or eliminate the stressors. The nurse

should then prevent other stressors and advise the client to follow stress-reduction and stress management techniques.

16. Answers: b, c, a, e, d
RATIONALE: At the immediate onset of the alarm stage of stress, the storage vesicles within the sympathetic nervous system neurons rapidly release norepinephrine. Shortly thereafter, the adrenal glands secrete additional norepinephrine and epinephrine. These stimulating neurotransmitters and neurohormones prepare the person for a fight-or-flight response. Almost simultaneously, the hypothalamus releases corticotropin-releasing factor, which triggers the pituitary gland to secrete adrenocorticotropic hormone. The result is the release of cortisol, a stress hormone, from the adrenal cortex.

SECTION IV: REVIEWING WHAT YOU HAVE LEARNED

Activity H
1. Stress
2. Serotonin

Activity I
1. False. Coping strategies are stress-reduction activities selected consciously to help people deal with challenges; coping mechanisms are unconscious tactics for defending the psyche.
2. True

Activity J
1. Homeostasis
2. Endorphins

Activity K

	Sympathetic Nervous System	Parasympathetic Nervous System
1. Function	It prepares the body for fight or flight when the mind perceives a dangerous situation.	It restores equilibrium after danger is no longer apparent.
2. Effect on Physiologic Functions	It accelerates the physiologic functions that ensure survival through enhanced strength or ability for rapid escape.	It inhibits the physiologic stimulation created by the sympathetic nervous system; however, it does not produce an opposite reaction for every sympathetic effect.
3. Example	• It causes the pupils to dilate. • It increases heart rate.	• It causes the pupils to constrict. • It decreases heart rate.

Activity L

1. See Figure 5-2 in your textbook.

Activity M

1. Homeostasis is a relatively stable state of physiologic equilibrium that the body maintains by adjusting and readjusting its responses to disruptions in the internal and external environment. Disruptions that affect homeostasis may be physiologic, psychological, social, or spiritual.
2. Factors that affect stress response include intensity of the stressor, number of stressors, duration of the stressor, physical health status, life experience, coping strategies, social support, personal beliefs, and attitudes and values.

Activity N

1. When a client is experiencing stress, the nurse can (1) identify the stressors; (2) assess the client's response to stress; (3) eliminate or reduce the stressors; (4) prevent additional stressors; (5) promote the client's physiologic adaptive responses; (6) support the client's psychological coping strategies; (7) assist in maintaining a network of social support; and (8) implement stress-reduction and stress management techniques.
2. When caring for a client scheduled for surgery who is experiencing stress, the nurse can provide adequate explanations in understandable language. They can demonstrate confidence and expertise when providing care and remain calm during crises. The nurse should respond promptly to the client's signal for assistance and encourage family interaction.

Activity O

There are no definite answers to this activity. Students may choose to discuss their thoughts with peers or instructors.

SECTION V: GETTING READY FOR NCLEX

Activity P

1. **Answer: d**
   RATIONALE: The client is displaying the denial coping mechanism by rejecting information provided by the nurse. A person using displacement takes out anger on someone or something else. A person using projection attributes unacceptable feelings or attitudes in him or herself onto others. Sublimation involves channeling one's energies into an acceptable alternative, such as turning to sports broadcasting when an athletic career is not realistic.
2. **Answer: c**
   RATIONALE: Per the social readjustment rating scale, experiencing a personal injury contributes the most to stress. Contributors in order of increasing severity thereafter are change in financial state, change to a different line of work, and change in living conditions.

CHAPTER 6

SECTION I: ASSESSING YOUR UNDERSTANDING

Activity A

1. Minority
2. Mediterranean
3. Subcultures
4. Generalization
5. Ethnocentrism
6. Lactase
7. Folk
8. Shaman
9. Hyperpigmentation
10. Bilingualism

Activity B

1. The figure shows a keloid (irregular, elevated, thick scars).
2. Keloids (irregular, elevated, thick scars) are common among dark-skinned people. They are thought to form from a genetic tendency to produce excessive transforming growth factor-β, a substance that promotes fibroblast proliferation during tissue repair.

Activity C

1. c   **2.** d   **3.** b   **4.** a

Activity D

1. Culture refers to the values, beliefs, and practices of a particular group. It incorporates the attitudes and customs learned through socialization with others. It includes, but is not limited to, language, communication style, traditions, religion, art, music, dress, health beliefs, and health practices. A group's culture is passed from one generation to the next.
2. The term "minority" is used when referring to those people who, collectively, differ from the dominant group in terms of cultural characteristics such as language, physical characteristics like skin color, or both. Minority does not necessarily imply that there are fewer group members in comparison with others in the society. Rather, it refers to the group's status in regard to power and control.
3. Generalization is the supposition that a person shares cultural characteristics with others of a similar background. Generalization is different from stereotyping. Stereotyping is a negative attitude that prevents a person from seeing and treating another person as unique, whereas generalizing suggests possible commonalities that may or may not be individually valid. Assuming that all people who affiliate themselves with a particular group behave alike or hold the same beliefs is always incorrect. Diversity exists even within cultural groups.
4. Ethnocentrism, the belief that one's own ethnicity is superior to all others, also interferes with intercultural relationships. Ethnocentrism is manifested

by treating anyone "different" as deviant and un-desirable. This form of cultural intolerance was the basis for the Holocaust, during which the Nazis attempted to carry out genocide, the planned ex-tinction of an entire ethnic group. Ethnocentrism continues to play a role in the ethnic rivalries be-tween pro-Russian separatists in Ukraine; Arabs and Jews in the Middle East; the Boko Haram in Nige-ria; Islamic State of Iraq and Syria (ISIS) militants in the Middle East; and other regions where culturally diverse groups live in close proximity. Similar con-flicts also occur among U.S. ethnic groups.

5. There are four major subcultures that exist in the United States. In addition to Anglo-Americans, there are African Americans, Latinos, Asian Amer-icans, and Native Americans. The term "African Americans" is used to identify those whose an-cestral origin is Africa. It is sometimes used in-terchangeably with Black Americans. Latinos are sometimes referred to as Hispanics, a term coined by the U.S. Census Bureau, or Chicanos when speaking of people from Mexico. Asian Americans are those who come from China, Japan, Korea, the Philippines, Thailand, Cambodia, Laos, and Viet-nam; these make up the third subculture. Native Americans are from Indian nations found in North America, including the Eskimos and Aleuts. They include approximately 2.3 million American Indi-ans and Alaskan natives belonging to 566 federally recognized tribes in the United States.

SECTION II: APPLYING YOUR KNOWLEDGE

Activity E

1. The nurse should keep the following points in mind while interviewing the client:
   - Native Americans tend to be private and may hesitate to share personal information with strangers. They may interpret questioning as prying or meddling.
   - The nurse should be client when awaiting an an-swer and listen carefully because people of this culture may consider impatience disrespectful.
   - Because Native Americans traditionally pre-served their heritage through oral rather than written history, they may be skeptical of nurses who write down what they say. If possible, the nurse should write notes after, rather than during, the interview.
   - Native Americans believe that lingering eye contact is an invasion of privacy or a sign of disrespect.
2. The nurse can demonstrate culturally sensi-tive nursing care by applying the following recommendations:
   - Learn to speak a second language.
   - Use culturally sensitive techniques to improve interactions such as sitting in the client's com-fort zone and making appropriate eye contact.

- Become familiar with physical differences among ethnic groups.
- Perform physical assessments, especially of the skin, using techniques that provide accurate data.
- Learn or ask clients about cultural beliefs con-cerning health, illness, and techniques for healing.
- Consult the client on ways to solve health problems.
- Never verbally or nonverbally ridicule a cultural belief or practice.
- Integrate helpful or harmless cultural practices within the plan of care.
- Modify or gradually change unsafe practices.
- Avoid removing religious medals or clothes that hold symbolic meaning for the client. If they must be removed, keep them safe and replace them as soon as possible.
- Provide customarily eaten food.
- Advocate routine screening for diseases to which clients are genetically or culturally prone.
- Facilitate rituals by a person the client identifies as a healer within their belief system.
- Apologize if cultural traditions or beliefs are violated.

SECTION III: PRACTICING FOR NCLEX

Activity F

1. **Answer: b**
   RATIONALE: While interviewing the Latino client, the nurse should go slowly when asking questions because many Latinos have difficulty with English, and they may be embarrassed to stop the nurse and ask them to repeat themselves. The nurse may sit close to the client if the client is comfortable with it. The nurse should not use too much medical terminology because the client may have problems understanding it. Latino men may be poor at emotionally expressing themselves be-cause of their cultural beliefs.
2. **Answer: c**
   RATIONALE: Keeping in mind that Asian Amer-icans feel threatened by physical closeness, the nurse should explain to the client the purpose of the care and physical closeness, which should not be mistaken as a threat. The nurse should not leave the client if the client feels uneasy. Leaving the room without any explanation would probably make the client feel more uneasy. The nurse should not instruct the client to feed themselves because they are not capable of doing it alone.
3. **Answer: d**
   RATIONALE: The nurse should ask the client to use nondairy creamers, which are lactose free, in-stead of cream. The nurse could ask the client to drink Lactaid because lactose is preconverted into other absorbable sugars in this product. The nurse should also suggest the client use kosher food, which can be identified by the word "pareve" on

the label. The client should avoid having milk, dairy products, and packaged food such as bread, cereals, puddings, chocolate, and caramels that have milk as one of the ingredients in it.

4. **Answer: b**
   RATIONALE: The nurse should consider it normal in a dark-skinned person. The brown discoloration is the result of shedding of the dead skin. The client does not need to be bathed again. It is not a sign of poor hygiene; therefore, educating the client about personal hygiene is not appropriate. Brown discoloration is not a sign of a disease condition.

5. **Answer: d**
   RATIONALE: The nurse should consider the dark-blue spots on the lower back of the child normal in this ethnicity. These spots are called Mongolian spots and are hyperpigmented areas on the lower back of the infant. Informing the police is not appropriate because the spots are not a sign of injury or abuse. They also do not need to be shown to the physician. Mongolian spots will not produce pain when pressure is applied.

6. **Answer: a**
   RATIONALE: The symptoms experienced by the client indicate a lactase deficiency. A lactase deficiency causes intolerance to dairy products. Glucose-6-phosphate dehydrogenase (G-6-PD) is an enzyme that helps red blood cells to metabolize glucose. When a person consumes alcohol, a process of chemical reactions involving enzymes, one of which is ADH, eventually breaks down the alcohol into acetic acid and carbon dioxide. The symptoms of the client are not thyroid deficiency.

7. **Answer: c**
   RATIONALE: The nurse should consider keloids normal in dark-skinned people. Keloids are irregular, elevated, thick scars found commonly among dark-skinned clients. They are thought to form from a genetic tendency to produce excessive transforming growth factor-β, a substance that promotes fibroblast proliferation during tissue repair. The nurse should not consider it pathologic or inform the physician about it. Ordering a biochemical test is not relevant in this case.

8. **Answers: a, b, e**
   RATIONALE: Nurses who are men should provide an explanation to the client to relieve the client's anxiety. The nurse may seek permission from the client's husband and allow him to be present in the room during the procedure. This act may alleviate the insecurity of the client and her husband. Keeping a woman attendant in the room may not be liked by the client because she may not want to expose her body in front of others. Instructing the husband to do the procedure is not an appropriate option because it does not ensure the correctness of the procedure.

9. **Answers: a, b, c**
   RATIONALE: African American clients have been victims of discrimination. Therefore, to make the client comfortable the nurse should address clients by their last names and follow up thoroughly with requests. The nurse should respect the client's privacy and not maintain eye contact during communication. African Americans believe that lingering eye contact is an invasion of privacy or a sign of disrespect. The nurse should ask open-ended rather than direct questions until trust has been established with the client.

10. **Answers: b, c, d**
    RATIONALE: To comb the curly hair of an African American client, the nurse should use a wide-toothed comb or pick. The nurse should apply a moisturizing cream or gel or can wet the hair with water before combing. It makes combing easy and the hair more manageable. However, asking the client to assist the nurse to comb their hair or letting the hair remain in its current state is unethical on the nurse's part.

SECTION IV: REVIEWING WHAT YOU HAVE LEARNED

Activity G

1. Ethnicity
2. Generalization

Activity H

1. True
2. True

Activity I

1. Lactase
2. Alcohol dehydrogenase (ADH)

Activity J

1. b   2. c   3. d   4. a

Activity K

Transcultural nursing care involves providing nursing care within the context of another's culture. Nurses must become skilled at managing language differences, understanding biologic and physiologic variations, promoting health teaching that will reduce prevalent diseases that are common within a particular cultural group, and respecting alternative health beliefs or health practices to provide culturally sensitive care.

SECTION V: APPLYING YOUR KNOWLEDGE

Activity L

1. Using untrained interpreters, volunteers, or family increases the risk for undermining the client's confidentiality and privacy. It may violate family roles and boundaries. It also may increase the potential for modifying, condensing, omitting, or adding information or projecting the interpreter's own values during communication between client and health care provider.
2. These areas contain the least pigmentation and are less likely to be tanned.

Activity M

1. The nurse assessing a client who is not fluent in English can:
   - speak slowly, not loudly, using simple words and short sentences.
   - avoid using technical terms, slang, or phrases with a double meaning.
   - ask direct questions to avoid elaborate explanations.
   - repeat the question if the client appears confused.
   - give the client sufficient time to respond.
2. The process of interpreting what has been said in English and then converting the response from the native language back to English requires extra time. Moreover, the nurse may communicate impatience nonverbally, which will increase the client's frustration.

Activity N

1. During assessment the nurse should obtain data that may be unique to the client's culture. These findings will enable the nurse to provide culturally sensitive care. Areas to cover are as follows:
   - Language and communication style
   - Hygiene practices, including feelings about modesty and accepting help from others
   - Special clothing or ornamentation
   - Religion and religious practices
   - Rituals surrounding birth, illness, and death
   - Family and gender roles including child-rearing practices and kinship with older adults
   - Proper forms of greeting and showing respect
   - Food habits and dietary restrictions
   - Methods for making decisions
   - Health beliefs and medical practices
2. The nurse is likely to find variations in language and communication, eye contact, space and distance, touch, emotional expression, dietary customs and restrictions, time, and beliefs about the causes of or approaches to treating illnesses.
3. There are no definite answers to this activity. Students may choose to discuss their thoughts with peers or instructors.

SECTION VI: GETTING READY FOR NCLEX

Activity O

1. **Answer: d**
   RATIONALE: Asian American clients are likely to believe that lingering eye contact is an invasion of privacy or a sign of disrespect; hence, it would be appropriate for the nurse to avoid lingering eye contact with the client. Some Asians consider the head to be a sacred part of the body and may be offended by the nurse touching the client's head gently. The nurse should not provide personal care in the presence of a family member because this is a violation of privacy. The client would likely not consider it offensive if the nurse gently touches the hand to convey reassurance or emotional support.

2. **Answer: a**
   RATIONALE: A skilled interpreter explains their role to the client, which helps the client to speak freely and explain problems. A skilled interpreter does not express views on the client's statement. The interpreter should maintain confidentiality and not inform the client's family about the client's condition. The interpreter should attempt to preserve the emphasis and emotions that the nurse and client express instead of simply translating, which will help to convey the essence of the conversation.

CHAPTER 7

SECTION I: ASSESSING YOUR UNDERSTANDING

Activity A

1. Relationship
2. Empathy
3. Collaboration
4. Delegator
5. Therapeutic
6. Introductory
7. Nonverbal
8. Paralanguage
9. Active listening
10. Terminating

Activity B

1. Therapeutic verbal communication refers to using words and gestures to accomplish a particular objective. It is extremely important, especially when the nurse is exploring problems with the client or encouraging expression of feelings.
2. Active listening is as important during communication as speaking. Giving attention to what clients say provides a stimulus for meaningful interaction. It is important to avoid giving signals that indicate boredom, impatience, or the pretense of listening. For example, looking out a window or interrupting is a sign of disinterest. When communicating with most people, it is best to position oneself at the person's level and make frequent eye contact unless their culture dictates otherwise.

Activity C

1. b   2. e   3. d   4. c   5. a

Activity D

| 1 | → | 4 | → | 3 | → | 2 |

Activity E

1. In providing effective care to the client, the nurse performs four basic roles: caregiver, educator, collaborator, and delegator. A caregiver is one who performs health-related activities that a sick person cannot perform independently. Caregivers provide physical and emotional services to restore or maintain functional independence. Being an educator is a necessity in today's complex health care arena. Nurses provide health teaching pertinent to each client's needs and knowledge base. The nurse also acts as a collaborator. The most obvious example of collaboration occurs between the nurse responsible for managing care and those to whom they delegate care. Before the nurse performs the role of delegator, they must know what tasks are legal and appropriate for particular health care workers to perform.

2. The nurse–client relationship can also be called a therapeutic relationship because the desired outcome of the association is almost always moving toward restored health. A therapeutic relationship is client centered, with a focus on goal achievement. It is also time limited; the relationship ends when goals are achieved.

3. Nurse–client relationships are ordinarily brief. They begin when people seek services that will maintain or restore health, or prevent disease. They end when clients can achieve their health-related goals independently. This type of relationship generally is described as having three phases: introductory, working, and terminating.

4. Many factors affect the ability to communicate by speech or in writing. Examples include the following:
   • Attention and concentration
   • Language compatibility
   • Verbal skills
   • Hearing and visual acuity
   • Motor functions involving the throat, tongue, and teeth
   • Sensory distractions
   • Interpersonal attitudes
   • Literacy
   • Cultural similarities

5. Nonverbal communication is the exchange of information without using words. It involves what is not said. The manner in which a person conveys verbal information affects its meaning. A person has less control over nonverbal than over verbal communication. Words can be chosen with care, but a facial expression is harder to control. As a result, people often communicate messages more accurately through nonverbal communication.

SECTION II: APPLYING YOUR KNOWLEDGE

Activity F

1. The client is grieving the loss of their limb and is emotionally unstable. At this stage, the best nursing response is to allow the client to express their emotions. It is never appropriate to probe and pry; rather, it may be advantageous to wait and be patient. If the client is angry and crying, allow the client to display their feelings without fear of retaliation or censure; this contributes to a therapeutic relationship. It is not unusual for reticent clients to share their feelings and concerns after they conclude that the nurse is sincere and trustworthy.

2. The nurse should help the client deal with the loss of their limb. The nurse may introduce them to other clients who have lost limbs to diabetes and are still optimistic about life (support groups). The nurse could show the client various kinds of prostheses if they wish to have one.

SECTION III: PRACTICING FOR NCLEX

Activity G

1. **Answer: b**
   RATIONALE: A client who is recovering from a cerebrovascular accident has many limitations of activity and resultant dependency, which could make the client angry and irritable. The nurse should use supportive statements to keep the client going. Ignoring the client's behavior may be disregarding their feelings. Increasing family visits likewise may not be a good idea because the family is also grieving and their visits would again demotivate the client. It is nontherapeutic to boast about the nurse's contribution.

2. **Answer: d**
   RATIONALE: The nurse should ask the client if they are feeling tired and frustrated with the recovery from surgery. The nurse should show empathy toward the client and encourage them to verbalize their feelings. It helps the client to express their feelings, which leads to problem-solving. The nurse should not show disapproval by telling them that they would keep on vomiting if they do not allow insertion of the tube. By suggesting a call to the physician, the nurse appears to be defensive, which blocks therapeutic communication. Telling the client that they would feel better with a nasogastric tube is giving false reassurance. All these are barriers to effective communication.

3. **Answer: c**
   RATIONALE: The nurse uses therapeutic communication to encourage the client to express their feelings. The nurse listens to the client and uses clarifying and focusing to assist the client in expressing feelings. The nurse should not give false reassurance by stating that they may improve with surgery. Additionally, the nurse should not try to relate the client's condition to another client's condition. By suggesting calling the physician, the nurse seems to be defensive, which blocks therapeutic communication.

4. **Answer: a**
   RATIONALE: Asking the parents to first read the pamphlet and then ask questions if they have any

doubts would be the most appropriate response because it enables the parents to become informed and then make their decision. The nurse should provide appropriate materials and answer their questions. The nurse should not give any personal opinion by saying that the physician is the best person to help or describing their own experience.

5. **Answer: c**
   RATIONALE: The nurse should address the parents' fears and encourage them to verbalize their feelings of anxiety. Telling the parents about the baby's condition may generate more anxiety in the parents. Also, talking about the highly specialized equipment in the nursing unit is inappropriate and may block further communication. Finally, the nurse should not generalize by saying that the condition is common in babies.

6. **Answer: d**
   RATIONALE: The nurse should gain the group's confidence by conveying the rule of confidentiality, which helps build a trusting relationship. Giving a formal introduction may not generate interest in the group. Filling out a survey questionnaire at the end of the session would not be an incentive for the group to attend the session. Telling the group that they may share their experience will indicate that there is no confidentiality of the discussion and may not encourage students to participate.

7. **Answer: b**
   RATIONALE: The nurse's response should reflect the client's feelings to provide them insight to their condition. For this, the nurse asks open-ended questions to encourage the client to explain and explore their feelings. Reflection is one of the therapeutic communication techniques. The nurse should try to divert the client's attention from the family. The nurse should not be judgmental and tell the client that they are pessimistic; doing so would negatively affect the therapeutic relationship. Asking the client to share their feelings with the family may not be appropriate at this time.

8. **Answer: b**
   RATIONALE: The nurse should ask the client whether they want to speak to their physician. The nurse uses reflection to validate the client's remarks and focus on the client's desire to talk to the physician. The nurse should not get angry at the client because anger is a nontherapeutic response. Telling the client that the physician has placed the client in the nurse's care would reinforce the client's behavior.

9. **Answer: a**
   RATIONALE: The nurse's response should be open-ended so that it gives scope to the client to verbalize and express their feelings. The client may then elaborate on what they said. Telling the client

that they always does right and everything will be good will block the communication and stop the conversation. This would not encourage the client to explore further.

10. **Answer: b**
    RATIONALE: Asking the client what they mean would be the most appropriate way to assess the client's further thoughts. It would be helpful to the client to share their personal thoughts. The nurse should avoid giving false reassurance, which is inappropriate and puts an end to the communication. Also, the nurse should avoid closed-ended questions, which have little role in facilitating communication.

11. **Answer: d**
    RATIONALE: The nurse should encourage the mother to speak by asking open-ended questions and providing an opportunity for the mother to express her feelings. The nurse should avoid giving false reassurance that a seizure will not occur and can be prevented. Telling the mother not to worry may block further communication.

12. **Answer: b**
    RATIONALE: The nurse should explore whether the client feels comfortable talking to the physician. The nurse should not sound accusing or irritated because it may hinder further communications if the nurse disagrees with the client.

13. **Answer: a**
    RATIONALE: The nurse should facilitate communication by asking open-ended questions and encouraging the client to discuss their concerns and feelings. Unnecessary reasoning and complimenting may block communication, thus preventing problem-solving.

14. **Answer: c**
    RATIONALE: By commenting that the client sounds discouraged, the nurse may encourage the client to talk. The nurse uses reflection technique on the client to help them evaluate themselves. The nurse should encourage further expression of emotions. Additionally, the nurse should not give false reassurance. By asking the client what they were thinking, the nurse may sound demanding and the client may not express their feelings. The nurse should avoid statements that devalue the client's concerns.

15. **Answer: b**
    RATIONALE: Asking the client if they are worried that the disease condition would extend into the wedding is the most appropriate statement and encourages the client to express their concerns and feelings. This is an example of therapeutic communication. The nurse should not make promises that cannot be kept. Telling the client that the disease condition could be the result of prewedding tension is correct, but inappropriate at this time.

SECTION IV: REVIEWING WHAT YOU HAVE LEARNED

Activity H

1. Kinesics
2. Paraphrasing

Activity I

1. True
2. False. Therapeutic verbal communication involves the use of words and gestures to accomplish a particular objective.
3. True

Activity J

1. Delegator
2. Caregiver

Activity K

1. c
2. a
3. b

Activity L

1. Task-oriented touch is the personal contact required to perform nursing procedures. Affective touch is personal contact that demonstrates feelings and concern.
2. Factors that affect verbal and written communication include attention and concentration; language compatibility; verbal skills; hearing and visual acuity; motor functions involving the throat, tongue, and teeth; sensory distractions; interpersonal attitudes; literacy; and cultural similarities.

SECTION V: APPLYING YOUR KNOWLEDGE

Activity M

The desired outcome of the association is almost always moving toward restored health. This client-centered relationship focuses on goal achievement.

Activity N

1. The nurse should speak at a lower pitch because hearing loss is generally in higher-pitch ranges. The nurse should rephrase rather than repeat instructions when the client does not understand. They should try to avoid words that begin with "F," "S," "K," and "Sh," because the client may find it difficult to distinguish these sounds. The nurse can use pamphlets or writing pads to supplement verbal instructions.
2. The nurse should explain procedures to the client before performing them and ensure that the client is properly draped or covered. A woman nurse could ask a man staff person to be present during examinations or procedures (and vice versa if the nurse is a man and the client is a woman).
3. Affective touch has different meanings to different people depending on their personal life experiences and cultural background. Nursing

care involves frequent touching; hence, the nurse should be sensitive about how clients may perceive it.

Activity O

There are no definite answers to this activity. Students may choose to discuss their thoughts with peers or instructors.

SECTION VI: GETTING READY FOR NCLEX

Activity P

1. **Answer: b**
   RATIONALE: The nurse should build therapeutic verbal communication by allowing the client to express emotions. The nurse should avoid asking "why" questions because the client may not always have an explanation. Furthermore, the client may not answer truthfully, but may respond just to appease the questioner. The nurse should not ask the client to stop complaining or tell the client to keep calm and take medication; this will not help build a therapeutic nurse–client relationship.
2. **Answer: c**
   RATIONALE: The nurse should maintain a distance of 6 inches to 4 feet (called personal space) when providing client teaching. A distance of 12 or more feet (public space) is maintained when speaking to a gathering of strangers. A distance of 4 to 12 feet (social space) is maintained during group interactions that are not meant to be private. A distance of 6 inches or less (intimate space) is too close for a client's comfort.

CHAPTER 8

SECTION I: ASSESSING YOUR UNDERSTANDING

Activity A

1. Motivation
2. Dietary
3. Functionally
4. Individualized
5. Telehome
6. Learning
7. Informal
8. Age
9. Net
10. Capacity

Activity B

1. The figure describes the cognitive domain. The cognitive domain is a style of processing information by listening or reading facts and descriptions.
2. There are three styles of learning, including the cognitive domain. The other two styles are the affective domain, which is a style of processing that appeals to a person's feelings, beliefs, or values; and

the psychomotor domain, which is a style of processing that focuses on learning by doing.

Activity C

1. c   **2.** a   **3.** b

Activity D

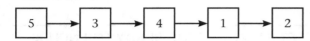

Activity E

1. The four stages of learning are as follows:
   - Recognition of what has been taught
   - Recollection or description of information to others
   - Explanation or application of information
   - Independent use of new learning
2. To implement effective teaching, the nurse should determine the client's
   - Preferred learning style
   - Age and developmental level
   - Capacity to learn
   - Motivation
   - Learning readiness
   - Learning needs
3. Learning styles mean how a person prefers to acquire knowledge. Learning styles fall within three general domains: cognitive, affective, and psychomotor. The cognitive domain is a style of processing information by listening or reading facts and descriptions. The affective domain is a style of processing that appeals to a person's feelings, beliefs, or values. The psychomotor domain is a style of processing that focuses on learning by doing.
4. There are three major categories of teaching learners of different age groups: pedagogy, androgogy, and gerogogy. Pedagogy is the science of teaching children or those with a cognitive ability comparable to children. Androgogy includes the principles of teaching adult learners. Gerogogy includes the techniques that enhance learning among older adults.
5. Although most clients with health problems are in their later years, nurse educators are advised to prepare themselves to teach adults who belong to Generation X, Generation Y, and Generation Z as they age. Generation X refers to those born between 1961 and 1981; Generation Y, millennials, refers to people who were born after 1981 through the latter part of the 20th century; and Generation Z, the Net Generation or "cyberkids," refers to those born at the beginning of the 21st century. In general, Generations X, Y, and Z may share many learning characteristics:
   - They are or will be technologically literate, having grown up with computers, smart phones, and tablet devices.
   - They crave stimulation and quick responses.
   - They expect immediate answers and feedback.
   - They become bored with memorizing information and doing repetitive tasks.
   - They like a variety of instructional methods from which they can choose.
   - They respond best when they find the information to be relevant.
   - They prefer visualizations, simulations, and other methods of participatory learning.
6. Functionally illiterate people possess minimal literacy skills, which means they can sign their name and perform simple mathematical tasks (e.g., make change) but read at or below fifth-grade level. For example, functionally illiterate people are those who cannot comprehend written instructions on prescription bottles and who are less likely to use screening procedures, follow medical regimens, keep appointments, or seek help early during the course of a disease. Functional illiteracy may be the consequence of a learning disability, not a below-average intellectual capacity.

SECTION II: APPLYING YOUR KNOWLEDGE

Activity F

1. Nurses can ask the following questions to assess the learning needs of the client:
   - What does being healthy mean to you?
   - What things in your life interfere with being healthy?
   - What do you not understand as fully as you would like?
   - What activities do you need help with?
   - What do you hope to accomplish before being discharged?
   - How can we help you at this time?
2. Providing the client with adequate support materials, encouraging the client to self-administer the medications, and providing tips to the client for applying knowledge are good practices to be followed to ensure that the health teaching is complete before the discharge of the client.

SECTION III: PRACTICING FOR NCLEX

Activity G

1. **Answer: a**
   RATIONALE: Because the nurse helps the client in self-administration of medications, the client is made to learn a task by performing it. By giving the client a pamphlet to clear nasal debris, or showing how to measure body temperature, or explaining to the client how to use a nebulizer, the nurse is not making the client perform the task to learn the correct way of doing it.
2. **Answer: b**
   RATIONALE: The affective domain is a style of processing that appeals to a person's feelings, beliefs, or values and therefore will be most effective because the client is low on motivation and feels that they cannot be cured. The cognitive domain

is a style of processing information by listening or reading facts and descriptions. The psychomotor domain is a style of processing that focuses on learning by doing. The interpersonal domain is a style of processing that focuses on learning through social relationships. These learning styles will not suit this client.

3. **Answer: a**
   RATIONALE: The cognitive domain is a style of processing information by watching, listening, or reading facts and descriptions and will be most effective for the client who likes watching videos and demonstrations and is an avid reader. The affective, psychomotor, and interpersonal domains would not be the best learning styles for this client. The affective domain is a style of processing that appeals to a person's feelings, beliefs, or values. The psychomotor domain is a style of processing that focuses on learning by doing. The interpersonal domain is a style of processing that focuses on learning through social relationships.

4. **Answer: c**
   RATIONALE: Teaching the client the self-administration of insulin is a part of the psychomotor domain, which is a style of processing that focuses on learning by doing. The cognitive domain is a style of processing information by listening or reading facts and descriptions. The affective domain is a style of processing that appeals to a person's feelings, beliefs, or values. The interpersonal domain is a style of processing that focuses on learning through social relationships.

5. **Answer: b**
   RATIONALE: A child will be more interested if the nurse uses colorful materials while teaching. Showing enthusiasm, varying tone and pitch, and using the client's name frequently are helpful but are more effective for adult clients than children.

6. **Answer: d**
   RATIONALE: Assessing previous learning and literacy abilities is helpful in teaching an adult client. Limiting the teaching session to no longer than 15 to 20 minutes and offering praise and encouragement for accomplishments help in teaching children. Focusing attention is a method that is helpful for older clients.

7. **Answer: b**
   RATIONALE: For an older client, the teaching session should be implemented when the client is most alert and comfortable. Involving the client helps more in the case of child or younger adult learners. Using diagrams is best suited for children; motivation helps a young adult client to learn.

8. **Answer: a**
   RATIONALE: Large print will help the client to read the pamphlets without stressing their eyes. Do not speak in a loud tone unless the client has a hearing impairment. Using flash cards is more helpful to a client with sensory impairment, and

select black print on white paper for clarity instead of red print on white paper.

9. **Answer: c**
   RATIONALE: Learning that builds from simple to complex is the best strategy. Therefore, when teaching an adult client, the nurse should begin from the basic concepts. Collaborating with the client on content and dividing information into manageable amounts are actions to be performed during the planning phase. Determining the client's learning style should be done at the beginning, before implementing the teaching.

10. **Answer: c**
    RATIONALE: It is better to involve the client actively by encouraging feedback and handling of equipment because adult learners prefer active rather than passive learning situations. This takes place when the teaching is implemented. Assessment, planning, and evaluation do not include this involvement.

11. **Answer: b**
    RATIONALE: The affective domain is a style of processing that appeals to a person's feelings, beliefs, or values and contains supporting, accepting, refusing, and defending. The cognitive domain is a style of processing information by listening or reading facts and descriptions. The psychomotor domain is a style of processing that focuses on learning by doing. The interpersonal domain is a style of processing that focuses on learning through social relationships. The client's behavior indicates that they do not fall into any of these learning styles.

12. **Answer: a**
    RATIONALE: The client in this case is a child. Children respond better when they are praised and rewarded for accomplishments. Adults, senior adults, and those of the Net Generation are more concerned about the relevance of information than being rewarded and praised.

13. **Answer: a**
    RATIONALE: In general, these groups share learning characteristics, such as they crave stimulation and quick responses, they become bored with memorizing information and doing repetitive tasks, they like a variety of instructional methods from which they can choose, and they prefer visualizations, simulations, and other methods of participatory learning.

14. **Answer: c**
    RATIONALE: The client is an older adult. In older adults, attention is affected by low energy level, fatigue, and anxiety. Children have a short attention span; however, adults and those of the Net Generation tend to have longer attention spans.

15. **Answer: d**
    RATIONALE: Asking the client about their needs and what they wish to accomplish after the training helps the nurse to assess the learning needs of the client. The preferred learning style, capacity to

learn, and learning readiness cannot be determined by knowing what the client hopes to accomplish at the end of the training.

16. Answers: a, c, d
   RATIONALE: A pedagogic learner lacks experience, prefers rote learning, and responds to competition. An androgogic learner is physically mature, whereas a gerogogic learner is a crisis learner.

17. Answers: a, b, d
   RATIONALE: A gerogogic learner has vast experience, has self-centered learning, and responds to family encouragement. A pedagogic learner needs direction and supervision, and an androgogic learner has long-term retention.

18. Answers: b, e, f
   RATIONALE: An androgogic learner prefers simulation, is physically mature, and has long-term retention. A gerogogic learner has vast experience and responds to family encouragement. A pedagogic learner needs direction and support.

19. Answers: b, e, f
   RATIONALE: Young clients have short attention spans; therefore, they learn better during short sessions instead of long ones. Using colorful materials and offering praise and encouragement for accomplishments will motivate them and keep them interested. Assessing their previous learning, being enthusiastic, varying tone and pitch, and addressing the client frequently will help in teaching adults.

SECTION IV: REVIEWING WHAT YOU HAVE LEARNED

Activity H
1. Affective
2. Readiness

Activity I
1. True.
2. False. People belonging to the Net Generation are technologically literate, having grown up with computers.

Activity J
1. Cognitive domain
2. Pedagogy

Activity K
1. b   2. a   3. d   4. c

Activity L

	Informal Teaching	Formal Teaching
1. Definition	It is unplanned and can occur spontaneously (e.g., at the client's bedside).	It requires a complete plan.
2. Requirements	It involves few people and can be completed quickly.	A student may work with the staff nurse or an instructor in developing a teaching plan. Usually one or more nurses carry out certain specific parts of teaching. It requires time, depending on the complexity of the topic.
3. Disadvantages	Without some organization of time and content, reaching goals and providing adequate information can be jeopardized.	The plan needs ongoing monitoring and possible amendments, which can be time- and labor-intensive.

Activity M

1. The nurse is teaching the client using pamphlets and books.
2. The client may prefer the cognitive domain, which is processing information by listening or by reading facts and descriptions.

Activity N

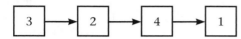

Activity O

1. The nurse should focus on combinations of the following subject areas when teaching a client:
   - Self-administration of medications
   - Directions and practice in using equipment for self-care
   - Dietary instructions
   - Rehabilitation programs
   - Available community resources
   - Plan for medical follow-up
   - Signs of complications and actions to take
2. To implement effective teaching, the nurse must determine the client's preferred learning style, age and developmental level, capacity to learn, motivation, learning readiness, and learning needs.

SECTION V: APPLYING YOUR KNOWLEDGE

Activity P

This combination provides maximum contrast and makes letters more legible.

Activity Q

1. The child may be in postoperative pain, so the nurse needs to first restore the child's comfort and then attend to teaching.
2. The nurse should:
   - Begin the session with a reference to the client's actual experience with which they can connect the new learning.
   - Use aids such as books, manuals, images, and charts to create awareness about the skin as a location where microorganisms reside and that microorganisms can cause infections.
   - Explain the importance of keeping the dressing clean and intact and how to change the dressing. Perform an actual demonstration or use a simulation model of the wound.

Activity R

There are no definite answers to this activity. Students may choose to discuss their thoughts with peers or instructors.

SECTION VI: GETTING READY FOR NCLEX

Activity S

1. **Answer: a**

RATIONALE: The nurse should provide pamphlets in 12- to 16-point type and serif lettering because words are usually more distinct when set in large type. The nurse should avoid glossy paper, which reflects light and can cause a glare that makes reading uncomfortable. A lamp should shine over the client's shoulder rather than from directly above, which tends to diffuse light instead of concentrating it on a small area where the client needs to focus. The nurse should avoid standing in front of a window letting in bright sunlight because it is difficult to look directly into the bright light.

2. **Answers: a, b, e**
RATIONALE: Pedagogic learners are physically immature and lack experience; hence, they need direction, supervision, and immediate feedback. They generally respond to competition. Pedagogic learners think concretely, not abstractly. They learn by rote, not analytically. Androgogic or adult learners are capable of abstract thinking and analytical learning.

CHAPTER 9

SECTION I: ASSESSING YOUR UNDERSTANDING

Activity A

1. Narrative
2. Computerized
3. Military
4. Abnormal
5. HIPAA
6. Reimbursement
7. Focus
8. Checklists
9. Beneficial
10. Encrypted

Activity B

1. The figure shows nurses exchanging reports on their clients during a change of shift.
2. A change-of-shift report is a discussion between a nursing spokesperson from the shift that is ending and personnel coming on duty. It includes a summary of each client's condition and current status of care. This helps the nurse on the next shift to provide uninterrupted care to their clients. To maximize the efficiency of change-of-shift reports, nurses should do the following:
   - Be prompt so that the report can start and end on time.
   - Come prepared with a pen and paper or clipboard.
   - Avoid socializing during reporting sessions.
   - Take notes.
   - Clarify unclear information.
   - Ask questions about pertinent information that may have been omitted.

Activity C

1. b   **2.** c   **3.** e   **4.** a   **5.** d

Activity D

$$ 4 \rightarrow 1 \rightarrow 2 \rightarrow 3 $$

Activity E

1. Medical records are written collections of information about a person's health, the care provided by health practitioners, and the client's progress. They also are referred to as health records or client records. Besides serving as a permanent health record, the medical record of a client provides a means of sharing information among health care workers, thus ensuring client safety and continuity of care. Occasionally, medical records are also used to investigate quality of care in a health agency, to demonstrate compliance with national accreditation standards, to facilitate reimbursement from insurance companies, to facilitate health education and research, and to provide evidence during malpractice lawsuits.

2. The Joint Commission requires the following documentation evidence to justify accreditation:
- Initial assessment and reassessments of physical, psychological, social, environmental, and self-care; education; and discharge planning
- Identification of nursing diagnoses or client needs
- Planned nursing interventions or nursing standards of care for meeting the client's nursing care needs including the education and training provided to the client and fall precaution strategies (The Joint Commission, 2012)
- Nursing care provided
- A client's response to interventions and outcomes of care including pain management, discharge planning activities, and the client's and/or significant other's ability to manage continuing care needs

3. The medical record may consist of various agency-approved paper forms, or the forms may be stored on the hard drive of a computerized record. The hard-copy paper forms are placed in a chart (binder or folder that promotes the orderly collection, storage, and safekeeping of a person's medical records). The paper forms in the chart are color coded or separated by tabbed sheets. Each person who writes in the client's medical record is responsible for the information they record and can be summoned as a witness to testify concerning what has been written. An electronic medical record stored on a computer is accessed by using a password and selecting the desired form from a menu. Electronic records can be printed if a hard copy is desired. All personnel involved in a client's health care contribute to the medical record by charting, recording, or documenting (the process of entering information).

4. When documenting a medical record the following points should be kept in mind:
- Each person who writes in the client's medical record is responsible for the information they record and can be summoned as a witness to testify concerning what has been written.
- Any writing that cannot be clearly read or that is vague, scribbled through, whited out, written over, or erased makes for a poor legal defense. If documentation is substandard, the Joint Commission may withdraw or withhold accreditation.

5. Although the medical record serves as an ongoing source of information about the client's status, nurses use other methods of communication to promote continuity of care and collaboration among the health personnel involved in the client's care. These methods are in written or verbal form. The written form of communication includes the nursing care plan, the nursing Kardex, checklists, and flow sheets. The verbal form includes change-of-shift reports, client assignments, team conferences, rounds, and telephone calls.

SECTION II: APPLYING YOUR KNOWLEDGE

Activity F

1. The nurse can ensure that client data are confidential by the following:
- Assigning an access number and password to authorized personnel who use a computer for health records. These are kept secret and are changed regularly.
- Using automatic save, using a screen saver, or returning to a menu if data have been displayed for a specific period
- Issuing a plastic card or key that authorized personnel use to retrieve information
- Locking out client information except to those who have been authorized through a fingerprint or voice activation device
- Blocking the type of information that personnel in various departments can retrieve. For example, laboratory employees can obtain information from the medical orders, but they cannot view information in the client's personal history.
- Storing the time and location from which the client's record is accessed in case there is an allegation concerning a breech in confidentiality
- Encrypting any client information transmitted via the internet

SECTION III: PRACTICING FOR NCLEX

Activity G

1. Answer: b
RATIONALE: The nurse is using the narrative charting method to record the medical records of the client. Narrative charting involves writing information about the client and client care in chronologic order, which resembles a log or

journal. SOAP charting, PIE charting, or focus charting do not contain much written information or lengthy narratives. The SOAP charting method demonstrates interdisciplinary cooperation because everyone involved in the care of a client makes entries in the same location in the chart. Focus charting is a modified form of SOAP charting. The PIE charting style prompts the nurse to address specific content in a charted progress note.

2. **Answer: a**
    RATIONALE: The nurse would need to enter the password to access the computerized medical record. Data are saved and password protected so that it is not easily accessible to everyone. The user name, employee ID, or name will not help the nurse to access the details from the computer.

3. **Answer: a**
    RATIONALE: A medical record can be used without the client's permission for sharing information among the client's health care personnel. Medical records serve as a permanent health record, which also provides a means of sharing information among health care workers, thus ensuring client safety and continuity of care. A medical record cannot be used to share information with personnel involved in research, the client's relatives, or insurance agencies without the client's permission.

4. **Answer: c**
    RATIONALE: The nursing Kardex is used to obtain information on the health care provided to clients and serves as legal evidence during malpractice lawsuits. The client's nurse, other staff, or the client's physician cannot serve as legal evidence for malpractice lawsuits.

5. **Answer: b**
    RATIONALE: The nurse should check the client's medical records to determine when the last pain-relieving drug was administered. The nurse should not rely on the client's statement regarding the administration of the last dose of medication for pain. The nurse should not provide medication as requested by the client. The nurse cannot make a decision regarding the need for medication by checking for the severity of pain experienced by the client.

6. **Answer: d**
    RATIONALE: The Joint Commission is a private association that has established criteria reflecting high standards for institutional health care. Representatives of the Joint Commission periodically inspect health care agencies to determine whether they demonstrate evidence of quality care. Representatives are not in the clinic to discuss any employee's health problem or to discuss the career growth plan of the staff. They are also not present to inspect the facilities. The Joint Commission representatives are present to inspect the quality of care given to the clients.

7. **Answer: b**
    RATIONALE: A health record is particularly useful for the client because it helps the client in verifying their health status. It also helps when they have to apply for an employment or disability application. Verifying care through quality assurance programs, meeting standards of care set by the government, and helping in providing safe and effective care help the health care agency meet its regulatory requirements, not the client.

8. **Answer: a**
    RATIONALE: The reimbursement of medical expenses incurred by the client can be denied if signatures of health care personnel are missing. The other possible reasons for refusal could be that the document was inconsistent or the expenses were undocumented. Sharing the documents with the family or researchers, or the presence of abbreviated instructions are not reasons to refuse reimbursement.

9. **Answer: b**
    RATIONALE: The client's medical record has been organized in the source-oriented recording method. This type of record contains separate forms on which physicians, nurses, dietitians, physical therapists, and so on make written entries about their own specific activities in relation to the client's care. The problem-oriented record is organized according to the client's health problems. PIE charting is a method of recording the client's progress under the headings of problem, intervention, and evaluation. Focus charting follows a DAR model.

10. **Answer: a**
    RATIONALE: The clinic is using the problem-oriented method to organize the data. The problem-oriented record is organized according to the client's health problems. In this type of record, the information is compiled and arranged to emphasize goal-directed care, to promote recording of pertinent information, and to facilitate communication among health care professionals. In the source-oriented record, data are organized according to the source of documented information. Narrative charting involves writing information about the client and client care in chronologic order.

11. **Answer: b**
    RATIONALE: The nurse is using the SOAP charting method, in which everyone involved in the care of a client makes entries in the same location in the chart. Documentation following SOAP charting has four components. Narrative, focus, and PIE charting are not used in this case. Narrative charting involves writing information about the client and client care in chronologic order. Focus charting follows a DAR model, whereas PIE charting is a method of recording the client's progress under the headings of problem, intervention, and evaluation.

12. **Answer: a**
    RATIONALE: When nurses use the PIE charting method, they document assessments on a separate form (not on one form) and give the client's

problem a corresponding number. They use the numbers subsequently in the progress notes when referring to interventions and the client's responses. Problem-oriented records organize data according to the client's health problems. The SOAP charting technique is used to make entries in the same location in the chart.

13. Answers: a, c, e
RATIONALE: The health agency requires the identification of nursing diagnoses or client needs, planned nursing interventions or nursing standards of care for meeting the client's nursing care needs, and client response to interventions and outcomes of care, including pain management, to justify accreditation. There is no fixed rule that the number of people working in the health agency should be more than 50. There is also no rule stating that the latest equipment should be used in the agency.

14. Answers: a, b, d, e
RATIONALE: Computerized charting has many advantages, such as the information is always legible, it automatically records the date and time of the documentation, the abbreviations and terms are consistent with agency-approved lists, and it saves time because it eliminates delays in obtaining the chart. The major disadvantage is the initial expense of purchasing a computer system. Electronic data also require less storage space and are quickly retrievable.

15. Answer: a
RATIONALE: The abbreviation "a.c." means before meals. The medication needs to be administered before the client eats a meal. The abbreviation "p.c." means after meals, "p.o." means by mouth, "HS" means hour of sleep or bedtime.

16. Answer: a
RATIONALE: Some hospitals use traditional time (time based on two 12-hour revolutions on a clock), which is identified with the hour and minute, followed by AM or PM. Other agencies prefer military time (time based on a 24-hour clock), which uses a different four-digit number for each hour and minute of the day. The use of military time avoids confusion because no number is ever duplicated, and the labels AM, PM, midnight, and noon are not needed. Military time begins at midnight (2400 or 0000). One minute after midnight is 0001. A zero is placed before the hours of one through nine in the morning; for example, 0700 refers to 7 AM and is stated as "oh seven hundred." After noon, 12 is added to each hour; therefore, 2 PM is 1400. Minutes are given as 1 to 59.

SECTION IV: REVIEWING WHAT YOU HAVE LEARNED

Activity H
1. Abnormal
2. Kardex
3. Focus

Activity I
1. False. PIE charting is a method of recording the client's progress under the headings of Problem, Intervention, and Evaluation.
2. True.

Activity J
1. Medical records
2. Narrative charting

Activity K

	Source-Oriented Records	Problem-Oriented Records
1. Definition	Client records are organized according to the source of documented information.	Client records are organized according to the client's health problems.
2. Components	They include separate forms on which physicians, nurses, dietitians, and physical therapists make written entries about their own specific activities in the client's care.	The forms have data organized in four major sections: database, problem list, plan of care, and progress notes.

Activity L

1. A team of caregivers with various types of expertise interacting with a client in the group process is known as making rounds.
2. When done as a group, the client is a witness to and often an active participant in the interaction. Observing and conversing in the client's presence provides an opportunity to survey the client's condition and determine the status of equipment used in their care. It also tends to boost client confidence and security in their care. Since the passage of HIPAA regulations, however, agencies avoid this type of communication if another client shares the room or if the client has not authorized family members or friends who may be visiting to have access to their health information.

Activity M

1. Medical records have the following seven uses:
   a. Permanent account—Medical records are filed and maintained for all future references so that client health histories can be reviewed during subsequent admissions.
   b. Sharing information—Documentation serves as a way to inform others about the client's status and plan for care.
   c. Quality assurance—Medical records help to promote quality assurance, also known as continuous quality improvement or total quality improvement.
   d. Accreditation—Documentation in randomly selected medical records is examined during an accreditation visit.
   e. Reimbursement—Auditors survey medical records to determine if documented care meets established criteria for reimbursement.
   f. Education and research—Examining the medical records of clients with specific disorders provides a valuable supplement that enhances learning and future problem-solving.
   g. Legal evidence—Portions of the medical record can be subpoenaed as evidence by attorneys to prove or disprove allegations of malpractice.
2. Military time is based on the 24-hour clock, which uses a different four-digit number for each hour and minute of a day. It begins at midnight (2400 or 0000). One minute after midnight is 0001. A zero is placed before the hours of one through nine in the morning; for example, 0700 refers to 7 AM and is stated as "oh seven hundred." After noon, 12 is added to each hour; therefore, 1 PM is 1300. Minutes are given as 1 to 59. The first two digits indicate the hour within the 24-hour period, whereas the last two digits indicate the minutes.

SECTION V: APPLYING YOUR KNOWLEDGE

Activity N

1. Such documentation provides a written record of the client's progress and avoids omissions or duplications during future teaching sessions.
2. Consistency in charting is important for legal purposes; deviating from the charting policy reduces a nurse's protection if the record is subpoenaed.
3. Military time prevents confusion because no number is ever duplicated; furthermore, it does not require the use of AM, PM, midnight, and noon.

Activity O

1. The nurse should prepare a change-of-shift report that summarizes each client's condition and current status of care.
2. The nurse receiving the shift report should do the following:
   • Be prompt so that the report can start and end on time.
   • Come prepared with a pen and paper or clipboard.
   • Avoid socializing during reporting sessions.
   • Take notes.
   • Clarify unclear information.
   • Ask questions about pertinent information that may have been omitted.
3. When using the telephone, the nurse should do the following:
   • Answer as promptly as possible.
   • Speak in a normal tone of voice.
   • Identify him or herself by name, title, and nursing unit.
   • Obtain or state the reason for the call.
   • Discreetly identify the client being discussed to avoid being publicly overheard.
   • Spell the client's name if there is any chance of confusion.
   • Converse in a courteous and businesslike manner.
   • Repeat information to ensure it has been heard accurately.
4. The nurse should document in the client's chart the information reported and the instructions received.

Activity P

There are no definite answers to this activity. Students may choose to discuss their thoughts with peers or instructors.

SECTION VI: GETTING READY FOR NCLEX

Activity Q

1. **Answer: d**
   RATIONALE: A checklist is a form of documentation in which the nurse indicates with a check mark or initials the performance of routine care. The nursing Kardex is a quick reference for current information about the client and their care.

A flow sheet is a form of documentation with sections for recording frequently repeated assessment data. A care plan is a written list of the client's problems, goals, and nursing orders for client care.

2. **Answer: c**
   RATIONALE: The nurse should note NPO, which indicates nothing by mouth, for a client who may not consume anything orally. AMA is used to denote a client leaving the health care facility against medical advice. NKA indicates that the client does not have any known allergies. NSS indicates a normal saline solution.

CHAPTER 10

SECTION I: ASSESSING YOUR UNDERSTANDING

Activity A

1. Hand washing or hand antisepsis
2. Microorganisms
3. Nonpathogens
4. Fimbriae
5. Infections
6. Systemic
7. Cestodes
8. Susceptible host
9. Lipping

Activity B

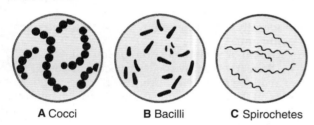

A Cocci   **B** Bacilli   **C** Spirochetes

1. The figure shows round (cocci), rod-shaped (bacilli), and spiral (spirochetes) bacteria.
2. There are two types of bacteria. Aerobic bacteria require oxygen to live, whereas anaerobic bacteria exist without oxygen.
3. The chemical actions of antibacterials, which consist of antibiotics and sulfonamides, alter the metabolic processes of bacteria but not viruses. They damage or destroy bacterial cell walls or the mechanisms that bacteria need to grow. They also, however, destroy normal bacterial flora.

Activity C

1. d   **2.** c   **3.** e   **4.** b   **5.** a

Activity D

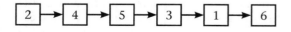

Activity E

1. Factors that cause infection or an infectious disease in the human body include the following:
   • The type and number of microorganisms present in the body
   • The characteristics of the microorganism (such as its virulence, the ability to overcome the immune system)
   • The person's state of health
2. Three types of viruses can exist in the human body. Some can remain dormant in a human and reactivate sporadically, causing recurrence of an infectious disorder, such as herpes simplex virus. Some are minor and self-limiting and terminate with or without medical treatment, such as the common cold. Some others are more serious or fatal, such as rabies, poliomyelitis, hepatitis, and AIDS.
3. Rickettsiae resemble bacteria. Like viruses, however, they cannot survive outside another living species. Consequently, an intermediate life form, such as fleas, ticks, lice, or mites, transmits rickettsial diseases to humans.
4. Protozoans are classified according to their ability to move. Some use amoeboid motion, by which they extend their cell walls and their intracellular contents flow forward. Others move by cilia (hair-like projections) or flagella (whip-like appendages). Some cannot move independently at all.
5. Mycoplasmas lack a cell wall. They are referred to as pleomorphic because they assume various shapes.
6. Biologic defense mechanisms are anatomic or physiologic methods that stop microorganisms from causing an infectious disorder. The two types of biologic defense mechanisms are mechanical and chemical. Mechanical defense mechanisms are physical barriers that prevent microorganisms from entering the body or expel them before they multiply. Examples include intact skin and mucous membranes, reflexes such as sneezing and coughing, and infection-fighting blood cells called phagocytes or macrophages. Chemical defense mechanisms destroy or incapacitate microorganisms through natural biologic substances. Examples include lysozymes, gastric acid, and antibodies.

SECTION II: APPLYING YOUR KNOWLEDGE

Activity F

1. To break the chain of infection, a nurse should acknowledge and follow the measures or principles of medical asepsis presented here:
   • Microorganisms exist everywhere except on sterilized equipment.
   • Frequent hand washing and maintaining intact skin are the best methods for reducing the transmission of microorganisms.
   • Blood, body fluids, cells, and tissues are considered major reservoirs of microorganisms.

- Personal protective equipment, such as gloves, gowns, masks, goggles, and hair and shoe covers, serves as a barrier to microbial transmission.
- A clean environment reduces microorganisms.
- Certain areas—the floor, toilets, and insides of sinks—are more contaminated than others; therefore, cleaning should be done from cleaner to dirtier areas.

2. Antimicrobial agents are chemicals that destroy or suppress the growth of infectious microorganisms.
3. The nurse should use antimicrobial agents such as antiseptics, disinfectants, and antiinfective drugs. Antiseptics, also known as bacteriostatic agents, inhibit the growth of but do not kill microorganisms. Some are also used as cleaning agents. Disinfectants, also called germicides and bactericides, destroy active microorganisms but not spores. They are used to kill and remove microorganisms from equipment, walls, and floors. Antiinfective drugs are used to combat infections. The two groups of drugs used most often to combat infections are antibacterials and antivirals.

SECTION III: PRACTICING FOR NCLEX

Activity G

1. **Answer: b**
   RATIONALE: The nurse explains that the primary advantage of an alcohol-based hand rub is that it provides the fastest and greatest reduction in microbial counts on the skin. Other advantages include the fact that hand rubs are more accessible because they do not require sinks or water (which increases compliance because they are easier to perform), they reduce cost by eliminating paper towels and waste management, and they are less irritating and drying than soap because they contain emollients. Disinfectants destroy active microorganisms but not spores. Antivirals do not destroy the infecting viruses; rather, they control viral replication (copying) or release from the infected cells.

2. **Answer: b**
   RATIONALE: When decontaminating with an alcohol-based hand rub, the nurse should apply about a nickel- to a quarter-size volume of the product to the palm of one hand or the amount recommended by the manufacturer. Dipping hands in the product for 15 seconds, applying antiinfection drugs to the product, or removing the product from the clean utility room are not proper interventions in the process of hand antisepsis.

3. **Answer: c**
   RATIONALE: The nurse should suggest that the client avoid sharing soaps, towels, and washcloths with other family members. Antiseptics, also known as bacteriostatic agents, inhibit the growth of but do not kill microorganisms. There is no antiviral lotion available that will kill the microorganisms. Sterilized instruments are required at the

time of treatment or operation, not during home care.

4. **Answer: c**
   RATIONALE: The nurse should perform a surgical scrub because this medical aseptic practice is a type of skin and nail antisepsis that is performed prior to donning sterile gloves and garments when the nurse is actively involved in an operative or obstetric procedure. Alcohol-based hand rubs and hand washing with soap and water are not substitutes for a surgical scrub. Both of these are medical aseptic practices. Sterile technique is a surgical aseptic practice performed on medical equipment to avoid contaminating microbe-free items.

5. **Answer: c**
   RATIONALE: The nurse should check that housekeepers follow concurrent disinfection by cleaning the less-soiled areas before the grossly dirty ones, wet mopping floors, and damp dusting furniture to avoid distributing microorganisms on dust and air currents, discarding solutions used for mopping frequently in a "flushable" hopper, and never placing clean items on the floor. Scrubbing the mattress and the insides of drawers and bedside stands is a part of the terminal disinfection process, which is more thorough than concurrent disinfection and consists of measures to clean the client environment after discharge. Contaminated equipment needs to be boiled for 15 minutes at 212°F (100°C) or longer in places at higher altitudes to sterilize items used in the home setting and not for medical asepsis.

6. **Answer: d**
   RATIONALE: Nurses who are sensitive to latex can wear a double pair of vinyl gloves when the risk for contact with blood or body fluids is high. Wearing a pair of latex gloves or one pair of vinyl gloves will not help the nurse who is allergic to latex. The nurse should wear a double pair of vinyl gloves, not double pair of latex gloves.

7. **Answer: b**
   RATIONALE: The nurse should place rubber caps or screw tops upside down on a flat surface or hold it during pouring to avoid contamination. Before each use of a sterile solution, the nurse pours and discards a small amount to wash away airborne contaminants from the mouth of the container. This is called lipping the container. While pouring, the nurse holds the container in front of him or herself and avoids touching any sterile areas within the field. The nurse controls the height of the container to avoid splashing the sterile field, causing a wet area of contamination. Agencies replace sterile solutions daily even if the entire volume is not used.

8. **Answer: c**
   RATIONALE: The nurse should consider the surgical instrument in a dry sterile wrapper safe from contamination. Any partially unwrapped sterile package is considered contaminated. A

commercially packaged sterile item is not considered sterile past its recommended expiration date. A sterile wrapper, if it becomes wet, wicks microorganisms from its supporting surface, causing contamination.

9. **Answer: b**
   RATIONALE: Indwelling catheters should be avoided if at all possible because older people have increased susceptibility to urinary tract infections. If an indwelling catheter is necessary, meticulous daily care is required. The tubing should never be placed higher than the bladder to prevent any backflow of urine into the bladder. Keeping the tube at the same level as the bladder will not help with an easy flow of urine.

10. **Answer: a**
    RATIONALE: Those family members who are 65 years and older should receive an initial dose of the pneumococcal vaccine. Infections are often transmitted to vulnerable older adults through equipment reservoirs such as indwelling urinary catheters, humidifiers, and oxygen equipment or through incisional sites such as those used for intravenous tubing, parenteral nutrition, or tube feedings. Use of proper aseptic technique is essential to prevent the introduction of microorganisms. Daily assessment for any signs of infection is imperative. All family members need not wear masks. Multivitamin capsules between meals will not prevent the outbreak of infections.

11. **Answer: a**
    RATIONALE: Prevention of urinary tract infections is best accomplished by prompt attention to perineal hygiene. Women should always clean from the urinary area back toward the rectal area to prevent organisms from the stool entering the bladder. Maintaining intact skin is an excellent first-line defense against nosocomial infections. Using dry tissue or wearing gloves to clean the urinary area will not help prevent infections.

12. **Answer: b**
    RATIONALE: Clients with burn injuries should be moved first if there is an outbreak of infection at a health care facility. A susceptible host, the last link in the chain of infection, is one whose biologic defense mechanisms are weakened in some way. Ill clients are prime targets for infectious microorganisms because their health is already compromised. The clients who are more susceptible to infections include burn victims, clients who have suffered major trauma, or clients who required invasive procedures such as endoscopy. Clients who are infected with HIV are also at a high risk for infection. Clients who have been admitted for pathologic testing, are waiting for surgery, or have just given birth may not be very susceptible to infection.

13. **Answers: a, c, d, e**
    RATIONALE: Microorganisms and spores are destroyed physically through radiation or heat, boiling water, free-flowing steam, dry heat, and steam under pressure. A chemical-dipped cloth or airtight packages will not help sterilize the equipment.

14. **Answers: a, c, f, e, d, b**
    RATIONALE: The nurse should unwrap the cloth by supporting the wrapped item in one hand rather than placing it on a solid surface. The nurse then holds each of the four corners to prevent the edges of the wrap from hanging loosely. The nurse places the unwrapped item on the sterile field and discards the cloth cover. The paper cover usually has two loose flaps that extend above the sealed edges. After separating the flaps, the nurse drops the sterile contents onto the sterile field.

SECTION IV: REVIEWING WHAT YOU HAVE LEARNED

Activity H
1. Anaerobic
2. Superficial

Activity I
1. True.
2. False. Some pathogens have tiny hair called fimbriae that enable them to attach to the host's tissue and avoid expulsion.

Activity J
1. Asepsis
2. Reservoir

Activity K
1. c   **2.** a   **3.** d   **4.** b

Activity L

	Medical Asepsis	Surgical Asepsis
1. Definition	These practices limit or reduce the numbers of microorganisms.	These measures render supplies and equipment totally free of microorganisms.
2. Technique	Medical asepsis consists of measures that interfere with the chain of infection in various ways.	Surgical asepsis involves sterilization of equipment and the creation of sterile fields.
3. Methods of Obtaining Asepsis	Antimicrobial agents Hand washing Wearing hospital garments	Steam under pressure Radiation Boiling water

Activity M

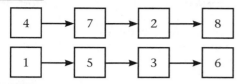

Activity N

1. A nosocomial infection is acquired while a person is receiving care in a health care facility.
2. The six components of the chain of infection are (1) an infectious agent, (2) a reservoir for growth and reproduction, (3) an exit route from the reservoir, (4) a mode of transmission, (5) a portal of entry, and (6) a susceptible host.

SECTION V: APPLYING YOUR KNOWLEDGE

Activity O

1. This action helps to wash away airborne contaminants from the mouth of the container (called "lipping" the container).
2. Chipped or peeling nail polish can contain many microorganisms, thus negating the aseptic environment that should be maintained during nursing care.

Activity P

1.
   a. The client's age, weakened condition, decreased activity, and exposure to many microorganisms from other clients and health care personnel may have led to increased susceptibility to infections such as pneumonia.
   b. Conscientious hand washing is necessary when caring for all clients, but it is especially important with older adults who are more susceptible to infections. Use proper aseptic techniques to prevent the introduction of microorganisms. Ensure that visitors with respiratory infections wear a mask or avoid contact with older adults until their symptoms have subsided. Take measures to maintain the client's intact skin.

2.
   a. The nurse should perform a surgical scrub and don sterile gloves and garments before active involvement in operative or obstetric procedures.
   b. A surgical scrub thoroughly removes transient microorganisms from the nails, hands, and forearms. Sterile gloves and garments provide a surface free of microorganisms that, if unsterile, could be transferred to the client.

Activity Q

There are no definite answers to this activity. Students may choose to discuss their thoughts with peers or instructors.

SECTION VI: GETTING READY FOR NCLEX

Activity R

1. Answers: a, c, d

RATIONALE: After leaving the client's room, the nurse should scrub the hands thoroughly, giving attention to the nails. They should avoid touching any part of the sink or faucets and discard paper towels appropriately after drying the hands. The nurse should use a dry, not wet, paper towel to turn off faucets because a wet paper towel can allow microorganisms to pass through. The nurse need not apply hand sanitizer to keep the hands free from odor.

2. **Answer: c**
RATIONALE: Alcohol-based rubs produce antisepsis as effectively as washing with soap and water when the hands are visibly clean. They do not remove dirt or soil with organic material and cannot be substituted for hand washing in this case. Alcohol-based rubs, when used for a minimum of 5 seconds, remove 99% of microorganisms on the hands. They have a brief antiseptic effect; therefore, the nurse must repeat the procedure several times within the course of a day.

CHAPTER 11

Activity A

SECTION I: ASSESSING YOUR UNDERSTANDING

1. Admission
2. Supervisor
3. Discharge
4. Admission
5. Transferring
6. 3
7. Intermediate
8. Referral
9. 60

Activity B

1. A client is having an ID bracelet applied.
2. The element contains information regarding the client's name, an ID number, and, in some cases, a bar code for computerized scanning purposes.
3. The element is used to identify the client and ensure their safety.

Activity C

1. c   **2.** b   3. e   **4.** a   **5.** d

Activity D

1.

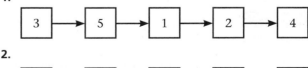

2.

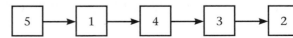

Activity E

1. After all admission data are collected, the nurse develops an initial plan for the client's care. The initial plan generally identifies priority problems and may include the client's projected needs for teaching and discharge planning.

2. The medical history and physical examination generally include identifying data, reason for seeking care, history of current illness, personal history, past health history, family history, review of body systems, and conclusions.

3. The discharge process generally consists of discharge planning, obtaining a written medical order, completing discharge instructions, notifying the business office, helping the client leave the agency, writing a summary of the client's condition at discharge, and requesting that the room be cleaned.

4. A transfer process may occur when a client's condition improves or worsens. Generally, a transfer has some advantage for the client. It may facilitate more specialized care in a life-threatening situation or it may reduce health care costs.

5. An extended care facility is a health care agency that provides long-term care. It is designed for people who do not meet the criteria for hospitalization. Examples of extended care facilities are group homes for assisted living, adult day care centers, senior residential communities, home health care agencies, and hospices.

SECTION II: APPLYING YOUR KNOWLEDGE

Activity F

1. When transferring a client to a different nursing unit within the health care facility, the nurse
   - Informs the client and family about the transfer
   - Completes a transfer summary briefly describing the client's current condition and reason for transfer
   - Speaks with a nurse on the transfer unit to coordinate the transfer
   - Transports the client and their belongings, medications, nursing supplies, and chart to the other unit

2. A transfer summary is a written review of the client's current status that briefly describes the client's current condition and reason for transfer.

SECTION III: PRACTICING FOR NCLEX

Activity G

1. **Answer: a**
   RATIONALE: Activities involved in discharge planning, which are incorporated within the plan of care, ideally begin at admission or shortly thereafter. If effective, discharge planning shortens the hospital stay, decreases the cost of in-hospital care, reduces the necessity for readmission, and eases the transition between the hospital and the next level of care.

2. **Answer: b**
   RATIONALE: Clients with terminal health conditions require special considerations and many details on their care in the discharge plan. Discharge planning usually is simple and routine for clients between the ages of 25 and 30 years, and clients living with their families or relatives.

3. **Answer: d**
   RATIONALE: The signed form releases the doctor and agency from future responsibility for any complications. The form does not contain any information about medications, client contact information, or billing details.

4. **Answer: a**
   RATIONALE: If the client refuses to sign, the nurse cannot prevent the client from leaving. The nurse can make a note in the client's medical record, however, that they presented the form to the client and they subsequently refused to sign it. The form cannot be signed by the nurse or the client's relatives. The form cannot be signed by the head of the facility.

5. **Answer: c**
   RATIONALE: Before the client leaves the agency and after briefing the client on the medication and self-care points, the nurse notifies the business office to complete the billing process. The nurse need not notify the physician, the head of the agency, or the housekeeping staff because they are not involved in the final steps of discharge.

6. **Answers: b, c**
   RATIONALE: In most cases, the client contacts a family member or friend for assistance with transportation. If no transportation is available, the client may use public transportation, a taxicab, or an ambulance to get home. Van transportation may be available for older adults through the local Commission on Aging, but 24-hour advance notification is usually required.

7. **Answers: a, b, c**
   RATIONALE: A client may be transferred to another health care facility to provide specialized care in life-threatening conditions, to provide care for a change in the client's condition, and to reduce the health care costs involved. A client cannot be transferred to another health care facility to provide room for another client at the facility. If a client requires long-term care at an extended care facility, the client is not transferred, but is referred to an extended care facility after discharge.

8. **Answers: a, b, d**
   RATIONALE: The level of care is determined at admission. Each client is assessed using a standard form developed by the Health Care Financing Association called a Minimum Data Set (MDS) for Nursing Home Resident Assessment and Care Screening. The MDS requires assessment of communication/hearing patterns, vision patterns, oral and nutritional status, continence patterns in the past 14 days, and mood and behavior patterns. The MDS does not require financial status of the client to decide the level of treatment.

9. **Answers: c, d, a, b**
   RATIONALE: The nurse should first inform the client and family about the transfer, then complete a transfer summary, briefly describing the client's current health and reason for transfer. Next, the nurse should speak to the nurse on the transfer unit to coordinate the transfer. Finally, the nurse should arrange to transport the client and their belongings, medications, nursing supplies, and chart to the other unit.

10. **Answer: c**
    RATIONALE: The nurse should provide the child with toys and books. These will not only calm the child but also provide important lessons. The nurse does not need to request a colleague's help in feeding or dressing the child. The nurse should not prevent the parents from fussing over the child. Instead, the nurse should ask the parents to assist with feeding and dressing the child.

11. **Answer: a**
    RATIONALE: The nurse should place the client's eyeglasses on the bedside table or drawer and inform them where they have been placed. Because they are personal items that may be required very often, the nurse does not need to hand them over to the client's family for safekeeping or keep them in the facility's safe along with other valuables. The nurse should not tell the client that the facility is not responsible for the client's belongings. Other valuables or possessions may be sent back with the family or kept in the facility's safe.

12. **Answer: a**
    RATIONALE: A client who has just delivered a baby would need to be transferred to another unit. The client would move into a postpartum care room. A client who is capable of going home to self-care, the client who returns after leaving the facility without information, or the client who is planning to leave the facility against medical advice will not be transferred to another unit. A client who is capable of going home to self-care is discharged from the facility. A client who returns after leaving the facility without information is readmitted to the facility as a new admission.

SECTION IV: REVIEWING WHAT YOU'VE LEARNED

Activity H
1. Referral

Activity I
1. Discharge
2. Transfer

Activity J
1. A Minimum Data Set (MDS) is a standard form containing various factors that require assessment when a client is admitted to an extended care facility to determine the appropriate level of care. The MDS is repeated every 3 months or whenever a client's condition changes. The nursing care plan reflects the problems identified on the MDS.
2. The nurse's duties when a client must be transferred within the same agency involve the following:
   - Informing the client and family about the transfer
   - Writing a transfer summary briefly describing the client's current condition and reason for transfer
   - Speaking with a nurse on the transfer unit to coordinate the transfer
   - Transporting the client and their belongings, medications, nursing supplies, and chart to the other unit
3. Physical assessment of the client upon admission to the health care facility is important to evaluate the client's current physical condition, to detect early signs of developing health problems, to establish a baseline for future comparisons, and to evaluate the client's responses to medical and nursing interventions.

Activity K
1. Losing a client's personal items can have serious legal implications for the nurse and health care agency; this measure fosters extra protection in case of liability.
2. Frequently, physical examinations take place with clients naked or wearing only a loose examination gown. A drape provides modesty and warmth while providing the examiner with access to the client's body.

Activity L
1. During admission, the nurse should prepare the client's room, welcome and orient the client, safeguard the client's valuables and clothing, help the client undress, and compile the nursing database.
2. The initial care plan generally identifies the client's priority problems and may include projected needs for teaching and discharge planning. The nurse revises the care plan as more data accumulate or the client's condition changes.

CHAPTER 12

SECTION I: ASSESSING YOUR UNDERSTANDING

Activity A

1. Pyrexia
2. Fahrenheit
3. Hypothalamus
4. Piloerection
5. Circadian
6. Emotions
7. Axilla
8. Electronic
9. Doppler
10. Korotkoff

Activity B

1. The equipment in the figure is a Doppler stethoscope.
2. A Doppler stethoscope helps to detect sounds created by the velocity of blood moving through a blood vessel.
3. The equipment in the figure is a digital thermometer.
4. A digital thermometer looks similar to a glass thermometer and can be used at oral, axillary, and rectal sites. It has a sensing tip at the end of the stem, an on/off button, and a display area that lights up during use.

Activity C

1. c   2. e   3. a   4. b   5. d

Activity D

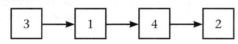

Activity E

1. Systolic pressure is the pressure within the arterial system when the heart contracts. It is higher than diastolic pressure.
2. If the client's temperature is above or below normal, the nurse should:
   - Record and report the temperature.
   - Implement appropriate nursing and medical interventions for restoring normal body temperature when appropriate.
   - Reassess the client frequently.
3. Objective assessment data include vital signs (body temperature, pulse rate, respiratory rate, and blood pressure) that indicate how well or how poorly the client's body is functioning.
4. Body temperature increases slightly in women of childbearing age during ovulation as a result of hormonal changes that affect metabolism or tissue injury and repair after release of an ovum (egg).
5. Emotions affect the metabolic rate by triggering hormonal changes through the sympathetic and parasympathetic pathways of the autonomic nervous system. People who tend to be consistently anxious and nervous are likely to have slightly increased body temperatures. Conversely, people who are apathetic or depressed are prone to have slightly lower body temperatures.
6. A paper chemical thermometer or plastic strip with chemically treated dots is used to assess the temperature of clients who require isolation precautions for infectious diseases. Some physician's offices use them also because they are disposable.

SECTION II: APPLYING YOUR KNOWLEDGE

Activity F

1. The nurse should insert the thermometer in the ear (tympanic membrane) to get the core body temperature. The ear is the peripheral site that most closely reflects core body temperature.
2. To evaluate trends in body temperature, the nurse should document the assessment site as O for oral, R for rectal, AX for axillary, TA for temporal artery, and T for tympanic membrane. The nurse should also take the temperature by the same route each time.

SECTION III: PRACTICING FOR NCLEX

Activity G

1. **Answer: c**
   RATIONALE: The chance of survival of a client is diminished when body temperatures exceed 110°F (43.3°C) or fall below 84°F (28.8°C). Temperatures above 105.8°F (41°C) and below 93.2°F (34°C) indicate impairment of the hypothalamic regulatory center.
2. **Answer: b**
   RATIONALE: The increase in the client's temperature could be the result of the amount and type of food the client consumed during lunch. This is known as thermogenesis. When a person consumes food, the body requires energy to digest, absorb, transport, metabolize, and store nutrients. Circadian rhythms are physiologic changes that are seen in people who work night shifts, whereas tachypnea is a rapid respiratory rate that may not lead to an increase in temperature. Medicines used generally do not lead to an increase in body temperature unless they are stimulant drugs.
3. **Answer: c**
   RATIONALE: Ephedrine, a stimulant used in the treatment for asthma, could have led to an increase in the client's body temperature. Stimulant drugs, such as those containing dextroamphetamine (Dexedrine) or ephedrine, increase metabolic rate and body temperature. Aspirin, acetaminophen, and ibuprofen directly lower body temperature instead of increasing it.
4. **Answer: d**
   RATIONALE: The nurse should preferably measure the temperature of the infant from the axilla

because infants can be injured internally with thermometers and because they lose heat through their skin at a greater rate than other age groups. The axilla and the groin, areas where there is skin-to-skin contact, are preferred sites for temperature assessment in this age group. The nurse should not measure infant temperature from oral, rectal, or ear sites.

5. **Answer: c**
   RATIONALE: Body temperature increases slightly in women of childbearing age during ovulation. This probably results from hormonal changes affecting metabolism or tissue injury and repair after release of an ovum (egg). Normal perspiration, or lack of it, affects temperature in infants and older adults only. People who are depressed are prone to have slightly lower body temperatures. Drugs such as aspirin lower body temperature by acting on the hypothalamus.

6. **Answer: b**
   RATIONALE: The client's pulse should be recorded as thready because it disappears with the slightest bit of pressure. A normal or strong pulse can be felt with mild pressure over the artery. A bounding or full pulse produces a pronounced pulsation that does not easily disappear with pressure.

7. **Answer: d**
   RATIONALE: Impaired muscle coordination is a common symptom of hypothermia. A client with hyperthermia is at extreme risk of brain damage or death from complications associated with increased metabolic demand. The breathing rhythm and pulse rate both drop to below normal and do not become irregular.

8. **Answer: b**
   RATIONALE: Antipyretics (drugs that reduce fever), such as aspirin, acetaminophen, or ibuprofen, are helpful when a temperature is 102° to 104°F (38.9° to 40°C). As long as a fever remains below 102°F (38.9°C) and the person does not have a chronic medical condition, fluids or rest may be all that is necessary. Physical cooling measures are used for temperatures between 104° and 105.8°F (40° and 40.6°C). If the temperature is higher than 105.8°F (40.6°C) or if a high temperature is unchanged after a sufficient response time with conventional interventions, more aggressive treatment is warranted.

9. **Answer: a**
   RATIONALE: In the case of dyspnea, the nurse should note how much and what types of activities bring on dyspnea in the client. Eating habits and sleeping hours should be noted, but it will give accurate results only if noted along with the duration and time of the activity. The nurse need not note the regularity with which dyspnea occurs in a client.

10. **Answer: a**
    RATIONALE: When using an aneroid manometer to measure blood pressure, the nurse should check that the needle of the gauge is positioned at zero to record the accurate and correct measurement. The gauge reading need not be positioned according to the client's body temperature. An aneroid manometer is not connected to an electric outlet, nor does it use an inflatable bladder.

11. **Answers: a, b, c, e**
    RATIONALE: When a Doppler ultrasound device is used to detect the movement of blood, the nurse first applies conductive gel over the arterial site. The nurse then moves the probe at an angle over the skin until a pulsating sound is heard. The pulsating sounds are then counted. The nurse documents the assessment site and the rate, followed by the abbreviation D to indicate use of a Doppler device.

12. **Answers: a, b, c**
    RATIONALE: The nurse should use an assessment site other than the brachial artery when the client's arms are missing or both breasts have been removed, or when the client has had a vascular surgery. Conditions such as hypothermia or hyperthermia do not determine the assessment site for measuring the blood pressure of a client.

13. **Answers: b, c, d**
    RATIONALE: A client could have a low blood pressure when sleeping at night, when in the prone position, or when the client is female. Blood pressure tends to be lowest after midnight, when a client is sleeping. Women tend to have lower blood pressure than men of the same age. A person has lower blood pressure when lying down than when sitting or standing, although the difference in most people is insignificant. Blood pressure tends to increase with age as a result of arteriosclerosis (a process in which arteries lose their elasticity and become more rigid) and atherosclerosis (a process in which the arteries become narrowed with fat deposits). However, blood pressure increases during exercise and activity.

14. **Answers: c, d, a, b, e**
    RATIONALE: The blood pressure of an older adult is assessed in each arm when collecting a baseline assessment and documenting subsequent trends. Also, older adults need to have their blood pressure assessed while lying and sitting to detect the possibility of postural hypotension. Begin with assessing the blood pressure with the client in a supine position; deflate and leave the blood pressure cuff in place. Have the older adult assume a sitting position and check the pressure. Deflate and leave the cuff in place; assist the client to stand and immediately check the pressure. Record each reading from the same arm, observing for a decrease on sitting or standing.

15. **Answer: d**
    RATIONALE: The nurse is listening to phase IV of Korotkoff's. This phase is characterized by a muffled, less-distinct sound that is softer with a blowing quality. Phase I is characterized by the

first appearance of faint, clear, repetitive, tapping sounds that gradually intensify for at least two consecutive beats. Phase II is characterized by muffled or swishing sounds that are softer and longer than phase I. Phase III is characterized by a return of distinct, crisp, and louder blood sounds.

SECTION IV: REVIEWING WHAT YOU HAVE LEARNED

Activity H

1. Homeothermic
2. Apnea
3. Bradycardia
4. Vesicular
5. Hypothalamus

Activity I

1. False. For every degree of Fahrenheit that temperature is elevated, heart and pulse rates increase 10 beats per minute.
2. True

Activity J

1. Transducer
2. Hyperventilation

Activity K

	Fever	Hyperthermia
1. Definition	Fever is an elevation of body temperature exceeding 99.3°F (37.4°C).	Hyperthermia is a state of excessively high core temperature (exceeding 105.8°F [40.6°C]).
2. Complications or Concerns	If the person does not have a chronic medical condition, fluids or rest may be all that is necessary.	The person is at extremely high risk for brain damage or death from complications associated with increased metabolic demands.

Activity L

1. One nurse is counting the radial pulse, whereas the other is counting the apical heart rate.
2. The apical heart rate is considered more accurate because the sound of each heartbeat is obvious and distinct. Also, sometimes the heart contraction is not strong enough to be felt at a peripheral pulse site.

Activity M

1. (1) In the prodromal phase, the client has nonspecific symptoms just before the temperature rises. (2) In the onset or invasion phase, obvious mechanisms for increasing body temperature, such as shivering, develop. (3) During the stationary phase, the fever is sustained. (4) With the resolution or defervescence phase, temperature returns to normal.
2. Postural or orthostatic hypotension is a sudden, temporary drop in blood pressure when rising from a reclining position. It causes dizziness and fainting. This type of hypotension is most common in clients who have circulatory problems, are dehydrated, or take diuretics or other drugs that lower blood pressure.

Activity N

Vital signs are very sensitive to alterations in physiology; therefore, nurses should measure them regularly or whenever appropriate to assess a client's health status.

Activity O

1. Because they lose heat through their skin at a greater rate than do other age groups, the axilla and groin (areas where there is skin-to-skin contact) are the preferred routes for temperature assessment in infants.
2. They have a three times greater surface area from which heat is lost and a metabolic rate twice that of adults.

Activity P

There are no definite answers to this activity. Students may choose to discuss their thoughts with peers or instructors.

SECTION V: GETTING READY FOR NCLEX

Activity Q

1. **Answer: a**
   RATIONALE: The nurse should document these squeaking sounds as wheezes. Crackles are intermittent, high-pitched, popping sounds heard in distant areas of the lungs, primarily during inspiration. Gurgles are low-pitched, continuous, bubbling sounds heard in larger airways; they are more prominent during expiration. Rubs are grating or leathery sounds caused by two dry pleural surfaces moving over each other.
2. **Answers: d, c, a, b**
   RATIONALE: The four phases of a fever are prodromal, invasion or onset, stationary, and resolution or defervescence.

3. **Answer: d**
   RATIONALE: The best site in this case is the right thigh. The right upper and lower arm areas are not appropriate because the client is receiving intravenous medication there. The left thigh would be uncomfortable for the client because the left lower leg is injured.

4. **Answer: a**
   RATIONALE: A pulse that is difficult to feel and is obliterated easily with slight pressure is called thready. A normal pulse is described as strong; it can be felt with mild pressure over the artery. A bounding or full pulse produces a pronounced sensation that does not easily disappear with pressure.

CHAPTER 13

SECTION I: ASSESSING YOUR UNDERSTANDING

Activity A

1. Objective
2. Ophthalmoscope
3. Audiologist
4. Lordosis
5. Edema
6. Cerumen
7. Jaeger
8. Rinne
9. Turgor
10. Weber

Activity B

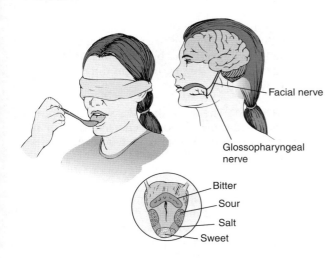

1. The figure shows taste assessment.
2. Assessment of taste is facilitated by placing substances on the tongue and asking clients to identify them with their eyes closed.
3. To ensure valid results, the nurse instructs the client to sip water between assessments.

4. The figure shows assessment of the muscle strength of the lower extremities.
5. The nurse assesses all four extremities separately to determine muscle strength. To test strength in the lower extremities, the nurse has the client push and pull against resistance. To assess strength in the upper extremities, the nurse asks the client to grasp, squeeze, and release their fingers. As the nurse pulls and pushes on the forearm and upper arm, they instruct the client to resist.

Activity C

1. c   **2.** a   **3.** e   **4.** b   **5.** d

Activity D

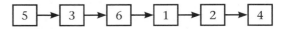

5 → 3 → 6 → 1 → 2 → 4

Activity E

1. A physical assessment is done for the following reasons:
   - To evaluate the client's current physical condition
   - To detect early signs of developing health problems
   - To establish a baseline for future comparisons
   - To evaluate the client's responses to medical and nursing interventions

2. Clients are examined in a special examination room or at the bedside. The examination area should have easy access to a restroom; a door or curtain that ensures privacy; adequate warmth for client comfort; a padded, adjustable table or bed; sufficient room for moving to either side of the client; adequate lighting; facilities for hand hygiene; a clean counter or surface for placing examination equipment; and a lined receptacle for soiled articles.

3. It is important for the nurse to document the client's weight and height because they provide more reliable data than a subjective assessment of body size. The recorded measurements help to assess trends in future weight loss or gain. Dosages of certain drugs are calculated on the basis of the client's weight and height.

4. The nurse assesses the scalp hair, eyebrows, and eyelashes during assessment of a client's hair. The nurse notes the color, texture, and presence or absence of hair in unusual locations for sex or age. They also inspect the hair for debris, such as blood in a client with head trauma; nits; or scales from scalp lesions. As the physical assessment progresses, the nurse also observes characteristics of body hair.

5. It is important for the nurse to document any unusual characteristics of the nails or surrounding tissues because changes in the shape and thickness of the fingernails and toenails are often signs of chronic cardiopulmonary disease or fungal infections.

6. For a basic physical assessment, a nurse requires gloves, examination gown, cloth or paper drapes, scale, stethoscope, sphygmomanometer, thermometer, penlight or flashlight, tongue blade, assessment form, and a pen.

SECTION II: APPLYING YOUR KNOWLEDGE

Activity F

1. The abdomen is always inspected and then auscultated before using palpation or percussion techniques. Touching or manipulating the abdomen can alter bowel sounds, producing invalid findings.

2. The nurse checks the abdominal girth daily by using a tape measure around the largest diameter. To ensure that they always measure from the same location, the nurse makes guide marks on the skin with an indelible pen.

3. The nurse should ask the client to examine the testes monthly during bathing or showering and to adhere to the following procedure:
   • Elevate the penis with one hand.
   • Gently roll each testicle within the scrotum between the thumb and the index finger.
   • Feel each testicle horizontally.
   • Feel each testicle vertically.
   • Check for any unusual lumps.

   • Continue palpation following the spermatic cord from the testicle to where it ascends into the abdomen.
   • Report any unusual findings to a physician as soon as possible.

SECTION III: PRACTICING FOR NCLEX

Activity G

1. **Answer: c**
   RATIONALE: The lesions should be documented as wheals. Wheals are lesions on the skin that are elevated, with an irregular border and no free fluid. Macules are skin lesions that are flat, round, colored, and nonpalpable. Papules are elevated, palpable, and solid lesions on the skin. Vesicles are elevated, round lesions filled with serum.

2. **Answer: a**
   RATIONALE: To assess skin turgor, the nurse gently pinches the client's skin over the sternum or below the clavicle in an attempt to lift it from the underlying tissue. The area over the chest is a good assessment location because the skin in other areas, such as the hand, forearm, and leg, tends to loosen with age. When the nurse releases the tissue, it should return quickly to its original position.

3. **Answer: d**
   RATIONALE: The nurse should document these sounds as crackles. Crackles are intermittent, high-pitched, popping sounds heard in distant areas of the lungs primarily during inspiration. Rubs are grating, leathery sounds caused by two dry pleural surfaces moving over each other. Wheezes are whistling or squeaking sounds caused by air moving through a narrowed passage; they may be audible without a stethoscope. Gurgles are low pitched, continuous, and bubbling and are heard in larger airways; they are more prominent during expiration.

4. **Answer: b**
   RATIONALE: The nurse should assess the appearance of raised sputum and the characteristics of any cough if adventitious sounds are heard when assessing the lung sounds of the client. The nurse need not assist the client to a supine position; the client is assisted to a sitting position to facilitate auscultating the anterior, posterior, and lateral aspects of the chest with minimal client exertion. The nurse should not move the diaphragm from the base of the lung to the top during auscultation; the diaphragm is moved from side to side, from the apices to the bottom of the lungs. The nurse should listen for one complete ventilation at each area auscultated, not just one inspiration or expiration.

5. **Answer: c**
   RATIONALE: The nurse is using the technique of palpation to assess the client. Palpation involves the use of the fingertips, the back of the hand, or the palm of the hand. Inspection involves examining

the body parts, looking for specific normal and abnormal characteristics. Percussion is striking or tapping part of the client's body with the fingertips to produce vibratory sounds that aid in determining the location, size, and density of underlying structures. Auscultation is the technique of listening to body sounds; it is used frequently, most often to assess the heart, lungs, and abdomen.

6. **Answer: a**
   RATIONALE: The nurse should check to see that the scale is calibrated at zero to ensure accuracy. The client should be asked to remove their shoes and stand barefoot on a paper towel placed on the scale. The nurse should not provide light slippers for this purpose. The paper towel helps to reduce contact with microorganisms, and standing barefoot facilitates measuring body weight. The nurse should move the lighter, not heavier, weight across the calibrations for individual pounds and ounces until the bar balances in the center of the scale. The nurse should position the heavier, not lighter, weight in a calibrated groove of the scale arm to provide a rough approximation of the gross body weight.

7. **Answers: a, b, e**
   RATIONALE: The nurse should perform an in-depth objective mental status assessment for clients with head injury, clients with psychiatric diagnoses, and clients who took an overdose of drugs to ensure that the mental status of these clients is not altered. Clients with impaired visual acuity or clients who are being treated with NSAIDs need not undergo an in-depth objective mental status assessment.

8. **Answer: b**
   RATIONALE: When examining the child's ear, the nurse should pull the ear down and back to straighten the ear canal for optimal visualization. The vibrating tuning fork is placed in the center of the client's head or on the mastoid area behind the ear to assess hearing. The nurse moves the skin behind and in front of the ears as well as underlying cartilage, not the external ear, to determine any tenderness. The nurse should shine a penlight or other light source within each ear to illuminate the ear canal. Positioning the client in front of a diffused source of light does not help to illuminate the ear canal.

9. **Answer: d**
   RATIONALE: The nurse should document the finding as ecchymosis, which is a purplish patch caused by trauma to soft tissue of the skin. Pallor is paleness of the skin; regardless of one's race, it is indicative of anemia or blood loss. Erythema is redness of the skin, possible causes of which could be superficial burns, local inflammation, or carbon monoxide poisoning. Cyanosis is bluish coloring of the skin caused by low tissue oxygenation.

10. **Answer: c**
    RATIONALE: The nurse should ask the client to squeeze the nipple gently to determine whether there is any clear or bloody discharge. The nurse

should ask the client to perform monthly breast self-examinations about 1 week after her menstrual period, not once every 2 months. The nurse should ask the client to place her hand on the side to be examined—behind the head and not alongside. The entire examination is not performed when lying down; it is partly done when standing in front of a mirror.

11. **Answer: b**
    RATIONALE: The nurse should document the edema as 2+ pitting edema because it depresses up to 4 mm and has a fairly normal contour. Pitting edema of 1+ is a slight indentation of 2 mm, with normal contours. Pitting edema of 3+ is a deep pit of 6 mm, which remains several seconds after pressing, and the swelling is obvious by general inspection. Pitting edema of 4+ is a deep pit of 8 mm; it remains for a prolonged time after pressing, possibly minutes.

12. **Answer: c**
    RATIONALE: The nurse should stroke the skin at various areas with a cotton ball to assess the client's ability to identify fine touch. The nurse places the stem of a vibrating tuning fork against the wrist to test the client's ability to sense vibration. The client is touched with pointed and curved ends of the safety pin to determine whether they can discriminate between sharp and dull sensations. The nurse touches the skin of the client at various areas with warm and cold containers to identify whether the client is able to identify the differences in the temperature.

13. **Answer: c**
    RATIONALE: The nurse should document the palpable mass as ovoid because it resembles an egg, and hard because it feels firm to the touch. If the mass is shaped like a ball, it is documented as round. A mass that feels bumpy to the touch is documented as having a nodular consistency.

14. **Answer: a**
    RATIONALE: The nurse should warm the diaphragm of the stethoscope before the procedure to promote comfort and prevent shock when the cold surface touches the abdomen. If no bowel sounds are heard initially, the nurse should listen for 2 to 5 minutes, not just 1 minute. The nurse should listen for bowel sounds in all four quadrants, not just one upper and one lower quadrant. The nurse should explain the procedure to the client before the assessment and avoid talking during the assessment to facilitate a quiet environment and accurate assessment.

15. **Answer: a**
    RATIONALE: The "lub" sound louder at the mitral area, also called the S1 sound, is a normal heart sound. S3, which sounds like "lub-dub-dub," is much more pronounced than a split-second sound; it is an abnormal heart sound. S4, which sounds like "lub-lub-dub," is another abnormal heart sound, heard just before S1. The soft "dub"

sound over the aortic area is also an abnormal sound. The normal "dub" sound is the second heart sound, S2, which can be heard in the mitral area; it is louder—not softer—over the aortic area.

SECTION IV: REVIEWING WHAT YOU HAVE LEARNED

Activity H

1. Fissure
2. Vesicular

Activity I

1. False. The nurse performs deep palpation by depressing tissue approximately 2.5 cm with the forefingers of one or both hands.
2. False. Kyphosis causes an increased curve in the thoracic area.

Activity J

1. Scoliosis
2. Auscultation

Activity K

	Head-to-Toe Approach	Body Systems Approach
1. Definition	This type of physical assessment of the client involves gathering data from the top of the body to the feet.	This type of physical assessment of the client involves collecting data according to the functional systems of the body.
2. Advantages	It prevents overlooking some aspect of data collection. It reduces the number of position changes required of the client. It generally takes less time.	Findings tend to be clustered, making problems more easily identifiable.
3. Disadvantages	Findings may be somewhat fragmented, taking longer to organize, cluster, and identify relationships.	Frequent position changes during the examination may tire the client. Some aspects of the examination may be inadvertently omitted or overlooked. The examination takes longer.

Activity L

1. Physical assessment of the client upon admission to the health care facility is important to evaluate the client's current physical condition, to detect early signs of developing health problems, to establish a baseline for future comparisons, and to evaluate the client's responses to medical and nursing interventions.
2. A Snellen eye chart is used to assess far vision. Each line on the chart is printed in progressively smaller letters or symbols. The client is asked to read the smallest line they can see comfortably from a distance of 20 feet with and without any corrective lenses. The client's vision is then compared with norms.

Activity M

1. Frequently, physical examinations take place with clients naked or wearing only a loose examination gown. A drape provides modesty and warmth while providing the examiner with access to the client's body.
2. The skin in other areas tends to loosen with age. "Tenting" could be misinterpreted as a sign of dehydration.

Activity N

There are no definite answers to this activity. Students may choose to discuss their thoughts with peers or instructors.

SECTION V: GETTING READY FOR NCLEX

Activity O

1. **Answer: d**
   RATIONALE: The nurse should document squeaking sounds as wheezes. Crackles are intermittent, high-pitched, popping sounds heard in distant areas of the lungs, primarily during inspiration. Gurgles are low-pitched, continuous, bubbling sounds heard in larger airways; they are more prominent during expiration. Rubs are grating or leathery sounds caused by two dry pleural surfaces moving over each other.
2. **Answer: c**
   RATIONALE: Percussion involves tapping or striking the examiner's fingers on the client's body to produce sounds that indicate the location and density of body tissues or organs. Auscultation is the technique of listening for sounds from within the body using a stethoscope or an ultrasound blood-flow detector. Palpation is the technique of feeling body tissues or parts with the hands or fingers. Observation is the technique of watching the client for general characteristics that do not require

closer scrutiny or use of measurement aids. These characteristics include overall appearance, skin color, grooming, body posture, gait, mood, and interactions with others.

CHAPTER 14

SECTION I: ASSESSING YOUR UNDERSTANDING

Activity A

1. Voluntariness
2. Lithotomy
3. Specimens
4. Roentgenogram
5. Iodine
6. Fluoroscopy
7. Endoscopy
8. Anesthesia
9. Constipation
10. Echography

Activity B

1. The figure shows a nurse arranging supplies and equipment in an endoscopic examination room.
2. The nurse should perform the following before the examination:
   - Cover the examination table with a sheet or paper dispensed from a roll.
   - Arrange a lined receptacle nearby for disposal of soiled items.
   - Ensure that sterile items remain wrapped or covered until just before their use.
   - Ensure that instruments that require electric power, batteries, or lights are functioning properly.
3. The figure shows a client wearing lead thyroid collar, apron, and skirt.
4. The items are used to shield vulnerable body parts or fetus during radiography.

Activity C

1. d   **2.** a   **3.** b   **4.** e   **5.** c

Activity D

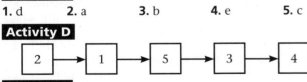

Activity E

1. A diagnostic examination is a procedure that involves physical inspection of body structures and evidence of their functions.
2. A culture is incubation of microorganisms performed by collecting body fluid or substances suspected of containing infectious microorganisms, growing the living microorganisms in a nutritive substance, and examining their characteristics with a microscope.
3. A contrast medium, such as barium sulfate or iodine, is a substance that adds density to a body

organ or cavity. It makes hollow body areas appear more distinct when imaged on X-ray film.

4. A lumbar puncture involves inserting a needle between lumbar vertebrae in the spine but below the spinal cord itself. The physician advances the tip of the needle until it is beneath the middle layer of the membrane surrounding the spinal cord. The physician then measures the spinal fluid pressure and withdraws a small amount of fluid.
5. A nurse's report may include information about whether or not the examination has been completed, the client's reactions during and immediately after the procedure, and any delayed reactions.
6. When attending to a client the nurse should take the following care:
   - Assist the client to a position of comfort and recheck vital signs to verify that the client's condition is stable.
   - Clean any substances from the client that caused soiling.
   - Offer a hospitalized client a clean gown or direct outpatients to dress in their own clothing.
   - Escort clients to their rooms or to the discharge area when it is safe to do so and provide instructions for follow-up care.

SECTION II: APPLYING YOUR KNOWLEDGE

Activity F

1. The nurse should obtain the following information prior to examination of the client:
   - Inquire about a woman's menstrual and obstetric history.
   - Find out whether the woman is pregnant or breast-feeding.
   - Ask about the client's allergy history because iodine is commonly used in radionuclide examinations, and the client may be allergic to it.
2. The nurse should provide the client with the following instructions after the examination:
   - Inform the client that they will be radioactive for a brief period (usually less than 24 hours), but body fluids (such as urine, stool, and emesis) can be safely flushed away.
   - Instruct premenopausal women to use effective birth control for the short period during which radiation continues to be present.

SECTION III: PRACTICING FOR NCLEX

Activity G

1. **Answer: c**
   RATIONALE: To examine the client's prostate gland, the nurse should assist the client to get into the genupectoral position. The dorsal recumbent position can be used for vaginal examination, whereas the lithotomy position is used during rectal examinations. The Sims position is used for rectal temperature assessment. These positions may

not be suitable for a prostate gland examination. However, a modified standing position can also be used for prostate gland examination.

2. **Answer: a**
   RATIONALE: The client is supposed to take a Pap smear test. A Pap smear test screens for abnormal cervical cells, the status of reproductive hormone activity, and normal or infectious microorganisms within the vagina or uterus. Both radiography and fluoroscopy are used to test bones, chest, and other such structures. Endoscopy is the visual examination of internal structures. These tests are not conducted for inspecting the vagina and cervix.

3. **Answer: d**
   RATIONALE: The nurse should withhold the client's food and fluids for at least 6 hours before any procedure in which an endoscope is inserted into the upper airway or upper gastrointestinal tract to prevent aspiration. The test will not show the correct result if food and fluids are withheld for less than 6 hours.

4. **Answer: a**
   RATIONALE: Endoscopic examinations that produce discomfort or anxiety are performed under a light, short-acting form of anesthesia sometimes referred to as conscious sedation. When conscious sedation is used, clients may have no memory of having had the test, even though they communicate and interact with staff during its performance. Conscious sedation will not affect the client's breathing nor will the client be under heavy sedation. This type of sedation also does not cause a sore throat.

5. **Answer: b**
   RATIONALE: One of the most important preprocedural steps before an endoscopic examination is to confirm that bowel preparation using laxatives and enemas has been completed. For an endoscopic procedure, clients are not allowed to have food or fluids for the past 6 hours. Checking the swallow, cough, and gag reflexes is a postprocedural check.

6. **Answer: b**
   RATIONALE: In addition to a written account of the client's examination, the nurse should report significant information to other nursing team members. This may include the fact that the examination was completed, the client's reactions during and immediately after the procedure, and any delayed reactions. The place and technique to transport the specimen, the details of the test performed, and the type and quantity of the specimen are some of the points covered in the written account of information.

7. **Answer: a**
   RATIONALE: When assisting a client who has to undergo a paracentesis procedure, the nurse should encourage the client to empty their bladder just before the procedure because an empty bladder prevents accidental puncture of the bladder. The nurse places a client in the sitting position to pool the abdominal fluids in the lower areas of the abdomen and displace the intestine posteriorly. The nurse holds the container of local anesthetic so that the physician can withdraw a sufficient amount to avoid contaminating the physician's sterile gloves.

8. **Answer: b**
   RATIONALE: To examine the anal region of the client, the nurse should help the client position themselves in the Sims position. The client will have to lie on their left side with the chest leaning forward, the right knee bent toward the head, the right arm forward, and the left arm extended behind the body. The dorsal recumbent position and the knee–chest position are used to facilitate gynecologic (reproductive organs of a woman) and urologic examinations. The modified standing position is used primarily for examining the prostate gland in men. These positions, however, may not be suitable for examining the anal regions of the client.

9. **Answer: a**
   RATIONALE: Before a client undergoes a radiographic examination, the nurse needs to ensure that the client removes any metal elements from their body, which includes hooks and eyes on a blouse. Metal produces a dense image that may be confused with a tissue abnormality. Endoscopy is a visual examination of internal structures, which is performed using optical scopes, whereas ECG is the examination of the electrical activity in the heart. Paracentesis helps in withdrawing fluid from the abdominal cavity. None of these examinations are affected by the presence of metal elements in the client's body.

10. **Answer: c**
    RATIONALE: During the pelvic examination the nurse folds back the drape just before the examination begins to expose the genitalia while minimizing client exposure. The nurse, however, covers the client with a cotton drape to maintain modesty and privacy, and introduces the physician to the client to reduce any anxious feelings. The nurse directs the examining light from behind the physician's shoulder toward the vaginal opening to illuminate the area to facilitate inspection.

11. **Answer: a**
    RATIONALE: Electroencephalography (or EEG) is an examination of the energy emitted by the brain. A client who has to undergo a sleep-deprived EEG is required to stay awake after midnight before the examination. Electrocardiography (or ECG or EKG) is an examination of the electrical activity in the heart. Electromyography (or EMG) is an examination of the energy produced by the stimulated muscles. These procedures, however, do not require the client to stay awake after midnight before taking the test.

12. Answer: d

RATIONALE: A paracentesis is performed to relieve abdominal pressure and to improve breathing, which generally becomes labored when fluid crowds the lungs. The lumbar puncture is a procedure that involves inserting a needle between lumbar vertebrae to withdraw spinal fluid. A pelvic examination is the physical inspection of the vagina and the cervix. A throat culture is the incubation of microorganisms, which is performed by collecting body fluid suspected of containing infectious microorganisms and examining their characteristics with a microscope.

13. Answer: b

RATIONALE: To enable the physician to perform a gynecologic examination, the nurse should assist the client to get into the lithotomy position. This position is a reclining position with the client's feet in metal supports called stirrups. The dorsal recumbent position is used to inspect the external genitalia, whereas the Sims position can be used for administration of enemas. The knee–chest position is used for rectal and lower chest examinations.

14. Answer: c

RATIONALE: The client will have to undergo a Papanicolaou test to determine the cause of irritation and itching in her vaginal area. The nurse collects a specimen of cervical secretions for a Pap (Papanicolaou) test. This test, also called a Pap smear, screens for abnormal cervical cells, the status of reproductive hormone activity, and normal or infectious microorganisms within the vagina or uterus. A blood test, ultrasound, and microorganism analysis need not be performed to check for any infectious microorganisms within the client's vagina.

15. Answer: a

RATIONALE: The best time to measure blood glucose level is about 30 minutes before eating and before bedtime to determine what are likely to be the lowest levels of glucose. This allows time for the client to increase or decrease food consumption or, if insulin dependent, to administer additional prescribed insulin, referred to as coverage. Checking the glucose level at any other time other than 30 minutes before eating and before bedtime will not give the lowest level of glucose.

16. Answers: b, d, e

RATIONALE: Many prescription and over-the-counter medications, as well as herbal therapies, may affect laboratory values. Therefore, nurses must take care to review and evaluate all medications and alternative therapies before any laboratory procedures. It is also important to know the client's previous results for the diagnostic test being done as a baseline for comparison. The nurse should also assess the urinary output, blood pressure, and mental status of an older adult to know how well an older adult is tolerating a fasting state. Older adults are likely to need additional clothing, slippers, and extra covers to keep them warm in waiting rooms and examination areas. The nurse scheduling the procedure before the client consumes the herbal medicines or telling the client to stop the medication is not a nurse's responsibility.

17. Answers: b, d, e

RATIONALE: Older adults, especially those who are medically frail, may not be able to tolerate the withholding of food or fluids for long periods before tests or examinations take place. The nurse should provide a bedside commode and hands-on assistance for older adults, especially those with impaired mobility, when they are undergoing preparation for gastrointestinal examinations. After a diagnostic examination, the nurse should offer older adults food, fluid, and a period of rest before they resume physically taxing activities. Suggesting the client fast 8 or 12 hours before the test is not a good idea and it will not help an older client in any way.

18. Answers: a, b, e

RATIONALE: The first step that the nurse takes when caring for the specimens and to ensure their accurate analysis is to collect the specimen in an appropriate container and label it. The nurse then attaches the proper laboratory request form and ensures that the specimen does not decompose before it can be examined. The nurse delivers the specimen to the laboratory as soon as possible. Changing the container of the specimen or refrigerating it is not advisable.

19. Answers: a, d, f, b, e, c

RATIONALE: While caring for a client who has come to the health agency for tests and examinations, the nurse should first help the client get into a comfortable position. The nurse should then check the client's vital signs to determine whether the client's condition is stable. The nurse then cleans any substances from the client that caused soiling. The nurse should then direct the client to dress in their own clothing. When it is safe to do so, the nurse escorts the client to their room or to the discharge area and provides instructions for follow-up care.

20. Answers: a, b, e

RATIONALE: In the Sims position, the client lies on the left side with the chest leaning forward, the right knee bent toward the head, the right arm forward, and the left arm extended behind the body. This type of position is used by clients with restricted joint movements such as that caused by arthritis. The client in a reclining position with the feet in metal supports is used in the lithotomy position. The knee–chest position is when the client rests on the knees and chest with their head supported to one side on a small pillow.

SECTION IV: REVIEWING WHAT YOU HAVE LEARNED

Activity H

1. Paracentesis
2. Spinal tap

Activity I

1. True
2. False. Electromyography is an examination of the energy produced by stimulated muscles; electro-encephalography is an examination of the energy emitted by the brain.

Activity J

1. Magnetic resonance imaging
2. Transducer

Activity K

1. The equipment shown in the figure includes the following:
   a. Glucometer
   b. Control solution
   c. Lancet
   d. Lancet holder
   e. Test strip
   f. Container of test strips
2. This equipment is used to perform capillary blood glucose testing.

Activity L

1. A culture is performed by collecting body fluids or substances suspected of containing infectious microorganisms, growing the living microorganisms in a nutritive substance, and examining their characteristics with a microscope. Cultures are commonly performed on urine, blood, stool, wound drainage, and throat secretions.
2. A lumbar puncture or spinal tap may be performed (1) to diagnose conditions that increase pressure within the brain, such as brain or spinal cord tumors or infections like meningitis; (2) before instilling contrast media for X-rays of the spinal column; or (3) to instill drugs directly into the spinal fluid after the withdrawal of a similar amount.

SECTION V: APPLYING YOUR KNOWLEDGE

Activity M

Metal produces a dense image on radiography, which examiners may confuse with a tissue abnormality.

Activity N

1. The nurse should perform a surgical scrub and don sterile gloves and garments before active involvement in operative or obstetric procedures.
2. A surgical scrub thoroughly removes transient microorganisms from the nails, hands, and forearms. Sterile gloves and garments provide a surface free of microorganisms that, if unsterile, could be transferred to the client.

3. The nurse should tell the client that the machine will record electrical impulses from the heart. Electrodes will be attached to the skin to detect electrical activity. Except for an awareness of the electrodes, the client will not experience any other sensations.
4. The nurse should:
   • Clean the skin and clip hair if necessary in the area where the electrode tabs will be placed to ensure adherence and reduce discomfort on removal.
   • Attach the adhesive electrode tabs to the skin where the electrode wires will be fastened.
   • Attach the adhesive tabs to areas other than over bones, scars, or breast tissue.

SECTION VI: GETTING READY FOR NCLEX

Activity O

1. **Answer: c**
   RATIONALE: The nurse should inform the client that the procedure is painless unless it touches a terminal nerve. The client need not stay awake after midnight before undergoing an EMG. Clients undergoing a sleep-deprived electroencephalography (EEG) are asked to stay awake after midnight before the examination. A client who is to undergo an EEG is asked to avoid cola beverages for 8 hours before the procedure and consult with the physician about withholding scheduled medications, especially those that affect neurologic activity. These measures are not necessary for clients undergoing an EMG.

CHAPTER 15

SECTION I: ASSESSING YOUR UNDERSTANDING

Activity A

1. Malnutrition
2. Calories
3. Kilocalorie
4. Lipoproteins
5. Cellulose
6. Minerals
7. Essential
8. Unsaturated
9. Dementia
10. Flatus

Activity B

1. The figure shows a sample of nutritional information.
2. The figure displays the amounts of each nutrient per serving in household measurements.
3. DVs are calculated percentages of set standards for total fat, saturated fat, cholesterol, sodium, carbohydrate, and fiber in a 2,000-calorie diet. The standards are as follows:

- Total fat: less than 65 g
- Saturated fat: less than 20 g
- Cholesterol: less than 300 mg
- Sodium: less than 2,400 mg
- Total carbohydrate: 300 g
- Dietary fiber: 25 g

Activity C

1. b   **2.** a   **3.** d   **4.** e   **5.** c

Activity D

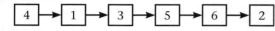

4 → 1 → 3 → 5 → 6 → 2

Activity E

1. The parameters for individual nutritional needs are as follows:
   - Age
   - Weight and height
   - Growth periods
   - Activity
   - Health status
2. Water-soluble vitamins (B complex, C) are eliminated with body fluids and thus require daily replacement. Fat-soluble vitamins (A, D, E, and K) are stored in the body as reserves for future needs.
3. Eating habits are influenced by cultural, economic, emotional, and social factors, including the following:
   - Food preferences
   - Established meal patterns
   - Nutritional attitudes and knowledge
   - Income level
   - Time available for food preparation
   - Number of people in the household
   - Access to food markets
   - Food as comfort, celebration, reward
   - Attitude toward body weight
   - Religious beliefs
4. While making a physical assessment of a client, the nurse would assess the following:
   - General appearance
   - Integrity of the mouth
   - Condition of the teeth
   - Ability to chew and swallow
   - Gag reflex
   - Characteristics of skin and hair
   - Joint flexibility
   - Hand strength
   - Attention and concentration
5. While feeding a visually impaired client, the nurse takes the following measures:
   - Place a thick towel across the client's chest and over the lap.
   - If the client can eat independently, consider using dishes with rims or bowls to prevent spilling.
   - Arrange as much as possible to have finger foods (foods that may be eaten with the hands) prepared for the client.
   - Describe the food and indicate its location on the tray.
   - Guide the client's hand to reinforce the location of food and utensils.
   - Prepare the food by opening cartons, cutting bite-size pieces, adding salt and pepper, buttering bread, and pouring coffee.
   - Use the analogy of a clock when describing where the client may find food on the plate. For example, "The potatoes are at 3 o'clock."
   - If the client needs to be fed, tell them what kind of food you are offering with each mouthful.
   - Devise a system by which the client can indicate when they are ready for more food or drink, such as asking or raising a finger.
6. The nutritional status of older adults is affected by the following:
   - Medical conditions
   - Adverse medication effects
   - Functional impairments
   - Psychosocial conditions such as dementia, depression, and social isolation
   - Oral and dental problems

SECTION II: APPLYING YOUR KNOWLEDGE

Activity F

1. The nurse should take the following measures when serving a client with impaired swallowing:
   - Always have equipment for oral and pharyngeal suctioning at the bedside.
   - Remain with the client throughout eating when there is a potential for aspiration.
   - If the client has a tracheostomy tube or endotracheal tube, make sure the cuff is inflated.
   - Place the client in a sitting position.
   - Ensure that the client is rested and that you have their attention.
   - Give short, simple instructions to prompt the client to eat and swallow.
   - Limit distracting stimuli; turn off the television and reduce or eliminate activities taking place in the area.
   - Request a full liquid or mechanically soft diet for the client who has missing teeth or has recently had oral surgery.
   - Provide small frequent meals if efforts to eat and swallow tire the client.
   - Modify eating or feeding equipment to facilitate the client's safety and independence.
   - Determine that the client has swallowed one portion of food before offering another.
   - Encourage repeated swallowing attempts if there is wet, gurgly vocalization, a sign that food is in the esophagus and not the stomach.

SECTION III: PRACTICING FOR NCLEX

Activity G

1. **Answer: a**
   RATIONALE: The nurse should recommend animal sources of protein such as poultry. Animal sources provide complete proteins, which contain all the essential amino acids. Plant sources contain incomplete proteins, which contain only some essential amino acids.

2. **Answer: a**
   RATIONALE: Malnutrition is a condition resulting from a lack of proper nutrients in the diet. Evidence of malnutrition is common among people living in poor, developing countries; however, it also occurs among people living in countries known for their affluence, like the United States. People with eating disorders are at risk. Religious beliefs, family history, and emotional disorders may not be a cause of malnutrition.

3. **Answer: b**
   RATIONALE: The nurse should recommend vitamin C supplements to make up for the lack of water-soluble vitamins. Vitamin B complex and vitamin C are water-soluble vitamins that are eliminated with body fluids. Therefore, these vitamins need daily replacement. Vitamins A, D, and E are fat-soluble vitamins and are stored in the body as reserves for future needs.

4. **Answer: a**
   RATIONALE: Obesity is a condition in which a person's body mass index equals or exceeds 30 kg/m^2 or the triceps skinfold measurement exceeds 15 mm. Client A is obese because the client's body mass index is 30.2 kg/m^2.

5. **Answer: d**
   RATIONALE: The nurse should recommend that the client with a blood clot in their lower left leg include good sources of minerals in their diet to regulate the chemical processes. Minerals are noncaloric substances in food that are essential to all cells and help to regulate many of the body's chemical processes such as blood clotting and conduction of nerve impulses. Fats are sources of energy, whereas proteins are the building blocks of the body. Carbohydrates are also sources of quick energy. They do not, however, regulate the chemical processes in the client's body.

6. **Answer: c**
   RATIONALE: DV is a percentage of set standards for total fat, saturated fat, cholesterol, sodium, carbohydrate, and fiber in a 2,000-calorie diet; diets more or less than 2,000 calories need adjustment to the DV percentage. Excessive cholesterol will give rise to more problems than the other nutrients. Vitamin and mineral requirements are uniform to all consumers because they are independent of calories.

7. **Answer: c**
   RATIONALE: Eating habits are influenced by cultural, economic, emotional, and social factors, including food preferences, established meal patterns, religious beliefs, and so on. In this case, the client does not eat any meat or dairy products; therefore, the client is a vegan. Vegetarians do not consume animal products; however, they do eat dairy products. The client works in the city and has access to food markets. Pregnancy probably will not usually influence the eating habits of a client to a great extent. Therefore, the only probable factor that influences the client's eating habits seems to be veganism.

8. **Answer: c**
   RATIONALE: The client's diet is lacking in protein. A vegan diet is often inadequate in complete protein, calcium, riboflavin, vitamins B$_{12}$ and D, and iron. A vegan diet does not include animal or animal products, such as meat or dairy products, which may provide fats. Minerals and vitamin C are adequate in vegan diets.

9. **Answer: a**
   RATIONALE: Anthropometric data are used to measure body size and composition. They are obtained by measuring the client's height. The biceps skin thickness, wrist diameter, and chest width are not measured to obtain these data.

10. **Answer: a**
    RATIONALE: A dietary history includes all findings about a client's eating habits, such as the number of meals the client eats, likes and dislikes, time when the client prefers to have meals, and so forth. It does not include findings of the client's cholesterol level or the nutrient content in the food.

11. **Answer: c**
    RATIONALE: Physical assessment of the client would include the skin characteristics of the client. Diet, weight, and height would be included while collecting anthropometric data.

12. **Answer: d**
    RATIONALE: When feeding a client who is visually impaired, the nurse should arrange (as much as possible) to have finger food (food that may be eaten with the hands) prepared for the client. Requesting a full liquid or mechanically soft diet; providing small, frequent meals if eating efforts tire the client; and determining whether the client has swallowed food before offering another mouthful are tasks that the nurse should do when feeding a client with dysphagia.

13. **Answer: a**
    RATIONALE: A gag reflex in the client implies that the client may have difficulty swallowing. Dysphagia implies difficulty swallowing and chewing food. Nausea usually precedes vomiting, eructation (or belching) is discharge of gas through the mouth, and xerostomia results from medications and not a gag reflex.

14. **Answer: d**
    RATIONALE: A client is considered to be obese if the body mass index is 30 or more and the triceps skinfold measurement exceeds 15 mm.

15. Answer: d

RATIONALE: To lose 1 lb of weight per week, it is recommended that people reduce their food intake by 500 calories per day. A sustained loss of 1 to 2 lb per week is a healthy goal. Therefore, reducing 800 calories from the client's diet every day will help the client to lose weight safely. Reducing excess calories from the diet will be harmful and will lead to exhaustion and weakness. However, omitting 200 calories per day from the diet may not be sufficient to meet the goal.

16. Answers: a, c

RATIONALE: Dementia refers to the deterioration of previous intellectual capacity. To make sure that such clients eat, the nurse should place the tray close to the client and ensure that the client sees another person eating. This will stimulate the client to eat. The nurse should inform the client about the food if the client is visually impaired. Clients with dementia require gentle handling and persistence. When feeding a client with dysphagia, the nurse should provide small, frequent meals if efforts to eat and swallow tire the client.

17. Answers: a, d, e, f

RATIONALE: The nurse should prescribe supplements of vitamins A, D, E, and K for a client with a fat-soluble vitamin deficiency. Fat-soluble vitamins (A, D, E, and K) are stored in the body as reserves for future needs. Water-soluble vitamins (B complex, C) are eliminated with body fluids and thus require daily replacement.

18. Answers: a, b

RATIONALE: The nurse should increase the quantity of cereals and grains in the client's diet to make up for the carbohydrate deficiency. Carbohydrates are nutrients that contain molecules of carbon, hydrogen, and oxygen and are generally found in plant food sources. Carbohydrates, the chief component of most diets, are the body's primary source for quick energy. Cereals and grains such as rice, wheat and wheat germ, oats, barley, corn and corn meal; fruits and vegetables; and sweeteners are sources of carbohydrates. Egg white, yolk, and meat are sources of protein.

19. Answers: a, b, c

RATIONALE: Oral and dental problems are common in older adults and interfere with adequate nutrition. The nurse should encourage older adults to get dental care every 6 months and to practice good dental hygiene daily. In addition, people with a dry mouth should drink adequate noncaffeinated and nonalcoholic beverages to promote salivation. Increasing caloric intake or using herbal therapies will not help reduce dental pain.

20. Answer: b

RATIONALE: The body mass index for the client is calculated to be 28.2. A body mass index above 25 is considered to be overweight. Therefore, the client is overweight. To calculate the body mass index, the nurse performs the following steps: (1) divides weight in pounds by 2.2 to get weight in kilograms, (2) divides the height in inches by 39.4 to get height in meters, (3) squares the answer in step 2 by multiplying the number by itself, and (4) divides the weight in kilograms by the square of the height in meters.

SECTION IV: REVIEWING WHAT YOU HAVE LEARNED

Activity H

1. Anorexia
2. Emesis

Activity I

1. False. Eructation (belching) is a discharge of gas from the stomach through the mouth.
2. True.

Activity J

Midarm circumference

Activity K

1. c   **2.** d   **3.** a   **4.** b

Activity L

1. The six nutritional components in food are calories, proteins, carbohydrates, fats, minerals, and vitamins.
2. The seven common hospital diets include the following:
   • Regular or general: allows unrestricted food selections
   • Light or convalescent: differs from regular diet in preparation; typically omits fried, fatty, gas-forming, and raw foods and rich pastries
   • Soft: contains foods soft in texture; is usually low in residue and readily digestible; contains few or no spices or condiments; provides fewer fruits, vegetables, or meats than a light diet
   • Mechanical soft: resembles a light diet but is used for clients with chewing difficulties; provides cooked fruits and vegetables and ground meats
   • Full liquid: contains creamed or blended soups, milk, ice cream, yogurt without bits of fruit, pudding, milkshakes, custards, and cooked cereals
   • Clear liquid: consists of items that may be colored, but are generally transparent and do not contain any pulp or bits of food. Examples include water, broth, fruit juices, flavored gelatin, popsicles, clear soft drinks, tea, and coffee
   • Special therapeutic: consists of foods prepared to meet special needs, such as low in sodium, fat, calories, or fiber

SECTION V: APPLYING YOUR KNOWLEDGE

Activity M

High-density lipoprotein (HDL) is delivered to the liver for removal, rather than becoming deposited within the arterial walls, which can eventually result in cardiovascular disease.

Activity N

1.
   a. A full liquid or mechanically soft diet is best.
   b. The nurse should proceed as follows when feeding a client with difficulty chewing or swallowing:
      • Place the client in a sitting position.
      • Ensure that the client is rested and is giving their full attention to eating.
      • Give short, simple instructions to prompt the client to eat and swallow.
      • Limit distracting stimuli such as television or other activities.
      • Modify eating or feeding equipment to facilitate the client's safety and independence.
      • Determine that the client has swallowed one portion of food before offering another.
      • Encourage repeated swallowing attempts if there are wet, gurgly vocalizations, a sign that food is in the esophagus and not the stomach.
      • Remain with the client throughout eating when there is a potential for aspiration.
      • Always include equipment for oral and pharyngeal suctioning at the bedside.

SECTION VI: GETTING READY FOR NCLEX

Activity O

1. **Answers: a, d, e**
   RATIONALE: The nurse should encourage the client to walk if possible, which helps gas rise to its highest point in the stomach, making belching easier. The client should not chew gum because doing so increases salivation and results in swallowing both secretions and air. The nurse should suggest that the client eat with a closed mouth because laughing or talking while eating increases the intake of swallowed air. The client should restrict intake of carbonated drinks because such beverages distend the stomach. The client should not use a straw while drinking because each swallow of liquid also contains the air in the straw.

CHAPTER 16

SECTION I: ASSESSING YOUR UNDERSTANDING

Activity A

1. Infiltration
2. Intracellular
3. Extracellular
4. Interstitial
5. Prions
6. Ions
7. Dehydration
8. Vented
9. Venipuncture
10. Phlebitis

Activity B

1. The distribution method shown in the figure is osmosis.
2. During osmosis, water moves through a semipermeable membrane—like those surrounding body cells, capillary walls, and body organs and cavities—from an area where the fluid is more dilute to another area where the fluid is more concentrated.
3. Colloids are undissolved protein substances such as albumin and blood cells within body fluids that do not readily pass through membranes. The presence and quantity of colloids on either side of the semipermeable membrane influence osmosis. Their very presence produces colloidal osmotic pressure (force for attracting water), which influences fluid volume in any given fluid location.

Activity C

1. d   2. e   3. a   4. b   5. c

Activity D

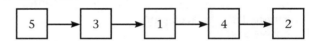

Activity E

1. Body fluid is a mixture of water, chemicals (electrolytes and nonelectrolytes), and blood cells. Body water normally is supplied and replenished from drinking liquids, consuming food, and metabolizing nutrients.
2. The donated blood is tested for syphilis, hepatitis, and HIV antibodies to exclude administering blood that may transmit these blood-borne diseases.
3. Electrolytes are chemical compounds, such as sodium and chloride, which are dissolved, absorbed, and distributed in body fluid. They are essential for maintaining cellular, tissue, and organ functions. For example, electrolytes affect fluid balance and complex chemical activities such as muscle contraction and the formation of enzymes, acids, and bases.
4. Type O blood is considered the universal donor because it lacks both A and B blood group markers on its cell membrane. Therefore, type O blood can be given to anyone because it will not trigger an incompatibility reaction when given to recipients with other blood types. Persons with type AB blood are referred to as *universal recipients* because their red blood cells have proteins compatible with types A, B, and O.

5. Nonelectrolytes are chemical compounds that remain bound together when dissolved in a solution and do not conduct electricity. The chemical end products of carbohydrate, protein, and fat metabolism—namely, glucose, amino acids, and fatty acids, respectively—provide a continuous supply of nonelectrolytes. In the absence of metabolic disease, a stable amount of nonelectrolytes circulates in body fluid as long as a person consumes adequate nutrients. Deficiency states occur when body fluid is lost or when the ability to eat is compromised.

6. There are several hundred differences among the proteins in the blood of a donor and the blood of a recipient. They can cause minor or major transfusion reactions. One of the most dangerous differences involves the antigens, or protein structures, on membranes of red blood cells. Antigens determine the characteristic blood group—A, B, AB, and O—and Rh factor. Rh positive means the protein is present; Rh negative means the protein is absent.

SECTION II: APPLYING YOUR KNOWLEDGE

Activity F

1. The client is showing signs of fluid deficit. The nurse should observe the following symptoms in the client:
   • Loss of body weight
   • Severe dehydration
   • Decreased skin turgor
2. The nurse should ensure that the client's fluid intake on an average is approximately 2,500 mL per day. It can also range from 1,800 to 3,000 mL per day. This will help the client's body maintain a match between fluid intake and output.

SECTION III: PRACTICING FOR NCLEX

Activity G

1. **Answer: b**
   RATIONALE: The nurse could consider blood type O, Rh negative for the client. Type O blood is considered the universal donor because it lacks both A and B blood group markers on its cell membrane. Therefore, type O blood can be given to anyone because it will not trigger an incompatibility reaction when given to recipients with other blood types. Persons with type AB blood are referred to as universal recipients because their red blood cells have proteins compatible with types A, B, and O, but this type of blood cannot be given to everyone. Rh-positive persons may receive Rh-positive or Rh-negative blood because the latter does not contain the sensitizing protein. Rh-negative persons, however, should not be given Rh-positive blood. So, the client with A, Rh-negative blood cannot be given A, Rh-positive or B, Rh-positive blood types.

2. **Answer: b**
   RATIONALE: The client with diarrhea would require fluid volume assessment. The client has been losing fluid from their body and would require intravenous fluid intake. Other clients who may need fluid volume assessment are those who have undergone surgery, those who have intravenous fluids with tube feedings, those with wound drainage or suction equipment, those who have urinary catheters, or those who are undergoing diuretic drug therapy. Clients with tonsillitis, viral infection, or jaundice may not be required to be placed on input-and-output tool immediately, although they may be given other intravenous fluids to help combat their illnesses.

3. **Answer: c**
   RATIONALE: The nurse should note hypovolemia as the possible cause of the client's condition. Hypovolemia is a low volume in extracellular fluid compartments. If untreated, hypovolemia may result in dehydration, which means a fluid deficit in both extracellular and intracellular compartments. Hypervolemia means a higher-than-normal volume of water in the intravascular fluid compartment and is another example of fluid imbalance. Edema develops when excess fluid is distributed to the interstitial space. Hypoalbuminemia is the result of a deficit of albumin in the blood. These, however, are not responsible for the client's condition.

4. **Answer: d**
   RATIONALE: The nurse should document the client's level of dehydration as mild. Mild dehydration is present when there is a 3% to 5% loss of body weight. Moderate dehydration is associated with a 6% to 10% loss of body weight; and severe dehydration, a life-threatening emergency, occurs with a loss of more than 9% to 15% of body weight.

5. **Answer: a**
   RATIONALE: To avoid the fluid and electrolyte imbalances that result from the administration of diuretic medication to older clients, the nurse should encourage the client to drink noncaffeinated drinks. As a part of nursing interventions and general care, the nurse should encourage older adults to drink noncaffeinated beverages because of the diuretic effect of caffeine or to replace the volume of caffeinated beverages by consuming the same volume of noncaffeinated fluids per day. Older adults may need to be encouraged to drink fluids, even at times when they do not feel thirsty because age-related changes may diminish the sensation of thirst. The nurse should not encourage the client to have more food or caffeinated drinks, or to avoid intake of salt in food.

6. **Answer: a**
   RATIONALE: Dextran 40 would help to increase the client's blood volume and blood pressure.

Dextran 40 (Rheomacrodex) and hetastarch (Hespan) are polysaccharides, which are large, insoluble complex carbohydrate molecules. They attract water from other fluid compartments and hence increase blood volume and blood pressure. Perfluorocarbons are used to restore oxygen to tissues with impaired circulation, such as the brain after a stroke. Microencapsulated hemoglobin is the product made from recycling outdated red blood cells in donated blood by sealing them within a lipid capsule. Hemosol is used to improve the treatment of disorders that previously required blood transfusions but are not used to increase blood volume and blood pressure.

7. **Answer: a**
   RATIONALE: The nurse should record the client condition as edema. Edema develops when excess fluid is distributed to interstitial spaces. Edema does not usually occur unless there is a 3-L excess in body fluid. Hypervolemia means a higher-than-normal volume of water in the intravascular fluid compartment. Hypovolemia is low volume in the extracellular fluid compartments. Hypoalbuminemia is a situation in which there is a deficit of albumin in the blood. These, however, are not related to the client's condition.

8. **Answer: b**
   RATIONALE: The nurse should ensure that the client is weighed at the same time daily, in the same clothing, and on the same scale to enable tracking of weight changes indicative of fluid volume fluctuations. There is no fixed rule that the client should wear light clothes, but it is mandatory that the client wear the same clothing when being weighed. The nurse need not weigh the client on different scales to avoid discrepancies. Also, the nurse needs to weigh the client every day and not three times a week at the same time.

9. **Answer: c**
   RATIONALE: The nurse should restrict the salt intake in a client with edema. When caring for a client with edema, the nurse should ensure that intake of oral fluids and salt consumption is restricted or limited. Hypovolemia or moderate dehydration is treated by increasing the oral intake, administering intravenous fluid replacements, controlling fluid losses, or a combination of these measures.

10. **Answer: b**
    RATIONALE: When administering the intravenous solution, the nurse should monitor the client for any circulatory overload. Clients with hypoalbuminemia have a deficit of albumin in their blood. The priority is to restore the circulatory volume by providing intravenous fluids, sometimes in large volumes at rapid rates. The nurse closely monitors clients who receive albumin replacement for signs of circulatory overload. The nurse would not check for dehydration, infuse fluids at smaller volumes at rapid rates, or infuse fluids at smaller volumes at slower rates.

11. **Answer: d**
    RATIONALE: The deficit of albumin in the blood may cause liver disease, chronic kidney disease, and disorders in which capillary and cellular permeability is altered, such as burns and severe allergic reactions. Dehydration is caused from excess of fluid output compared with fluid intake. Deficit of albumin will not cause heart or peritoneum infection.

12. **Answer: a**
    RATIONALE: The nurse would observe cyanosis as a symptom of adverse reaction to lipid infusion. Cardiac arrest, gallbladder enlargement, and anemia are not specific symptoms of adverse reactions to lipid infusion.

13. **Answer: b**
    RATIONALE: An isotonic solution generally is administered to maintain fluid balance in clients who may not be able to eat or drink for a short period. A hypotonic solution is administered to clients with fluid losses in excess of fluid intake. Hypertonic solutions are used when it is necessary to reduce cerebral edema or to expand the circulatory volume rapidly. An isotonic solution is not administered when the client is unable to urinate.

14. **Answer: c**
    RATIONALE: The nurse knows that Hespan is used to treat a client for hypovolemic shock. Plasma expanders such as dextran 40 (Rheomacrodex) and hetastarch (Hespan) are used as economic and virus-free substitutes for blood and blood products when treating hypovolemic shock. D10W (10% Detrose in water), TPN (total parenteral nutrition), and 3%NaCl (3% saline) are used for conditions other than hypovolemic shock.

15. **Answers: b, d, e**
    RATIONALE: The nurse needs to monitor the client receiving the intravenous solution for phlebitis, dehydration, and thrombus formation. These are complications associated with administration of intravenous solutions. Edema and hypervolemia are disorders resulting from a fluid imbalance.

16. **Answer: b**
    RATIONALE: During the blood transfusion the nurse should remain with the client for the first 15 minutes because serious transfusion reactions generally occur within the first 5 to 15 minutes of infusion. The nurse should infuse the blood within 4 hours (not 5 hours) after being released from the blood bank. The nurse can gently rotate the blood, but not squeeze and turn the container to avoid damaging intact cells. The nurse should assess the client at 15- to 30-minute intervals during the transfusion.

17. **Answer: c**
    RATIONALE: The nurse should weigh the wet diapers and subtract the weight of a similar dry item. An estimate of fluid loss is based on the equivalent 1 pound (0.47 kg) = 1 pint (475 mL). It is, however, not equivalent to 0.87 kg = 487 mL, 1.00 kg = 100 mL, or 0.37 kg = 337 mL.

18. **Answer: a**
    RATIONALE: The nurse uses 15 mL glucose, which is equivalent to 1 tablespoon. One teaspoon of sugar is equivalent to 5 mL sugar. One tablespoon is not equivalent to 20, 10, or 25 mL glucose.
19. **Answer: b**
    RATIONALE: Fluid volumes are recorded in milliliters. The approximate equivalent for 1 ounce is 30 mL. Therefore, the nurse should give 30 mL glucose to the client and not 10, 20, or 15 mL.

SECTION IV: REVIEWING WHAT YOU HAVE LEARNED

Activity H

1. Cations
2. Hypervolemia

Activity I

1. True.
2. False. Passive diffusion is the physiologic process in which dissolved substances such as electrolytes and gases move through a semipermeable membrane from an area of higher concentration to an area of lower concentration.

Activity J

Interstitial fluid

Activity K

1. b   **2.** c   **3.** d   **4.** a

Activity L

	Crystalloid Solution	**Colloid Solution**
Definition	This intravenous solution is made of water and other uniformly dissolved crystals.	This intravenous solution is made of water and molecules of suspended substances.
Effects	A crystalloid solution influences the osmotic distribution of body fluid.	A colloid solution ensures a circulating blood volume because the suspended molecules pull fluid from other compartments.
Example	Solution of salt and sugar	Blood, blood products, plasma expanders

Activity M

1. Parenteral nutrition is provided by a route other than oral. It may be administered through an intravenous catheter inserted into a peripheral vein or through a catheter that terminates in a central vein near the heart.

2. Intravenous solutions are administered to the client to:
   • Maintain or restore fluid balance when oral replacement is inadequate or impossible.
   • Maintain or replace electrolytes.
   • Administer water-soluble vitamins.
   • Provide a source of calories.
   • Administer drugs.
   • Replace blood and blood products.

SECTION V: APPLYING YOUR KNOWLEDGE

Activity N

The plastic bags of IV solutions collapse as the fluid infuses.

Activity O

1.
   a. Before preparing the IV solution, the nurse should determine that the solution is the one prescribed by the physician, it is clear and transparent, the expiration date has not elapsed, there are no apparent leaks, and a separate label is attached identifying the type and amount of other drugs added to the commercial solution.
   b. To remove bubbles from the IV tubing, the nurse should:
      • Flush the line with IV solution to purge air from the tubing before inserting the adapter into the venipuncture device.
      • Tighten the roller clamp if small bubbles are observed to prevent continued forward movement of the air.
      • Tap the tubing below the air bubbles to promote upward movement of the air above the fluid in the drip chamber.
      • Milk the air in the direction of the drip chamber or filter, if one is incorporated within the tubing. Doing so pushes the air physically to an area where it can be trapped and released.
      • Wrap the tubing around a circular object like a pencil, starting below the trapped air to move the air toward the drip chamber where it can escape from the liquid into the empty air space.
      • Remove the barrel from a syringe. Insert the needle on the syringe or the needleless adaptor on the syringe within a port below the air, and open the roller clamp to siphon fluid and air from the tubing as it passes by the syringe.

SECTION VI: GETTING READY FOR NCLEX

Activity P

1. **Answers: a, b, c, e**
   RATIONALE: The nurse should suggest rinsing the mouth without swallowing water because

rinsing reduces thirst and keeps the mouth moist. The nurse should provide fluids in a plastic squeeze bottle or spray atomizer because these devices provide small amounts of fluids. The nurse should explain to the client the purpose for fluid restrictions because knowledge facilitates client cooperation. The nurse should ask the client to restrict intake of salt in the food because this helps reduce thirst. The nurse should offer ice chips, which appear to contain more fluids than they actually do, and holding them in the mouth prolongs consumption time.

CHAPTER 17

SECTION I: ASSESSING YOUR UNDERSTANDING

Activity A

1. Keratin
2. Mucus
3. Deciduous
4. Caries
5. Cornea
6. Mouth
7. Feet
8. Cerumen
9. Optometrist
10. Subcutaneous

Activity B

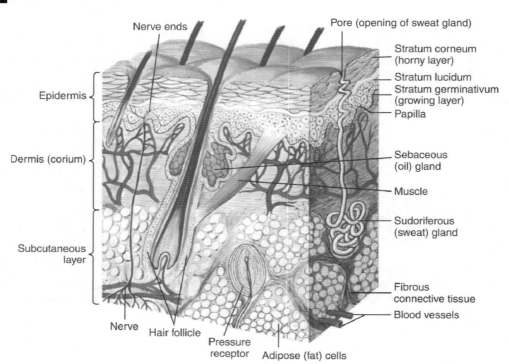

1. The figure shows a cross-section of the skin.
2. The functions of the different layers of the skin are as follows:
   - The epidermis contains dead skin cells that form a tough protein called keratin, which protects the layers and structures within the lower portions of the skin.
   - The dermis contains most of the secretory glands.
   - The subcutaneous layer separates the skin from skeletal muscles. It contains fat cells, blood vessels, nerves, and the roots of hair follicles and glands.
3. The figure shows a cross-section of a tooth.
4. Some common problems associated with the teeth are caries, gingivitis, and periodontal disease.

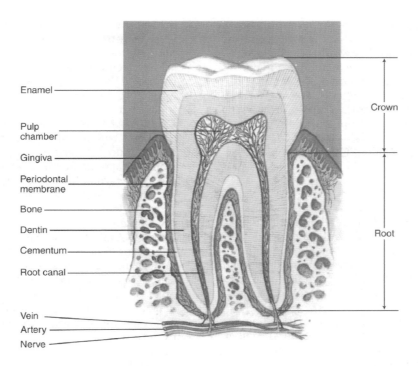

Enamel

Pulp chamber

Gingiva

Periodontal membrane

Bone

Dentin

Cementum

Root canal

Vein

Artery

Nerve

Crown

Root

1. d   **2.** b   **3.** e   **4.** a   **5.** c

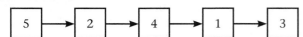

5 → 2 → 4 → 1 → 3

1. Toothbrushing is the preferred technique for providing oral hygiene to unconscious clients. In addition to toothbrushing, the nurse can also moisten and refresh the client's mouth with oral swabs.
2. A partial bath is washing only those body areas subject to greatest soiling or that are sources of body odor, such as the face, hands, axillae, and perineal area. Partial bathing is done at a sink or with a basin at the bedside.
3. The five main functions of the skin are to
   - Protect inner body structures from injury and infection.
   - Regulate body temperature.
   - Maintain fluid and chemical balance.
   - Provide sensory information such as pain, temperature, touch, and pressure.
   - Assist in converting precursors to vitamin D when exposed to sunlight.
4. When grooming a client's hair, the nurse should
   - Try to use a hairstyle the client prefers.
   - Brush the hair slowly and carefully to avoid damaging the hair.
   - Brush the hair to increase circulation and distribution of sebum.
   - Use a wide-toothed comb, starting at the ends of the hair rather than from the crown downward, especially if the hair is matted or tangled.
   - Apply a conditioner or alcohol to loosen tangles.
   - Use oil on the hair if it is dry. Many preparations are available, but pure castor oil, olive oil, and mineral oil are satisfactory.
   - Braid the hair to help prevent tangles.
   - If hair loss occurs from cancer therapy or some other disease or medical treatment, provide the client with a turban or baseball cap.
   - Avoid using hairpins or clips that may injure the scalp.
   - Obtain the client's or family's permission before cutting the hair if it is hopelessly tangled and cutting seems to be the only solution to provide adequate grooming.
5. When cleaning eyeglasses, the nurse should
   - Hold the eyeglasses by the nose or ear braces.
   - Run tepid water over both sides of the lenses (hot water damages plastic lenses).
   - Wash the lenses with soap or detergent.
   - Rinse with running tap water.
   - Dry with a clean, soft cloth such as a handkerchief.
   - Avoid use of paper tissues because some contain wood fibers and pulp can scratch the lenses.

SECTION II: APPLYING YOUR KNOWLEDGE

1. The nurse can suggest the client undergo partial bathing. A partial bath means washing only those body areas subject to greatest soiling or that are sources of body odor: generally the face, hands, axillae, and perineal area. Partial bathing is done at a sink or with a basin at the bedside.

2. When providing perineal care, the nurse must
   • Prevent direct contact between themselves and any secretions or excretions by wearing clean gloves.
   • Clean so that they remove secretions and excretions from less soiled to more soiled areas.
   • Use these principles to help prevent the transfer of infectious microorganisms to the nurse and to uncontaminated areas on or within the client.

SECTION III: PRACTICING FOR NCLEX

Activity G

1. **Answer: a**
   RATIONALE: The nurse removes the prosthetic eye by depressing the lower eyelid until the lid margin is wide enough to allow the eye to slide free. The nurse uses an ophthalmic suction cup to remove the lens from the eyes. Extending the eyelid will not help the prosthetic eye to come out. Irrigating the eye socket is a method of cleaning the eye.

2. **Answer: c**
   RATIONALE: A partial bath is the most suitable for the older client with arthritis because the client cannot move too much and the client also does not perspire much. During a bed bath, the client needs to assist the nurse with some aspects of bathing. With a towel bath, the nurse uses a single large towel to cover and wash a client. A towel bath is used on those clients who are incapable of assisting the nurse in bathing. Clients who can bathe independently may use a tub or shower bath, which may not be applicable in this case.

3. **Answer: a**
   RATIONALE: Removing the lens from the cornea to the sclera by sliding it into position is the easiest and safest way to remove the lens. To remove a hard contact lens, the nurse places the thumb and a finger on the center of the upper and lower lids. The nurse applies slight pressure to the lids while instructing the client to blink, which separates the hard lens from the cornea. Depressing the lower eyelid or using a finger to remove the lens will damage the soft lens and the eyes as well.

4. **Answer: b**
   RATIONALE: The best bath for a client with a fever is a sponge bath using tepid water. A Sitz bath removes blood, serum, stool, or urine and reduces swelling. Medicated baths relieve itching or a rash, and whirlpool baths improve circulation, increase joint mobility, relieve discomfort, and remove dead tissue.

5. **Answer: c**
   RATIONALE: Body aid devices will be best suited for the client because they have electrical components enclosed in a case carried somewhere on the body to deliver sound via a wire connected to an ear mold receiver. Use of body aids is most common for those with severe hearing loss or for those who cannot care for a small device. A behind-the-ear device is a very small device that consists of a microphone and amplifier worn behind the ear that delivers sound to an internal receiver. Infrared listening devices resemble earphones attached to a handheld receiver. Canal aids fit deep within the ear canal and are largely concealed. Because of their small size, they may be difficult to remove and adjust.

6. **Answer: b**
   RATIONALE: The nurse should always clean the eyeglasses with a clean, soft handkerchief or cloth so that it does not damage the glasses. A woolen cloth or paper tissue can scratch the lenses because it contains wood fibers and pulp. A dryer is not a good option because it ejects hot air, which may crack the lens.

7. **Answer: a**
   RATIONALE: Because the client has cancer, the hair needs to be covered by a turban or cap to protect the scalp and hair. Chemotherapy might lead to hair loss; therefore, the client need not cut or keep his hair short. The nurse should comb the hair slowly with a wide-tooth comb and should comb starting at the ends of the hair rather than from the crown.

8. **Answer: d**
   RATIONALE: The nurse should use oral swabs to keep the client's mouth moist because the client is in coma and there is no secretion of saliva to keep the mouth moist. Waxed floss is used by clients who can take care of their oral hygiene independently. The nurse need not use sterile solutions or liquids for oral care because these could predispose clients to pneumonia from aspiration.

9. **Answer: d**
   RATIONALE: For clients who cannot remove their own dentures, the nurse dons gloves and uses a dry gauze square or a clean facecloth to grasp and free the dentures from the mouth. The nurse should clean the dentures with a toothbrush, toothpaste, and cold or tepid water. The nurse should take care to hold the dentures over a plastic basin or towel so they will not break if dropped. The nurse should store the dentures in a covered cup. Plain water is used most often to cover dentures when they are not in the mouth, but some denture wearers add mouthwash or denture cleaner to the water. Antiseptic solution, hot water, or cotton swabs are not used to clean dentures.

10. **Answer: a**
    RATIONALE: When providing personal hygiene care, the nurse should take care of the client's personal preference and assist them in taking a full shower or tub bath. The nurse should provide nonskid mats on floor and ensure that there are handles and grab bars at arm level. Insisting on a partial bath, bag bath, or towel bath will only make the client uncomfortable.

11. **Answer: d**
    RATIONALE: The nurse should request the services of a podiatrist. Clients who have diabetes, impaired circulation, or thick nails are at risk for

vascular complications secondary to trauma. The nurse should refrain from cleaning and filing the nails before the client consults a podiatrist. The nurse should clean under the nails with a wooden orange stick or other sturdy but blunt instrument, not with a clean towel.

12. Answer: c
RATIONALE: The nurse should advise the client to avoid injuring the feet and instruct the client to wear sturdy slippers. Flip-flops, heeled shoes, or leather slippers should not be used by the client because these may further aggravate the problem.

13. Answer: b
RATIONALE: Skin lesions such as senile lentigines show symptoms like brown, flat patches on the face, hands, and forearms. Seborrheic keratoses are benign skin lesions that look like tan-to-black raised areas on the trunk. Scleroderma is caused by collagen deposits on the skin, whereas acne occurs from excess secretion of the sebaceous glands, mostly in young age.

14. Answers: a, c, d
RATIONALE: The nurse, while grooming the client's hair, should brush the hair slowly and carefully to avoid damaging it, use a wide-tooth comb, and start at the ends of the hair rather than from the crown downward if the hair is matted or tangled. The nurse should braid the hair rather than tie it in a bun, to help prevent tangles. The nurse should also brush the hair for a longer time to increase circulation and distribution of sebum.

15. Answers: c, d, a, b, e
RATIONALE: The nurse cleans glass and plastic lenses by first holding the eyeglasses by the nose or ear braces and running tepid water over both sides of the lenses. The nurse then washes the lenses with soap or detergent and rinses them with running tap water to clean them. Last, the nurse dries the glasses with a clean, soft cloth such as a handkerchief.

16. Answers: d, b, e, c, a
RATIONALE: Before removing contact lenses, the nurse should obtain an appropriate storage container. The nurse should then elevate the client's head and place a towel over the client's chest to prevent loss or damage to the contact lenses. To remove a soft contact lens, the nurse moves the lens from the cornea to the sclera by sliding it into position with a clean, gloved finger. When repositioning the lens, the nurse compresses the lid margins together toward the lens. Compression bends the pliable lens, allowing air to enter beneath it. The air releases the lens from the surface of the eye. The nurse then gently grasps the loosened lens between the thumb and forefinger for removal.

SECTION IV: REVIEWING WHAT YOU HAVE LEARNED

Activity H
1. Caries
2. Ophthalmologist

Activity I
1. True
2. True

Activity J
1. Hygiene
2. Sordes

Activity K
The figure shows a cross-section of the skin.

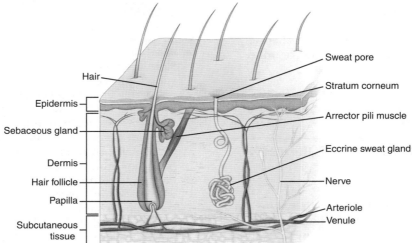

Activity L
1. An infrared listening device (IRLD) helps improve the ability to hear by converting sound into infrared light and sending it via a wall- or ceiling-mounted receiver to the person wearing the listening device. The light is converted back into an auditory stimulus.
2. The nurse should wear gloves and use dry gauze square or clean face cloth to grasp and free the dentures from the client's mouth. They should

clean the dentures and removable bridges with a toothbrush, toothpaste, and cold or tepid water. The nurse should hold the dentures over a plastic basin or towel so they will not break if dropped. If removing the bridge or dentures at night, the nurse should store them in a covered cup filled with plain water and mouthwash or denture cleanser.

SECTION V: APPLYING YOUR KNOWLEDGE

Activity M

The nurse needs to make sure that bathing does not interfere with other components of care and treatment and that bathing preferences are individualized to the client's needs and minimize unnecessary interruptions.

Activity N

1.
   a. Comatose or unconscious clients are at risk for pneumonia if they aspirate saliva or liquid oral hygiene products into their lungs during oral care.
   b. The nurse should position the client on the side with the head slightly lowered to prevent liquids from draining into the airway. They should use a tongue blade to open the mouth and separate the teeth. The nurse should suction the mouth with a bulb syringe or Yankauer suction device to remove debris and reduce the potential for aspiration.

2.
   a. When providing perineal care, nurses must take the following precautions:
     • Wear clean gloves.
     • Prevent direct contact with any secretions or excretions.
     • Cleanse from less soiled to more soiled areas when removing secretions and excretions.
     • Rinse and pat the skin dry to prevent infection from soap residue and retained moisture.
   b. Sitz baths help reduce local swelling and discomfort. They also clean the perineal area by removing any blood, serum, stool, or urine.

Activity O

1. There are no definite answers to this activity. Students may choose to discuss their thoughts with peers or instructors.

SECTION VI: GETTING READY FOR NCLEX

Activity P

1. **Answer: b**
   RATIONALE: Rinsing the lenses with running tap water ensures that they are easily cleaned without any scratches. The nurse should not use paper tissue, which might contain wood fibers and pulp that could scratch the surface. The nurse should not immerse the lenses in hot soapy water, which could damage the plastic surface. The nurse need not allow the lenses to air-dry; instead, the nurse could use a clean, soft cloth such as a handkerchief to wipe them dry.

CHAPTER 18

SECTION I: ASSESSING YOUR UNDERSTANDING

Activity A

1. Thermoregulation
2. Paradoxical
3. Parasomnias
4. Stimulants
5. Insomnia
6. Phototherapy
7. Rest
8. Sundown
9. Hypersomnia

Activity B

1. The figure shows characteristic ECG waveforms by sleep stage.
2. Sleep is divided into two phases: NREM sleep and REM sleep. These names derive from the periods during sleep when eye movements are either subdued or energetic. NREM sleep is characterized as quiet sleep; REM sleep is characterized as active sleep.
3. A photosensitive light system influences the sleep–wake cycle.
4. Wakefulness corresponds with sunrise and daylight. Cycles of wakefulness followed by sleep are linked to a photosensitive system involving the eyes and the pineal gland in the brain. Without bright light, the pineal gland secretes melatonin, the hormone that induces drowsiness and sleep. Light triggers suppression of melatonin secretion. Seasonal affective disorder results from excessive melatonin. To counteract these symptoms, phototherapy is prescribed, which suppresses melatonin by stimulating light receptors in the eye.

Activity C

1. d   **2.** a   **3.** b   **4.** c

Activity D

1. Sleep promotes emotional well-being and enhances various physiologic processes. Sleep is believed to play a role in reducing fatigue, stabilizing mood, improving blood flow to the brain, increasing protein synthesis, maintaining the disease-fighting mechanisms of the immune system, promoting cellular growth and repair, and improving the capacity for learning and memory storage.
2. Progressive relaxation is a therapeutic exercise during which a person actively contracts then relaxes muscle groups to break the worry–tension cycle that interferes with relaxation. Clients can learn to perform progressive relaxation exercises independently using self-suggestion. Some clients eventually omit the muscle contraction phase and go directly to the progressive relaxation of muscle groups.
3. Factors that affect sleep are light, activity, environment, motivation, emotions and moods, food and beverages, illness, and drugs.

4. Nocturnal polysomnography is a diagnostic assessment technique in which a client is monitored for an entire night's sleep to obtain physiologic data. It generally takes place in a sleep disorder clinic, but it is now possible to conduct the study at the client's home. A technician monitors a computerized recording system up to 60 feet away. The diagnostic data are compared with the patterns and characteristics of normal sleep cycles to help diagnose sleep disorders.

5. Seasonal affective disorder is characterized by hypersomnolence, lack of energy when awake, increased appetite accompanied by cravings for sweets, and weight gain. The symptoms begin during the darker winter months and disappear as daylight hours increase in the spring. In some ways, the disorder resembles the hibernation patterns in bears and other animals. Some suggest that seasonal affective disorder results from excessive melatonin.

SECTION II: APPLYING YOUR KNOWLEDGE

Activity E

1. During the apneic or hypopneic periods, ventilation decreases and blood oxygenation decreases. The accumulation of carbon dioxide and the decrease in oxygen cause brief periods of awakening throughout the night. This disturbs the normal transitions and periods of NREM and REM sleep. Consequently, clients with sleep apnea/hypopnea syndrome feel tired after having slept, or worse, their symptoms may cause a heart attack, stroke, or sudden death from hypoxia of the heart, brain, and other organs.

2. The nurse should implement the following interventions to promote sleep in the client:
   - Suggest that the client sleep in positions other than the supine position.
   - Encourage the client to lose weight.
   - Ask the client to avoid substances that depress respiration, such as alcohol and sleeping medication.
   - In severe cases, provide the client with a continuous positive airway pressure (CPAP) mask that keeps the alveoli inflated at all times.
   - Surgery on the tonsils, uvula, pharynx, tongue, or epiglottis is another treatment option when conservative measures are ineffective.

SECTION III: PRACTICING FOR NCLEX

Activity F

1. **Answer: b**
   RATIONALE: The nurse should keep the stair gates and doors locked when caring for a client with somnambulism. Keeping the client restrained is not a justified action. Keeping a call bell within reach of the client may not help because sleepwalking happens during sleep and the client is not aware of it. Administering sedatives is not an appropriate intervention.

2. **Answer: c**
   RATIONALE: The nurse should provide the client with extra pillows. It would help to position the client comfortably as well as elevate the fractured leg. A mattress, blanket, and headboard are important in providing comfort to the client; however, taking into consideration the client's fractured leg, pillows would be the most suitable option in providing comfort to this client.

3. **Answer: d**
   RATIONALE: The headboard in the client's room can be used to improve the effectiveness of CPR given to the client. Placing the headboard under the client's upper body allows more effective cardiac compression than is possible on a mattress. An over-the-bed table, a side stand, and a bedside chair have no specific function when performing CPR.

4. **Answer: c**
   RATIONALE: The nurse should place a mattress overlay on the client's bed to keep the skin intact. Providing extra pillows and a draw sheet does not contribute to the prevention of bedsores. The nurse should not provide a soft mattress because it may strain the muscles and joints.

5. **Answer: a**
   RATIONALE: The nurse should elevate the limb with pillows to reduce swelling in the leg. Immobilizing the limb may not reduce the swelling associated with the leg ulcer. Changing the dressing of the wound does not relieve swelling. Restricting fluid intake is not an appropriate intervention in this case.

6. **Answer: b**
   RATIONALE: For a client with urinary incontinence, the nurse should place an absorbent pad between the client and the bottom sheet. Restricting fluids is not appropriate because of the risk for dehydration. Adding an extra draw sheet or bottom sheet may not help to prevent the frequent changing of linens.

7. **Answer: b**
   RATIONALE: The nurse should draw the privacy curtain around the client when examining the mastectomy site to maintain the privacy of the client. Providing an explanation for the procedure, placing the client in a comfortable position, and using soft strokes when palpating the site are appropriate interventions, but do not contribute to the maintenance of client dignity.

8. **Answer: a**
   RATIONALE: To prevent hypoxia in a client with sleep apnea, the nurse should provide a continuous positive airway pressure (CPAP) mask to keep the alveoli inflated at all times. Physical exercise, drinking milk before sleeping, and back massages promote sleep but do not prevent sleep apnea.

9. **Answer: c**
   RATIONALE: The nurse should ask the client to avoid drinking alcohol before going to sleep. Alcohol is a depressive drug that promotes sleep, but it tends to reduce normal REM and deep-sleep stages

of NREM sleep. As alcohol is metabolized, stimulating chemicals that were blocked by the sedative effects of the alcohol surge forth from neurons, causing early awakening. Engaging in diversional activities, exercising, or avoiding listening to music may not affect early awakening.

10. Answer: a

RATIONALE: The nurse should administer the diuretic in the morning so that its effect diminishes by the time the client goes to bed. Reducing the dosage of the diuretic may not help because the client would still have to get up to urinate. Catheterization is associated with infection; therefore, it is not an appropriate intervention. Restriction of fluids may cause dehydration in the client.

11. Answer: a

RATIONALE: The nurse should suggest that the client avoid driving vehicles. Clients with narcolepsy experience excessive sleepiness during the daytime and are at risk of motor vehicle and occupational hazards. Performing moderate exercise and practicing relaxation techniques are helpful for promoting good sleep, so they are not prohibited. The client can watch nonstimulating television before sleep.

12. Answer: d

RATIONALE: The client is experiencing seasonal affective disorder. Phototherapy is the most appropriate therapy for the client in this case. Tranquilizers are not effective for treating seasonal affective disorders. Relaxation and back massage promote good sleep but are not effective treatments for this condition.

13. Answer: c

RATIONALE: The appropriate nursing diagnosis that the nurse should record for the client is relocation stress syndrome. Most people sleep best in their usual environment. They develop a preference for a particular pillow, mattress, and blanket. They also tend to adapt to the unique sounds of where they live, such as traffic, trains, and the hum of appliance motors or furnaces. Alterations in the environment or the activities performed before bedtime negatively affect a person's ability to fall and remain asleep. Impaired bed mobility is an inappropriate diagnosis because the client is not confined to bed. Disturbed sleep pattern is incorrect because the sleep pattern is not impaired. Impaired gas exchange is an inappropriate diagnosis because the client has normal breathing.

14. Answer: b

RATIONALE: The nurse should omit stimulatory strokes if the purpose of the back massage is relaxation. Giving circular and firm strokes is part of a back massage. Taking shallow breaths is not part of the procedure.

15. Answers: a, c, e

RATIONALE: Promoting physical exercise, providing milk before sleeping, and encouraging the client to practice relaxation techniques promote sleep.

Physical exercises increase fatigue and the need for sleep. Milk has a hypnotic effect as a result of the L-tryptophan present in it. Relaxation techniques also promote sleep. Administering sedatives should be used as a last resort and not the first approach.

16. Answers: a, b, c

RATIONALE: The nurse should tell the client to avoid coffee, cola, and chocolates before bedtime to promote sleep. Caffeine, which is a stimulant and causes wakefulness, is present in coffee, tea, chocolate, and most cola drinks. Fish and legumes contain L-tryptophan, which promotes sleep.

SECTION IV: REVIEWING WHAT YOU HAVE LEARNED

Activity G

1. Rest
2. Parasomnia

Activity H

1. False. Some sedatives tend to produce restlessness and wakefulness instead of sleep in older clients.
2. False

Activity I

1. Melatonin

Activity J

1. Sleep promotes emotional well-being and enhances various physiologic processes by reducing fatigue, stabilizing mood, improving blood flow to the brain, increasing protein synthesis, maintaining the disease-fighting mechanisms of the immune system, promoting cellular growth and repair, and improving the capacity for learning and memory storage.
2. The four categories of drugs that affect sleep are sedatives, tranquilizers, hypnotics, and stimulants.

SECTION V: APPLYING YOUR KNOWLEDGE

Activity K

1. Diuretics increase urine formation. If given too close to bedtime, the need to urinate may awaken the client from sleep. Peak effect of diuretics diminishes by bedtime if administered early in the morning.
2. Caffeine, a central nervous system stimulant, interferes with relaxation and sleep.

Activity L

1.
   a. The nurse should encourage the client to develop comforting sleep rituals, reduce the intake of stimulating chemicals, engage in daytime exercise, and adhere to a regular schedule for retiring and awakening.
   b. The nurse should teach the client progressive relaxation exercises, in which the client actively contracts then relaxes muscle groups to break the worry–tension cycle that interferes with relaxation. The nurse should provide back massages to promote relaxation of tense muscles and improve circulation.

Activity M

There are no definite answers to this activity. Students may choose to discuss their thoughts with peers or instructors.

SECTION VI: GETTING READY FOR NCLEX

Activity N

1. **Answer: d**

RATIONALE: The client should repeat exposure to artificial light up to 3 to 6 hours a day until spring to relieve symptoms of seasonal affective disorder. The client should not wear eyeglasses or contact lenses with ultraviolet filters during therapy to allow the light to stimulate the light receptors in the eye. The client should sit 3, not 5, feet away for approximately 2 hours soon after awakening from sleep. The client can glance away from the light occasionally while reading or doing crafts.

CHAPTER 19

SECTION I: ASSESSING YOUR UNDERSTANDING

Activity A

1. Thermal
2. Asphyxiation
3. Macroshock
4. Restraints
5. Contact
6. Conductor
7. Protocol
8. Osteoporosis
9. Ground
10. Microshock

Activity B

1. The figure shows a decision tree for treating ingested poison.
2. The initial treatment for a victim of suspected poisoning involves maintaining breathing and cardiac function. After that, rescuers attempt to identify what was ingested, how much, and when. Definitive treatment depends on the substance, the client's condition, and whether the substance is still in the stomach. For ingestions of commercial products containing multiple ingredients, the poison control center is consulted.
3. The figure shows examples of restraint alternatives.
4. Restraints are methods of restricting a person's freedom of movement, physical activity, or normal access to their body. Restraint alternatives are protective or adaptive devices that promote client safety and postural support, but which the client can release independently. Restraint alternatives are generally appropriate for clients who tend to need repositioning to maintain their body alignment or to improve their independence and

functional status. Although the use of restraints is intended to prevent falls and other injuries, in many cases their risks outweigh their benefits.

Activity C

1. d   2. a   3. b   4. c

Activity D

1.

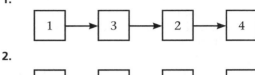

2.

Activity E

1. Latex reactions are of two types—contact dermatitis and immediate hypersensitivity. Contact dermatitis is a delayed, localized skin reaction that occurs within 6 to 48 hours and lasts several days. Immediate hypersensitivity is an instantaneous or fairly prompt systemic reaction manifested by swelling, itching, respiratory distress, hypotension, and death in severe cases.
2. To prevent thermal burns, stay away from flames and use hot liquids with care. Exits must be identified, lighted, and unlocked. Most fire codes require that public buildings, including hospitals and nursing homes, have a functioning sprinkler system.
3. Carbon monoxide, an odorless gas, is released during the incomplete combustion of carbon products, such as fossil fuels, that are commonly used to heat homes. When inhaled, carbon monoxide binds with hemoglobin and interferes with the oxygenation of cells. Without adequate ventilation, the consequences can be lethal. This is called carbon monoxide poisoning.
4. The following measures should be practiced to prevent drowning:
   - Learn to swim.
   - Never swim alone.
   - Wear an approved flotation device.
   - Do not drink alcohol when participating in water-related sports.
   - Notify a law enforcement officer if boaters appear unsafe.
5. Restraint alternatives are protective or adaptive devices that promote client safety and postural support, but that the client can release independently. Restraint alternatives are generally appropriate for clients who tend to need repositioning to maintain their body alignment or to improve their independence and functional status. Some examples include seat inserts or gripping materials that prevent sliding, support pillows, seat belts or harnesses with front-releasing Velcro or buckle closures, and commercial or homemade tilt wedges.

SECTION II: APPLYING YOUR KNOWLEDGE

Activity F

1. The nurse should not use conventional restraints because the client has a steady gait and there is no risk associated with their ambulation. The nurse can use restraint alternatives and other supplementary measures like assistive ambulatory devices, and use an electronic seat and bed monitors.
2. Conventional restraints have many disadvantages. Restrained clients become increasingly confused; suffer chronic constipation, incontinence, infections such as pneumonia, and pressure ulcers; and experience a progressive decline in their ability to perform activities of daily living. Restrained clients are more likely to die during their hospital stay than those who are not restrained.

SECTION III: PRACTICING FOR NCLEX

Activity G

1. **Answer: b**
   RATIONALE: The nurse should provide the client with prefilled containers for separate drugs to ensure that the client does not take the wrong medicines. Instructing the client to see the blister pack, giving the orders in writing, and explaining the drug regimen may not help the senior client who is experiencing cognitive impairment.
2. **Answer: c**
   RATIONALE: The first priority of the nurse should be to assess and maintain the breathing and cardiac function of the child. After that, rescuers should attempt to identify what was ingested, how much, and when. Definitive treatment depends on the substance ingested, the client's condition, and whether the substance is still in the stomach.
3. **Answer: d**
   RATIONALE: The nurse should move the client to a quiet room and let them air their concerns. Moving the client to a quiet room decreases environmental stimulus. Restraint or isolation is not required because the client is not a threat to themselves or others. Anxiolytics can be administered, but this is a secondary method.
4. **Answer: a**
   RATIONALE: The nurse should educate the parents to keep the baby restrained in the automobile. Infants rely on the safety consciousness of their adult caretakers. They are especially vulnerable to injuries resulting from falling off changing tables or being unrestrained in automobiles. The baby should not be prevented from moving around and should not be restrained while feeding. The baby can be made to sit in the chair, but under supervision.
5. **Answer: d**
   RATIONALE: The nurse should educate the parents to keep the cleaning solutions locked. Toddlers are naturally inquisitive and more mobile than infants. Labeling the solutions may not help because toddlers are inquisitive by nature and cannot read. Educating the kids is a secondary measure. Not keeping the cleaning solution at home is an inappropriate intervention.
6. **Answer: b**
   RATIONALE: Risk for injury is the most appropriate nursing diagnosis for the restrained client. Restrained clients become increasingly confused; suffer chronic constipation, incontinence, infections such as pneumonia, and pressure ulcers; and experience a progressive decline in their ability to perform activities of daily living. Impaired mobility, impaired sensory perception, and altered consciousness are not appropriate for the client.
7. **Answer: c**
   RATIONALE: The nurse should emphasize the use of grounded equipment to prevent electrical hazards. The use of grounded equipment reduces the potential for electrical shock. A ground diverts leaking electrical energy to the earth. Grounded equipment is identified by the presence of a three-pronged plug. Unplugging the equipment after use, putting electrical cords under the carpet, and not operating the devices with wet hands are secondary measures.
8. **Answer: a**
   RATIONALE: The nurse's priority should be to protect the child from injury. Toddlers are naturally inquisitive and more mobile than infants, and they fail to understand the dangers that accompany climbing. Consequently, they are often the victims of accidental poisoning, falls down stairs or from high chairs, burns, electrocution from exploring outlets or manipulating electric cords, and drowning. Befriending the toddler, adapting, and preparing for the diagnostic test are not a priority.
9. **Answer: b**
   RATIONALE: Because the client has improved, the nurse should remove the restraints even if the restraint order has not expired. Waiting for the physician to inspect the client and revise the order, continuing the restraint until the order expires, and loosening the restraint to allow limited movement are not appropriate actions because restraints are not justified when the client has improved and is harmless to self and others.
10. **Answers: a, b, c**
    RATIONALE: In the case of carbon monoxide poisoning, the victim should be immediately removed from the site. The victim should be assessed for vital signs and should be administered oxygen. The windows and doors should not be kept closed, but should be opened to promote ventilation. Reorienting the client may not be immediately important.
11. **Answer: d**
    RATIONALE: The most appropriate action should be to evacuate the client from the room. According to RACE protocol, the client should be rescued

from the room followed by raising the alarm, confining the fire, and extinguishing it.

12. Answers: a, c, d
RATIONALE: The tilt wedges, seat belts with Velcro, and harnesses with buckles are restraint alternatives because these devices provide client safety and postural support and can be released by the client. Vest and elbow restraints are not restraint alternatives.

13. Answers: a, b, d
RATIONALE: To prevent accidental drowning, the parents should not allow the child to swim alone, should provide floatation devices, and should keep the swimming pool fenced when the child is unattended. The child should not be allowed to swim with their friends because the risk of drowning is high.

14. Answer: b
RATIONALE: The nurse should tell a family member to sit with the client to prevent them from removing the endotracheal tube. Applying elbow restraints and taking restraint orders from the physician are not appropriate because they are restrictive methods, and the nurse should first use nonrestrictive methods of restraining. Applying a waist restraint is a restrictive method and is not useful in restraining the hands.

15. Answer: a
RATIONALE: The mode of injury in the child may be play-related, taking into consideration their age. Automobile accidents are more common in adults and adolescents. Falls from beds are most commonly seen in infants, and toddlers have the tendency to fall down stairs.

16. Answers: a, b, c
RATIONALE: The nurse should attach an allergy-alert ID bracelet on the client, stock the client's room with latex-free equipment, and communicate with other personnel to use nonlatex equipment to protect the client from exposure to latex. Washing the hands before wearing gloves to provide care to the client does not solve the purpose because the gloves are made of latex. Instructing the client to wash the area in contact with latex immediately may not reduce a latex reaction.

17. Answer: b
RATIONALE: The nurse should place moist towels or blankets on the thresholds of doors to prevent smoke from escaping. Closing the door of the room on fire may not prevent the escape of smoke because smoke can escape through door thresholds. Switching on the fan may be dangerous because it could promote the spreading of the fire. It may be too late to control the fire if the nurse waits for the firemen to come and handle it.

18. Answer: d
RATIONALE: The nurse should tell the client to avoid keeping area rugs to help prevent falls. Wearing slippers at home is comfortable, but does not

provide appropriate support. Walking with a cane can lead to falls, especially if area rugs are present. Calling for assistance to ambulate may not be feasible all the time.

SECTION IV: REVIEWING WHAT YOU HAVE LEARNED

Activity H
1. Asphyxiation
2. Insulator

Activity I
1. False. Carbon monoxide is an odorless gas released during the incomplete combustion of fossil fuels commonly used to heat homes.
2. True.

Activity J
1. Drowning
2. A thermal burn is a skin injury caused by flames, hot liquids, or steam and is the most common form of burn.
3. Environmental hazards are potentially dangerous conditions in the physical surroundings. Examples include latex sensitization, thermal burns, asphyxiation, electrical shock, poisoning, and falls.

SECTION V: APPLYING YOUR KNOWLEDGE

Activity K
Cold lowers the metabolism of the victim and helps to conserve oxygen.

Activity L
1.
   a. The nurse should explain to the client that pulling the IV tubing and catheter within the vein could cause injury. The nurse could request a relative to sit beside the client to prevent the client from pulling the venipuncture device out. Before considering the use of physical restraints, the nurse must observe and document the client's response to other alternatives.
   b. The nurse should perform and document frequent and regular nursing assessments of the restrained client's vital signs, circulation, skin condition or signs of injury, psychological status and comfort, and, finally, readiness to discontinue the restraint. The nurse must record nursing care with regard to toileting, nutrition, hydration, and range of motion as per the health care facility's established protocol. The nurse must remove the restraint if the assessment findings indicate that the client is alert and cooperative.

Activity M
There are no definite answers to this activity. Students may choose to discuss their thoughts with peers or instructors.

SECTION VI: GETTING READY FOR NCLEX

Activity N

1. **Answer: c**
   RATIONALE: The client should keep the home ventilated when using aerosol sprays that leave lingering fumes in the air as this could have toxic effects on children if inhaled in large quantities. The client should not discard old medications in the wastebasket because they then could be accessible to children. The client should not refer to any medication as sweet, candy, or yummy, nor should medications be carried in purses.

CHAPTER 20

SECTION I: ASSESSING YOUR UNDERSTANDING

Activity A

1. Fifth
2. Modulation
3. Chronic
4. Rhizotomy
5. Biofeedback
6. Distraction
7. Transduction
8. Nociceptors
9. Nonopioid
10. Acupuncture

Activity B

1. The figure shows patient-controlled analgesia.
2. Patient-controlled analgesia is advantageous to both clients and nurses. Some of the advantages are as follows:
   - Pain relief is rapid because the drug is delivered intravenously.
   - Pain is kept within a constant tolerable level.
   - Less drug is actually used because small doses continuously control the pain.
   - Clients are spared the discomfort of repeated injections.
   - Anxiety is reduced because the client does not wait for the nurse to prepare and administer an injection.
   - Side effects are reduced with smaller individual doses and lower total doses.
   - Clients tend to ambulate and move more, reducing the potential for complications from immobility.
   - Clients take an active role in their pain management.
   - The nurse is free to carry out other nursing responsibilities.

Activity C

1. c   **2.** e   **3.** b   **4.** a   **5.** d

Activity D

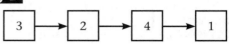

Activity E

1. Transmission of pain occurs when peripheral nociceptors form synapses with neurons within the spinal cord that carry pain impulses and other sensory information, such as pressure and temperature changes, via fast and slow nerve fibers.
2. Acute pain is a discomfort that can last for a few seconds to less than 6 months. It is associated with tissue trauma, including surgery or some other recent identifiable etiology. Although severe initially, acute pain eases with healing and eventually disappears.
3. Transduction refers to the conversion of chemical information at the cellular level into electrical impulses that move toward the spinal cord. Transduction begins when injured cells release chemicals such as substance P, prostaglandins, bradykinin, histamine, and glutamate. These chemicals excite nociceptors, sensory nerve receptors activated by around 20 neuropeptides and noxious chemicals released from damaged tissue such as substance P, serotonin, histamine, arachidonic acid, which is metabolized into prostaglandin, acetylcholine, and others. Nociceptors are located throughout the skin, bones, joints, muscles, and internal organs.
4. The PENS technique has been successful in research trials on clients with low back pain, pain caused by the spread of cancer to bones, shingles (acute herpes zoster viral infection), diabetic neuropathy, and migraine headaches.
5. A placebo is an inactive substance or treatment used as a substitute for an analgesic drug or conventional therapeutic measure. Placebos can relieve pain, especially when clients have confidence in their health care providers. The trust a client has in the nurse or physician probably has more to do with the efficacy of placebos than any other factor. Consequently, it is wrong to assume that a client whose pain is relieved with placebos is addicted or is a malingerer (someone who pretends to be sick or in pain). Using deception and withholding pain medication are considered unethical.
6. Pain tolerance (or the amount of pain a person endures) is influenced by genetics; learned behaviors specific to gender, age, and culture; and other biopsychosocially unique factors such as current anxiety level, past pain experiences, and overall emotional disposition.

SECTION II: APPLYING YOUR KNOWLEDGE

Activity F

1. When caring for a client in pain, the nurse should check and document the client's pain every time they assess the client's temperature, pulse,

respiration, and blood pressure. The overall goal of pain assessment is to gather objective data about a client.

2. When caring for clients, especially those who are often underassessed and undertreated, the nurse observes for behavioral signs that are common nonverbal indicators of pain, such as moaning, crying, grimacing, guarded position, increased vital signs, reduced social interactions, irritability, difficulty concentrating, and changes in eating and sleeping patterns.

SECTION III: PRACTICING FOR NCLEX

Activity G

1. **Answer: b**
   RATIONALE: The nurse should select the oral route for effective absorption of medication for senior clients. Senior clients may experience physiologic changes such as decreased gastric acid production, decreased gastrointestinal motility, changes in body fat ratio, and changes in organ function such as decreased liver blood flow and decreased glomerular filtration rate. The nurse should avoid the rectal or nasal route in senior clients because senior clients have diminished pain tolerance because they have less energy to cope with pain. Medication may be absorbed more slowly from the intramuscular route in senior clients, resulting in delayed onset of action, prolonged duration, and altered absorption with potential for toxicity. Dermal, oral, and sublingual routes may be more effective for senior clients.

2. **Answer: d**
   RATIONALE: Most nonopioids are very effective at relieving pain caused by inflammation. These drugs relieve pain by altering neurotransmission peripherally at the site of injury. They are not very effective on pain caused by injury, headache, and weak muscles. Botulinum toxin has been approved to treat painful musculoskeletal conditions and various types of headaches.

3. **Answer: a**
   RATIONALE: The EMG machine (or a pulse oximeter) is a machine that produces a visual or audible signal that correlates with the person's heart rate, skin temperature, or muscle tension. The client is encouraged to reduce or extinguish the signal using whatever mechanism they can—generally by physically relaxing. The feedback from the machine demonstrates to the client how well they are accomplishing the goal. The machine does not produce visual or audible signals correlating to a person's pain, intramuscular tension, age, or body mass index.

4. **Answer: b**
   RATIONALE: The nurse should ask the client if they are able to recollect the name and dosage of the pain medication that the client has taken. The main goal of pain assessment during admission is to gather objective data quickly about a client; hence, the nurse should ask direct and specific questions such as the nature of the pain, whether it changes on medications, and the name and exact dosage of the pain medicine. The nurse should avoid asking close-ended questions such as the client's ability to do strenuous activities or whether the client takes medicines in the morning because they do not add any value to the pain assessment data.

5. **Answers: b, c, d**
   RATIONALE: Clients with cardiac pacemakers (especially the demand type), clients prone to an irregular heartbeat, clients with previous heart attacks, and pregnant clients are not candidates for TENS. TENS is a non-narcotic, noninvasive method and has no toxic side effects. It is contraindicated in pregnant women because its effect on the unborn fetus has not been determined. Young adults and clients involved in sports activities are not contraindicated from TENS; on the contrary, many sports persons undergo TENS when they are in acute pain.

6. **Answer: a**
   RATIONALE: The intraspinal analgesic is administered several times per day or as a continuous low-dose infusion. Intraspinal analgesia is a method of relieving pain by instilling a narcotic or local anesthetic via a catheter into the subarachnoid or epidural space of the spinal cord. It relieves pain while producing minimal systemic drug effects. The intraspinal analgesic is not administered once a day in a high-dose infusion, twice a day in a low-dose infusion, or once in 6 months with continuous low-dose infusion because it will not produce the desired effect.

7. **Answer: d**
   RATIONALE: The nurse should use a FACES scale to assess the pain in a 3-year-old client. The Wong–Baker FACES scale is best suited for children and clients who are culturally diverse or mentally challenged. Children as young as 3 years of age can use the FACES scale. Regardless of the assessment tool used, many clients underrate or minimize their pain intensity. A numeric scale, word scale, and linear scale are the most commonly used tools when assessing adults and people from different cultural backgrounds.

8. **Answers: a, b, c**
   RATIONALE: The longer chronic pain exists, the more likely it is that people associated with clients in chronic pain will begin to show negative reactions to the client. They may say that they are tired of hearing about the client's pain, ignore the client's concerns and complaints, or criticize the client for using drugs as a crutch. They usually do not say that they are eager to know about the client's pain or are concerned about the client's pain.

9. **Answer: d**
   RATIONALE: The client is experiencing neuro-pathic pain in the amputated limb. Neuropathic pain or functional pain is often experienced days, weeks, or even months after the source of the pain has been treated and resolved. The client is not experiencing somatic pain because somatic pain develops from injury to structures such as muscles, tendons, and joints. In acute pain, the pain lasts for a few seconds to less than 6 months; although severe initially, acute pain eases with healing and eventually disappears. With chronic pain, the discomfort lasts longer than 6 months.

10. **Answers: a, c, e**
    RATIONALE: The nurse can administer the me-peridine, an opioid, to the client through oral, rectal, transdermal, or parenteral routes. When pain is no longer controlled with a nonopioid, the nonopioid is combined with an opioid. The nurse, however, does not administer the drug through the sublingual or the intramuscular routes.

11. **Answer: a**
    RATIONALE: The antidepressants may produce their analgesic-enhancing effect by increasing nor-epinephrine and serotonin levels, augmenting the release of endorphins in the client. The antidepressant will not regulate the inhibitory neurotransmitter γ-aminobutyric acid because that is done by anticon-vulsants. NMDA drugs interfere with the function of nociceptive nerve fibers, perhaps blocking the release of substance P, its nerve-sensitizing properties, and other inflammatory chemicals. Antidepressants do not stimulate the body to release endogenous opi-oids, which is done by the TENS technique.

12. **Answers: a, c, d, e**
    RATIONALE: Nondrug and nonsurgical interven-tions in pain management include independent nursing education, imagery, distraction, relaxation techniques, and applications of heat or cold. Other interventions, such as TENS, acupuncture and acu-pressure, PENS, biofeedback, and hypnosis, require collaboration with people who have specialized training and expertise. A cordotomy is surgical inter-ruption of pain pathways in the spinal cord. A mas-sage may provide only a temporary relief of the pain.

13. **Answer: a**
    RATIONALE: The client's body may have devel-oped a tolerance to the prescribed medicine dose or frequency of administration. Senior clients have increased sensitivity to narcotics. Medication may be absorbed more slowly from the intramuscular route in older adults, resulting in delayed onset of action, prolonged duration, and altered absorption with potential for toxicity. The dosage prescribed by the physician or the medicine administered by the nurse is not responsible for the client's toler-ance to the drug.

14. **Answer: a**
    RATIONALE: The client has undertreated pain; therefore, apart from obvious behavioral signs like moaning and crying, the nurse should look for other autonomic nervous system responses such as tachycardia, hypertension, dilated pupils, perspira-tion, pallor, rapid and shallow breathing, urinary retention, reduced bowel motility, and elevated blood glucose levels. Dehydration, reduced glucose level, and convulsions are not responses of the au-tonomic nervous system.

15. **Answer: c**
    RATIONALE: Somatic pain develops from injury to structures such as muscles, tendons, and joints. It does not develop from skin irritation, traumatic head injury, or the effect of opioids and opiate analgesic drugs. Cutaneous pain is discomfort that originates at the skin level and is a commonly experienced sensation resulting from some form of trauma. Acute pain is associated with tissue trauma, including surgery. Opioids and opiate an-algesic drugs are narcotic drugs that are prescribed to clients when pain is no longer controlled with nonopioid drugs.

16. **Answer: b**
    RATIONALE: The nurse assesses the client's pain once per shift. Per The Joint Commission's pain assessment standards, client choices regarding pain management are respected. The nurse assesses pain whenever they consider it appropriate and does so routinely in the following circumstances:
    - When the client is admitted
    - Whenever the nurse takes vital signs
    - Once per shift when pain is an actual or poten-tial problem
    - When the client is at rest and when involved in a nursing activity
    - After each potentially painful procedure or treatment

17. **Answers: a, b, d**
    RATIONALE: Opioids and opiates cause seda-tion, nausea, constipation, and respiratory depres-sion. Because of an exaggerated fear of causing addiction, narcotics tend to be underprescribed even if clients can benefit from their use. When they are used, the treatment biases lead some nurses to administer the lowest dosage of a pre-scribed range or to delay administration until the maximum time between dosages has elapsed. Opioids and opiates do not lead to diarrhea and dilated pupils.

18. **Answer: c**
    RATIONALE: The nurse should document that the client's discomfort reduces gradually with medicine. Acute pain lasts for a few seconds to less than 6 months, whereas chronic pain discomfort lasts longer than 6 months. It is as-sociated with tissue trauma, including surgery or some other recent identifiable etiology. Cuta-neous pain is the discomfort that originates at the skin level. Clients with chronic pain are not as likely to manifest autonomic nervous system responses.

SECTION IV: REVIEWING WHAT YOU HAVE LEARNED

Activity H

1. Transduction
2. Visceral
3. Distraction

Activity I

1. False. Some sedatives tend to produce restlessness and wakefulness instead of sleep in older clients.
2. True.
3. False. Adjuvant drugs are never used as a first-line treatment for pain; they are administered in addition to pain medication to improve pain control.

Activity J

1. Placebo
2. Nociceptor
3. Endogenous opioids

Activity K

	Acute Pain	**Chronic Pain**
Duration	Lasts for a few seconds to less than 6 months	Lasts longer than 6 months
Cause	Associated with tissue trauma, including surgery or some other recent, identifiable etiology	May not be related to any primary injury or disease
Site of Pain	Specific and localized	Nonspecific and generalized
Relief of Pain	Eases with healing and eventually disappears	Has more far-reaching effects the longer it lasts

Activity L

1. A rhizotomy is surgical sectioning of a nerve root close to the spinal cord. A cordotomy is surgical interruption of pain pathways in the spinal cord.
2. Addiction is a pattern of compulsive drug use characterized by a continued craving for the drug.

Activity M

When the client's pain is continuous, administering analgesic drugs on a scheduled basis rather than irregularly controls pain better by maintaining a lower intensity of pain.

Activity N

There are no definite answers to this activity. Students may choose to discuss their thoughts with peers or instructors.

SECTION V: GETTING READY FOR NCLEX

Activity O

1. **Answer: b**
   RATIONALE: Patient-controlled analgesia (PCA) uses less drug overall because small doses continuously control pain. Pain relief is rapid because the drug is delivered intravenously; it is not slow and long lasting. Clients using a PCA do not find it difficult to ambulate and are not at risk from immobility. Clients tend to ambulate and move more, reducing the potential for complications from immobility.

CHAPTER 21

SECTION I: ASSESSING YOUR UNDERSTANDING

Activity A

1. Ventilation
2. Hypoxemia
3. Orthopneic
4. Deep
5. Flowmeter
6. Humidifier
7. Venturi
8. Tracheostomy
9. Calcification
10. Inspiration

Activity B

1. The figure shows a portable oxygen concentrator that extracts nitrogen and concentrates oxygen to enable clients who require oxygen therapy to travel or maintain their lifestyle without the need for multiple tanks of oxygen.
2. An oxygen concentrator eliminates the need for a central reservoir of piped oxygen or the use of bulky tanks that must be constantly replaced. This type of oxygen source is used in home health care and long-term care facilities primarily because of its convenience and economy. Oxygen concentrators typically provide oxygen flows of 1 to 5 L/min, with some that are capable of flows up to 10 L/min.

Activity C

1. d   **2.** a   **3.** b   **4.** e   **5.** c

Activity D

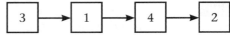

3 → 1 → 4 → 2

Activity E

1. The nurse physically assesses oxygenation by the following:
   - Monitoring the client's respiratory rate
   - Observing the breathing pattern and effort
   - Checking chest symmetry
   - Auscultating lung sounds
   - Additional assessments include the following:
   - Recording heart rate and blood pressure
   - Determining the client's level of consciousness
   - Observing the color of the skin, mucous membranes, lips, and nailbeds

2. An arterial blood gas assessment is a laboratory test using arterial blood to evaluate oxygenation, ventilation, and acid–base balance. It measures the partial pressure of oxygen dissolved in plasma (PaO_2), the percentage of hemoglobin saturated with oxygen (SaO_2), the partial pressure of carbon dioxide in plasma ($PaCO_2$), the pH of blood, and the level of bicarbonate (HCO_3) ions.

3. Pulse oximetry is a noninvasive, transcutaneous technique for periodically or continuously monitoring the oxygen saturation of blood.

4. Oxygen therapy is an intervention for administering more oxygen than present in the atmosphere to prevent or relieve hypoxemia. It requires an oxygen source, a flowmeter, in some cases an oxygen analyzer or humidifier, and an oxygen delivery device.

5. Although an oxygen concentrator is more economical than oxygen supplied in portable tanks, the device increases the client's electricity bill. The oxygen concentrator generates heat from its motor and produces an unpleasant odor or taste if the filter is not cleaned weekly. Clients have to keep a secondary source of oxygen ready in case of a power failure.

6. A non-rebreather mask is an oxygen delivery device in which all the exhaled air leaves the mask rather than partially entering the reservoir bag. It is designed to deliver an Fio_2 of 90% to 100%. This type of mask contains one-way valves that allow only oxygen from its source as well as the oxygen in the reservoir bag to be inhaled. No air from the atmosphere is inhaled. All the air that is exhaled is vented from the mask. None enters the reservoir bag.

SECTION II: APPLYING YOUR KNOWLEDGE

Activity F

1. Unless contraindicated by their condition, clients with hypoxia are placed in the high Fowler position. This position eases breathing by allowing the abdominal organs to descend away from the diaphragm. As a result, the lungs have the potential to fill with a greater volume of air. As an alternative, clients who find breathing difficult may benefit from variations of Fowler position. One option is a tripod position in which the client is in a seated position with the arms supported on pillows or the arm rests of a chair. The tripod position increases a client's breathing capacity by using the arms to lift the chest upward. Another option is an orthopneic position in bed. In the orthopneic position, the client leans forward over the bedside table or a chair back. The orthopneic position allows room for maximum vertical and lateral chest expansion and provides comfort while resting or sleeping.

2. The nurse could teach the client the following techniques to help them breathe efficiently:
   - Deep breathing, which is a technique for maximizing ventilation that involves taking in a large volume of air that fills the alveoli to greater capacity, thus improving gas exchange
   - Pursed-lip breathing, which is a form of controlled ventilation in which the client consciously prolongs the expiration phase of breathing
   - Diaphragmatic breathing, which is breathing that promotes the use of the diaphragm rather than the upper chest muscles
   - Use of a nasal strip, which is adhesive, available for commercial purchase, and used to reduce airflow resistance by widening the breathing passageways of the nose

SECTION III: PRACTICING FOR NCLEX

Activity G

1. **Answer: a**
   RATIONALE: The arterial blood gas test measures the partial pressure of oxygen dissolved in plasma. It assesses oxygenation, ventilation, and acid–base balance and also measures the percentage of hemoglobin saturated with oxygen, the partial pressure of carbon dioxide in plasma, the pH of blood, and the level of bicarbonate. During a physical assessment of the client, the nurse measures the blood pressure of the client and monitors the client's level of consciousness. The pulse oximeter measures the oxygen saturation in the blood.

2. **Answer: c**
   RATIONALE: The nurse should teach the client with emphysema the pursed-lip breathing technique, which is a form of controlled ventilation in which the client consciously prolongs the expiration phase of breathing. This helps to eliminate more than the usual amount of carbon dioxide from the lungs. Deep breathing is therapeutic for clients who tend to breathe shallowly, such as those who are inactive or in pain. Incentive spirometry, a technique for deep breathing using a calibrated device, encourages clients to reach a goal-directed volume of inspired air. Adhesive nasal

strips are used to reduce airflow resistance by widening the breathing passageways of the nose.

3. **Answers: a, b, c**
   RATIONALE: The nurse should inform the client using a liquid oxygen unit that the unit may leak during the warm weather, and frozen moisture may occlude the outlet of the unit. The nurse should also inform the client that the liquid oxygen unit is more expensive than other portable sources. An oxygen concentrator increases the electricity bill of the client and may emit a bad taste or odor if the filters are not cleaned weekly.

4. **Answer: b**
   RATIONALE: The nurse would use an oxygen analyzer to determine whether the client is getting the prescribed amount of oxygen. An oxygen analyzer measures the percentage of delivered oxygen to determine whether the client is receiving the amount prescribed by the physician. A flowmeter, humidifier, and nasal cannula are not used to determine whether the client is getting the prescribed amount of oxygen. A flowmeter is a gauge used to regulate the amount of oxygen delivered to the client and is attached to the oxygen source. A humidifier is a device that produces small water droplets and may be used during oxygen administration because oxygen dries the mucous membranes. A nasal cannula is a hollow tube with half-inch prongs placed into the client's nostrils, which provides a means of administering low concentrations of oxygen.

5. **Answer: b**
   RATIONALE: The nurse should use a face tent for the claustrophobic client with facial burn injuries. A face tent provides oxygen to the nose and mouth without the discomfort of a mask, and the client is less likely to feel claustrophobic. A nasal cannula is used for administering low concentrations of oxygen for clients who are not extremely hypoxic or who have chronic lung diseases. A tracheostomy collar delivers oxygen through an artificial opening. A T-piece fits securely onto a tracheostomy tube or endotracheal tube. It is similar to a tracheostomy collar but is attached directly to the artificial airway. The nasal cannula, tracheostomy collar, or the T-piece cannot be used to deliver oxygen to a client with burns.

6. **Answer: b**
   RATIONALE: The nurse should use an oxygen tent to deliver oxygen to the 2-year-old client with symptoms of bronchitis. An oxygen tent is a clear plastic enclosure that provides cooled, humidified oxygen and is useful for children, who are less likely to keep a mask or cannula in place. A nasal catheter is a tube for delivering oxygen that is inserted through the nose into the posterior nasal pharynx and is used for clients who tend to breathe through the mouth or experience

claustrophobia when a mask covers their face. A CPAP mask maintains positive pressure within the airway throughout the respiratory cycle and is used by clients who experience sleep apnea. Some clients who require long-term oxygen therapy may prefer its administration through a transtracheal catheter. However, a nasal catheter, a CPAP mask, and a transtracheal catheter are less likely to be used in this case.

7. **Answer: a**
   RATIONALE: When cleaning the opening and the tube of a transtracheal catheter, oxygen should be administered through a nasal cannula. When cleaning the transtracheal catheter, oxygen would not be administered with a Venturi mask, a face tent, or a partial breather mask.

8. **Answer: d**
   RATIONALE: The nurse should be aware that oxygen toxicity could occur when the client receives 60% oxygen concentration for 48 hours. Oxygen toxicity causes lung damage, which develops when oxygen concentrations of more than 50% are administered for longer than 48 to 72 hours.

9. **Answer: b**
   RATIONALE: The nurse could use hyperbaric oxygen therapy when treating a client with carbon monoxide poisoning. Hyperbaric oxygen therapy helps to generate new tissue at a faster rate; thus, it is used for promoting wound healing. It also is used to treat gangrene associated with diabetes or other conditions of vascular insufficiency. Water-seal chest tube drainage is a technique for evacuating air or blood from the pleural cavity, which helps to restore negative intrapleural pressure and reinflate the lung. A liquid oxygen unit is a device that converts cooled liquid oxygen to a gas by passing it through heated coils. An oxygen concentrator is a machine that collects and concentrates oxygen from room air and stores it for client use.

10. **Answer: d**
    RATIONALE: The nurse should understand that the chest walls become stiffer in older clients, thus affecting the respiratory system. In older adults, the alveolar walls become thinner and the lungs become less elastic, which also affects the respiratory system. More breathing from the mouth is a functional change that occurs in older adults.

11. **Answer: c**
    RATIONALE: To improve the condition of a client with lowered respiratory function, the nurse should suggest that the client maintain a liberal fluid intake. Unless contraindicated, older adults need encouragement to maintain a liberal fluid intake (to keep mucous membranes moist) and to engage in regular exercise to maintain optimal respiratory function. An adhesive nasal strip reduces

airflow resistance by widening nasal breathing passageways, promoting easier breathing. If a simple mask is used to deliver oxygen to the client, the nurse needs to maintain proper skin care.

12. Answer: d
RATIONALE: When administering oxygen using a T-piece, the nurse should drain the tube regularly. The moisture that collects within the tubing tends to condense and may enter the airway during position changes if it is not drained periodically. A nurse should remember that a T-piece does not normally interfere with eating or create a feeling of suffocation, or even deliver an inconsistent amount of oxygen. A simple mask affects eating and creates a feeling of suffocation. The amount of oxygen received using an oxygen tent may be inconsistent.

13. Answers: c, a, d, b, e
RATIONALE: During expiration, the respiratory muscles relax, the thoracic cavity decreases, the stretched elastic lung tissue recoils, intrathoracic pressure increases as a result of the compressed pulmonary space, and air moves out of the respiratory tract.

14. Answers: b, d, a, c
RATIONALE: The nurse should teach the client to breathe using the pursed-lip technique in the following order.

15. Answers: a, b, c
RATIONALE: When administering oxygen to toddlers using an oxygen tent, the nurse should tuck the edges of the tent securely under the mattress, limit the opening of the zippered access port, and monitor the oxygen levels in the tent using an analyzer. When using a face tent, the nurse should remember that the amount of oxygen the client actually receives may be inconsistent with what is prescribed because of environmental losses, and the amount of oxygen delivered may need to be regulated. A client using a simple mask may need skin care because of the effects of trapped moisture.

SECTION IV: REVIEWING WHAT YOU HAVE LEARNED

Activity H

1. Hypoxemia

Activity I

1. False. Carbon monoxide is an odorless gas released during the incomplete combustion of fossil fuels commonly used to heat homes.
2. True.
3. False. Oxygen toxicity is lung damage that develops when oxygen concentrations of more than 50% are administered for longer than 48 to 72 hours.

Activity J

1. Interstitial fluid

Activity K

	Inspiration	Expiration
Definition	In this process of breathing in, the lungs stretch and fill with air.	In this process of breathing out, the lungs return to a resting position.
Process	The dome-shaped diaphragm contracts and moves downward in the thorax. The intercostal muscles move the chest outward by elevating the ribs and sternum. This combination expands the thoracic cavity, which lowers the pressure inside the lungs and causes air to enter from the atmosphere.	The respiratory muscles relax, the thoracic cavity decreases in size, the stretched elastic lung tissue recoils, and intrathoracic pressure increases as a result of the compressed pulmonary space. Pressure inside the lungs increases, causing air to move out of the respiratory tract.
Additional Muscles Involved	When there is an acute need for oxygen, the pectoralis minor and sternocleidomastoid contract to assist with even greater chest expansion.	Additional air is exhaled by contracting abdominal muscles such as the rectus abdominis, transverse abdominis, and external and internal obliques.

Activity L

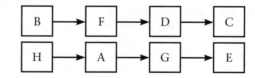

Activity M

Adhesive nasal strips reduce airflow resistance by widening the passageways of the nose, thus promoting easier breathing. They are appropriate for people with ineffective breathing, to reduce or eliminate snoring, and to increase oxygen requirements during sustained exercise.

Activity N

Oxygen dries mucous membranes. The small water droplets produced by the humidifier add moisture to the mucous membranes.

Activity O

The nurse should teach the client and family as follows:
- Lie down with knees slightly bent.
- Place one hand on the abdomen and the other on the chest.

- Inhale slowly and deeply through the nose while letting the abdomen rise more than the chest.
- Purse the lips.
- Contract the abdominal muscles and begin to exhale.
- Repeat the exercise for one full minute; rest for at least 2 minutes.
- Practice the breathing exercises at least twice a day for 5 to 10 minutes each time.
- Progress to practicing diaphragmatic breathing while upright and active.

Activity P

There are no definite answers to this activity. Students may choose to discuss their thoughts with peers or instructors.

SECTION V: GETTING READY FOR NCLEX

Activity Q

1. **Answer: d**
   RATIONALE: The client should lean forward over the bedside table in the orthopneic position, which enables maximum vertical and lateral chest expansion. Lying flat on the back or on the left side will not reduce airway resistance. Inclining the bed 15 degrees will not sufficiently help to improve the client's breathing.

CHAPTER 22

SECTION I: ASSESSING YOUR UNDERSTANDING

Activity A

1. Infection
2. Colonization
3. Gloves
4. Soiled
5. Intact
6. Tuberculosis
7. Blood-borne
8. More subtle
9. Contagious
10. Biodegradable

Activity B

1. The figure shows two nurses performing the double-bagging technique.
2. Double bagging is an infection control measure in which one bag of contaminated items, such as trash or laundry, is placed within another. This measure requires two people. One person bags the items and deposits the bag in a second bag, which is held by another person outside the client's room. The person holding the second bag prevents contamination by manipulating the bag underneath a folded cuff.

Activity C

1. d **2.** c **3.** b **4.** a **5.** e

Activity D

$$\boxed{5} \rightarrow \boxed{6} \rightarrow \boxed{2} \rightarrow \boxed{3} \rightarrow \boxed{1} \rightarrow \boxed{4}$$

Activity E

1. When transmission-based precautions are in effect, it is important to plan frequent contact with the client. Nurses encourage visitors to come as often as the agency's policies and the client's condition permit. They use every opportunity to emphasize that as long as visitors follow the infection control precautions, they are not likely to acquire the disease.
2. Senior clients are more susceptible to infections because of diminished immune system functioning and inadequate nutrition and fluid intake. Symptoms of infections tend to be more subtle among senior clients, who tend to have a lower normal or baseline temperature.
3. The three types of transmission-based precautions are airborne precautions, droplet precautions, and contact precautions. These three types replace the earlier categories of strict isolation, contact isolation, respiratory isolation, tuberculosis isolation, enteric precautions, and drainage/secretion precautions.
4. Direct contact involves skin-to-skin contact with an infected or colonized person. Indirect contact occurs by touching a contaminated intermediate object in the client's environment. Contact precautions are measures used to block the transmission of pathogens by direct or indirect contact.
5. Personal protective equipment includes cover gowns, face-protection devices (mask, respirator, goggles, face shield), and gloves. Infection control measures involve the use of one or more items for personal protection. These items are located just outside the client's room or in an anteroom.
6. Nurses wrap moist items such as soiled dressings so that, during their containment, flying or crawling insects cannot transfer pathogens. Eventually, the bag and its contents are destroyed by incineration or they are autoclaved. Autoclaved items can be safely disposed of in landfills.

SECTION II: APPLYING YOUR KNOWLEDGE

Activity F

1. To avoid the transmission of pathogens, the nurse should ensure that senior clients, family members in close contact with senior clients, and all personnel in health care settings obtain annual immunizations against influenza. Visitors with respiratory infections need to wear a mask or avoid contact with older adults in their homes or long-term care settings until their symptoms have subsided. In addition to the mask, frequent, thorough hand washing can help prevent the transfer of organisms.

Health care workers who are ill should take sick leave rather than expose susceptible clients to infectious organisms.

2. Symptoms of infections tend to be more subtle among older adults because senior clients have a lower normal or baseline temperature (a temperature in the normal range may actually be elevated for an older adult). Infections are more likely to have a rapid course and life-threatening consequences after they become established. Common manifestations of infections in senior clients include changes in behavior and mental status.

SECTION III: PRACTICING FOR NCLEX

Activity G

1. **Answer: a**
RATIONALE: The nurse should place the catheter tubing lower than the client's bladder. When indwelling catheters are absolutely necessary, the tubing should never be bent or placed higher than the client's bladder to prevent any backflow of urine into the bladder. Indwelling catheters should be avoided, if at all possible, because senior clients have increased susceptibility to urinary tract infections. Bladder training is much more desirable, but it is not a measure that nurses need to take when adjusting or fixing catheters. When indwelling catheters are absolutely necessary, they require meticulous daily care.

2. **Answer: d**
RATIONALE: When the client returns, the nurse should deposit the soiled linen in the linen hamper in the client's room, touching only the outside surface of the protective covers. Some agencies also spray or wash the transport vehicle with disinfectant before reuse. There is no need to line the edge of the client's bed with a clean sheet on the client's return or spray the X-ray department with disinfectant after the client leaves. Covering the client's body with a second sheet is done before transporting, not upon their return.

3. **Answer: a**
RATIONALE: The Centers for Disease Control and Prevention has relaxed its recommendation concerning double bagging. Its revised position is that one bag is adequate if the bag is sturdy and the articles are placed in the bag without contaminating the outside of the bag. Otherwise, double bagging is used. Biodegradable trash includes items such as unconsumed beverages, paper tissues, urine, and stool, which are flushed down the toilet. Wearing a nonsterile gown and spraying disinfectant on the contaminated material is not part of the double-bagging technique.

4. **Answer: b**
RATIONALE: Gloves should be changed between tasks on the same client after contact with material because they might contain a high concentration

of microorganisms. A nurse will remove the contaminated gown after they have finished assessing and cleaning the infected area of the client. Making contact between two contaminated surfaces or two clean surfaces is part of the sequence followed by nurses when removing their personal protective equipment. Nurses perform thorough hand washing before leaving a client's room and before touching any other client, personnel, environmental surface, or client care items.

5. **Answer: d**
RATIONALE: A powered air-purifying respirator is usually used when rescuing victims exposed to bioterrorist substances or hazardous chemicals, compared with an N-95 respirator, which is individually fitted for each caregiver. An atomizer is a device used to reduce liquid medication to fine particles in the form of a spray or aerosol; it is useful in delivering medication to the lungs, nose, and throat. A drinker respirator is a mechanical respirator in which the body, excluding the head, is encased within a metal tank.

6. **Answers: b, c, d**
RATIONALE: The nurse needs to take airborne precaution, contact precaution, and droplet precaution because the client has chickenpox (varicella) and common cold. Infectious diseases like smallpox (variola), chickenpox (varicella), and severe acute respiratory syndrome (SARS) require both airborne and contact precautions. Nurses are supposed to take standard and basic precautions at the health care facility on a daily basis.

7. **Answer: b**
RATIONALE: The most appropriate nursing diagnosis for the client is social isolation. Usually, clients with HIV and AIDS have the fear of being rejected by loved ones and are socially ostracized. The nurse should not only care for the client but also try to arrange for a counselor who will understand the client better. Clients with AIDS are at risk of developing other infections easily, but the nursing diagnoses such as powerlessness and ineffective protection may not be applicable to this client.

8. **Answer: c**
RATIONALE: Double bagging is an infection control measure in which one bag of contaminated items, such as trash or laundry, is placed within another. This technique requires two people, one to bag the items and deposit it in a second bag held by the other person outside the client's room. The person holding the second bag prevents contamination by manipulating the bag underneath a folded cuff. Emptying solid waste bags at the end of a shift and disposing off biodegradable and contaminated material in separate bags are not the steps involved in the double-bagging method.

9. **Answers: a, c, d**
RATIONALE: Health care personnel should follow standard precautions whenever there is the

potential for contact with blood and all body fluids except sweat, regardless of whether they contain visible blood, nonintact skin, and mucous membranes. The client has an infected wound, not an airborne infectious disease like tuberculosis or SARS; hence, the client's breath will not transmit the infection.

10. **Answer: a**
RATIONALE: Transmission-based precautions are required for various lengths of time, depending mostly on the nature of the infecting microorganisms. Acute rheumatic fever may be prevented with treatment within 10 days of onset of symptoms. Health care personnel base the decision to use one or a combination of precautions on the mechanism of transmission of the pathogen. Moreover, infections progress through distinct stages and, lastly, also depend on the effective treatment available for the infection.

11. **Answer: b**
RATIONALE: Transmission-based precautions are discontinued when a wound or lesion stops draining, with the exception of standard precautions, when culture findings are negative, or after the initiation of effective therapy. Sometimes, personnel use them throughout a client's treatment when culture findings are positive, when the client shows drug-resistant strains, or when the blood around a wound dries up.

12. **Answer: d**
RATIONALE: Specimens are delivered to the laboratory in sealed containers in a plastic biohazard bag. Wearing new gloves is part of the standard precautions, whereas leaving an air gap in the container when collecting specimens is not part of precautionary measures. Specimens are not collected and delivered in plastic biohazard bags.

13. **Answers: a, c, e**
RATIONALE: The housekeeping personnel should clean the infectious client's room last to avoid transferring organisms on the wet mop to other client areas. An instruction card stating that isolation precautions are required should also be posted on the door or nearby at eye level. When caring for clients with infectious diseases, the door to the room should be closed to control air currents and the circulation of dust particles. Any number of visitors can meet the client, provided they comply with the infection control measures. If disposable linen and equipment are not available, the used material should be thoroughly disinfected and sterilized before reuse.

14. **Answer: b**
RATIONALE: Droplet precautions are measures that block pathogens within moist droplets larger than 5 μm. They are used to reduce pathogen transmission from close contact (usually 3 feet or less) between an infected person or a person who is a carrier of a droplet-spread microorganism and others. Microorganisms carried on droplets commonly exit the body during coughing, sneezing, and talking and during procedures such as airway suctioning and bronchoscopy.

15. **Answer: a**
RATIONALE: Any trash item destroyed by incineration or autoclaved can be safely disposed of in landfills. Syringes, wrapped dressings, and sealed containers are not biodegradable trash. They can transfer pathogens easily; hence, they cannot be disposed of in landfills without incineration or autoclaving.

16. **Answers: a, b, c**
RATIONALE: Long-term care residents and senior hospitalized clients are at an increased risk for pneumonia, influenza, urinary tract and skin infections, and tuberculosis. AIDS is transmitted sexually or through blood transfusion, whereas glanders is a chronic debilitating disease of horses and cats, which is transmissible to humans.

17. **Answer: b**
RATIONALE: A powered air-purifying respirator is an alternative if a client has not been fitted for an N-95 respirator or has facial hair or a facial deformity that prevents a tight seal with an N-95 respirator. It blows atmospheric air through belt-mounted air-purifying canisters to the face piece via a flexible tube. An ultrasonic nebulizer is a high-frequency humidifier used during inhalation therapy. A nebulizer is a device used to deliver medication to deeper parts of the respiratory tract.

SECTION IV: REVIEWING WHAT YOU HAVE LEARNED

Activity H

1. Gloves

Activity I

1. True.
2. False. The nurse should apply a mask and hair cover before performing a surgical scrub to prevent contamination of the hands after they are washed.

Activity J

Medical cover gowns prevent contamination of clothing and protect the skin from contact with blood and body fluids. When they are removed after direct care of the infectious client, they reduce the possibility of transmitting pathogens from the client, the client's environment, or contaminated objects. Many types of cover gowns exist, but all have the following common characteristics:

- They open in the back to reduce inadvertent contact with the client and objects.
- They have close-fitting wristbands to help prevent contamination of the forearms.
- They fasten at the neck and waist to stay securely closed, thus covering all of the caregiver's clothing.

Activity K

Contact precautions block the transmission of pathogens directly via skin-to-skin contact with an infected or colonized person or indirectly via contaminated objects in an infected client's environment.

Activity L

1. a.
The nurse should follow these transmission-based precautions:
- **a.** Don gloves before entering the client's room; change gloves during client care after contact with infectious material that contains a high concentration of microorganisms and remove them before leaving the room.
- **b.** Perform hand washing immediately after removing the gloves and avoid touching potentially contaminated surfaces or items.
- **c.** Wear a gown when entering the room if there is a possibility that clothing will touch the client and remove it before leaving the room.
- **d.** Clean bedside equipment and client care items daily.
- **e.** Use assessment tools exclusively for one infected client and disinfect them before using for another client.
- **b.** The nurse can flush all biodegradable trash down the toilet in the client's room. Chemicals and filtration methods in sewage treatment centers are sufficient for destroying pathogens in human waste. The nurse should place bulkier items in a lined trash container and remove them from the room by single or double bagging. They should wrap moist items (such as soiled dressings) so that during their containment, flying or crawling insects cannot transfer pathogens. Eventually, the bag and its contents are destroyed by incineration or are autoclaved. Autoclaved items can be safely disposed of in landfills.

Activity M

There are no definite answers to this activity. Students may choose to discuss their thoughts with peers or instructors.

SECTION V: GETTING READY FOR NCLEX

Activity N

1. **Answers: a, b, e**
RATIONALE: The client should use paper tissues because they collect moist respiratory secretions, decrease airborne transmission, and are incinerated to destroy microorganisms present in secretions. A particulate air filter respirator worn by the nurse is much more efficient than a cloth or a paper mask because it can filter particles 1 μm in size with 95% efficiency. The nurse need not line the client's wheelchair or stretcher with a clean sheet unless the client is transported from their room. Because tuberculosis is an airborne disease, the nurse should place a mask on the client during transports. Once a skin test is positive, it is always positive and will not be repeatedly administered.

CHAPTER 23

SECTION I: ASSESSING YOUR UNDERSTANDING

Activity A

1. Disuse
2. Gravity
3. Spasms
4. Ergonomics
5. Trendelenburg
6. Transfer
7. Trochanters
8. Ambulation

Activity B

1. The figure shows a good standing posture.
2. A good posture, whether in a standing, sitting, or lying position, distributes gravity through the center of the body. It affects a person's appearance, stamina, and ability to use the musculoskeletal system efficiently.
3. The figure shows protective boots to avoid foot drop.
4. Footboards, boots, and splints are devices that prevent foot drop by keeping the feet in a functional position.

Activity C

1. c   **2.** a   **3.** d   **4.** b

Activity D

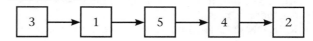

Activity E

1. In a good sitting position, the buttocks and upper thighs become the base of support. Both feet rest on the floor. The knees are bent, with the posterior of the knee free from the edge of the chair to avoid interfering with distal circulation.
2. The use of proper body mechanics increases muscle effectiveness, reduces fatigue, and helps to avoid repetitive strain injuries that result from cumulative trauma to musculoskeletal structures.
3. Health care workers are vulnerable to ergonomic hazards in the workplace as a direct consequence of lifting clients, reaching and lifting with loads far from the body, twisting while lifting, unexpected changes in load demand during the lift, reaching low or high to begin a lift, and moving or carrying a load at significant distance.
4. In an air-fluidized bed, fluid balance in the client may become a problem because of the accelerated

evaporation caused by the warm, blowing air. Puncturing or tearing the mattress is also a potential problem.

5. By the seventh or eighth decade of life, muscle strength, endurance, and coordination decline. Older adults need to maintain as much mobility as possible to prevent disability.

SECTION II: APPLYING YOUR KNOWLEDGE

Activity F

1. Before planning to turn and move the client, the nurse should assess the client and the situation as follows:
   - Assess for risk factors that may contribute to inactivity.
   - Determine the time of the client's last position change.
   - Assess their own physical, mental, and emotional ability to assist in turning, positioning, or moving.
   - Inspect for drainage tubes and equipment.
2. As part of planning before moving the client, the nurse should consider the following:
   - Explain the procedure to the client.
   - Remove all pillows and current positioning devices.
   - Raise the bed to a suitable working height (elbow height).
   - Secure two or three additional caregivers, positioning and moving devices (e.g., roller sheets, repositioning sling, mechanical lift), or both if the client cannot assist.
   - Close the door or draw the bedside curtain.

SECTION III: PRACTICING FOR NCLEX

Activity G

1. **Answer: c**
   RATIONALE: Maintaining the hips at an even level is a component of a good standing posture. A good standing posture includes keeping the feet about 4 to 8 inches (not 2 to 3 inches) apart from each other, bending the knees slightly to avoid straining the joints, and holding the chest slightly forward, not backward.
2. **Answer: d**
   RATIONALE: When working at the computer, the nurse should use wrist rests to keep the wrists in a neutral position. The nurse should work under lights that do not produce glare, not dim lights, which could strain the eyes. The elbows should be flexed no more than 100 to 110 degrees, not 120 degrees. The nurse should use a chair that is high enough so that they can place their feet firmly on the floor.
3. **Answers: a, b, c**
   RATIONALE: When caring for an inactive client, the nurse should raise the bed to the height of the caregiver's elbow to work at a comfortable height to avoid straining the back. The nurse should

remove pillows and positioning devices to enable easier movement. The nurse should change the inactive client's position at least every 2 hours to relieve pressure on bony areas of the body. The nurse should turn the client as a complete unit to avoid twisting the spine, rather than turn the upper part of the client's body and then the lower part. The nurse should not lift and drag the client when transferring to a stretcher; instead, the nurse should use a low-friction fabric or gel-filled plastic sheet, roller sheet with handles, or a repositioning sling to slide the client; this will also avoid injuring the client.

4. **Answer: b**
   RATIONALE: Placing the client in supine position for long could lead to skin breakdown at the end of the spine because the client is positioned on their back. In the prone position, the client lies on the abdomen, reducing skin breakdown from pressure ulcers. The lateral position is a side-lying position in which the spine is not in touch with the surface of the bed. The Sims position is a semiprone position in which the client's spine does not encounter pressure.
5. **Answer: c**
   RATIONALE: In the Fowler position, the abdominal organs drop away from the diaphragm, allowing for the exchange of a greater volume of air, which is especially useful for a client with dyspnea. Supine, Sims, and the lateral positions do not promote the exchange of a greater volume of air. In the supine position, the client lies on their back; the Sims and lateral positions are side-lying positions, which do not make breathing easier.
6. **Answer: a**
   RATIONALE: To elevate the upper part of the body, the nurse should use oversized pillows if an adjustable bed is not available. Contour pillows, triangular wedges, and bolsters are ideal for supporting and elevating the head, extremities, and shoulders.
7. **Answer: a**
   RATIONALE: The nurse uses hand rolls to prevent contracture of the fingers. Hand rolls are not used to hold the fingers in a tight fist, to keep the fingers and thumb together, or to prevent the wrist from turning outward. A hand roll keeps the thumb positioned slightly away from the hand and at a moderate angle to the fingers. The fingers are kept in a slightly neutral position rather than a tight fist.
8. **Answer: b**
   RATIONALE: The nurses should avoid stooping when turning the client by placing the sheet close to the client to ensure good body mechanics. Roller sheets are used to slide and roll, rather than to lift, a client. Roller sheets are not placed away from the client; they are placed close to the client when turning the client. After use, the sheets are not kept at the edge of the bed; the sheets are

removed and kept dry and free of wrinkles to prevent skin breakdown.

9. Answer: d

RATIONALE: The client should be provided with a trapeze to move around in bed. It is especially useful for the client who needs to develop strong arms to use a crutch later. A footboard, a bed board, and a trochanter roll are not used to help the client move around in bed. A footboard is used to prevent outward rotation of the lower leg and foot. A bed board is a rigid structure that provides support. Trochanter rolls are also used to prevent the legs from turning outward.

10. Answer: a

RATIONALE: Side rails are appropriate for the bed of a senior client who has undergone a surgery for cataracts because they serve as a restrictive device to prevent the client from falling off the bed. A cradle is often used for clients with burns, painful joint disease, and fractures of the leg; it is a metal frame that forms a shell over the client's lower legs to keep bed linen off the feet or legs. A transfer handle fits between the mattress and bed frame or box spring and serves as a combination grab bar and handrail to support the client's weight while exiting and returning to bed. A transfer board serves as a supportive bridge between two surfaces such as the bed and a wheelchair, bed and stretcher, wheelchair and car seat, or wheelchair and toilet; it is used to transfer the client.

11. Answer: c

RATIONALE: A water mattress requires filling and emptying, although it is done infrequently and is time-consuming. Water mattresses do not distribute water cyclically, contain inflated air sacs, or drain excretions away from the body. In an alternating air mattress, the wavelike redistribution of air cyclically relieves pressure over bony prominences. A low air loss bed contains inflated air sacs within the mattress. Excretions and secretions drain away from the body through the beds, thereby preventing skin irritation and maceration from moisture.

12. Answer: b

RATIONALE: The use of assistive devices helps the nurse reduce musculoskeletal injuries. The use of assistive devices allows the client to maintain their dignity and self-esteem and to relieve anxiety concerning safety and promotes faster recovery.

13. Answer: c

RATIONALE: The nurses should stand facing each other on opposite sides of the bed between the client's hips and shoulders, not on the same side of the client. The nurses should place the roller sheet beneath the client's shoulders and buttocks. The nurses should raise the bed to elbow height, rather than lowering it to the position of the waist, to reduce back strain.

14. Answer: b

RATIONALE: A functional status of level 4 indicates that the client needs total supervision. A client who needs total assistance has a functional status of level 5. A client who needs an assistive device is given a functional status of level 1, and a client who needs minimal help is given a functional status of level 2.

15. Answer: d

RATIONALE: A client with burns, who requires frequent dressing changes and topical applications, should be provided with a circular bed, which allows the client to remain passively immobilized during a position change. An oscillating support bed is best suited for a client who is at high risk for systemic effects of immobility, such as pneumonia and skin breakdown. A foam mattress and gel cushion can be provided to clients with intact skin and minimal risk for breakdown, so the client can change positions spontaneously or with minimal assistance.

SECTION IV: REVIEWING WHAT YOU HAVE LEARNED

Activity H
1. Gravity
2. Contracture

Activity I
1. False. The ability of the muscles to respond to stimulation is referred to as tone. Strength means the power of the muscles to perform.
2. False. A trapeze is a triangular piece of metal hung by a chain over the head of the bed.

Activity J
1. Ergonomics

Activity K
1. d   **2.** f   **3.** e   **4.** a   **5.** b   **6.** c

Activity L

$$2 \rightarrow 5 \rightarrow 1 \rightarrow 3 \rightarrow 4$$

Activity M
1.
- Keep the feet parallel, at right angles to the lower legs and approximately 4 to 8 inches (10 to 20 cm) apart.
- Distribute weight equally on both feet to provide a broad base of support.
- Bend the knees slightly to avoid straining the joints.
- Maintain the hips at an even level.
- Pull in the buttocks and hold the abdomen up and in to keep the spine properly aligned. This position supports the abdominal organs and reduces strain on both back and abdominal muscles.

- Hold the chest up and slightly forward; extend or stretch the waist to give internal organs more space and maintain good alignment of the spine.
- Keep the shoulders even and centered above the hips.
- Hold the head erect with the face forward and the chin slightly tucked.

2. Footboards, boots, and splints help prevent foot drop by keeping the feet in a functional position. Some footboards have supports that prevent outward rotation of the feet and lower legs. If the client is short and cannot reach a footboard, a foot splint may be used. Some clients are provided with ankle-high tennis shoes to wear in bed to prevent foot drop.

Activity N

1. Lying supine or prone promotes venous circulation, reduces stump edema, and prevents joint contractures.
2. Fowler position causes the abdominal organs to drop away from the diaphragm, thus enhancing the exchange of a greater volume of air.

Activity O

1. While assisting with this client transfer, the nurse should perform the following:
   - Evaluate the need for assistive equipment and devices such as a mechanical lift.
   - Assist the client to sit on the side of the bed.
   - Help the client don a bathrobe, shoes, or non-skid slippers.
   - Place the chair parallel to the bed on the client's stronger side.
   - Apply a transfer belt around the client's abdomen if the client is strong enough to assist in the transfer.
   - Grasp the transfer belt.
   - Practice good body mechanics by bending the hips and knees to reduce the potential for injury.
   - Brace the client's knees.
   - Rock the client to a standing position at an agreed signal while encouraging the client to straighten their knees and hips.
   - Pivot the client with their back toward the chair.
   - Tell the client to step back until they feel the chair at the back of the legs.
   - Instruct the client to grasp the arms of the chair while you stabilize their knees and lower the client into the chair.
   - Support the feet on the footrests.

Activity P

There are no definite answers to this activity. Students may choose to discuss their thoughts with peers or instructors.

SECTION V: GETTING READY FOR NCLEX

Activity Q

1. **Answers: b, c, d**
   RATIONALE: Keeping the feet apart lowers the center of gravity, which promotes stability and provides a broad base of support. Resting at intervals promotes work endurance. Bending the knees prepares the spine to accept the weight of the load. The nurse should avoid twisting and stretching, which causes muscle strain because the line of gravity is outside the body's base of support. The nurse should contract the abdominal muscles to avoid strain and injury to their abdominal walls.

CHAPTER 24

SECTION I: ASSESSING YOUR UNDERSTANDING

Activity A

1. Exercise
2. Composition
3. Submaximal
4. Target
5. Metabolic
6. Aerobic
7. Active

Activity B

1. The figure shows stationary cycling, which is an isokinetic exercise.
2. Isokinetic exercise combines movement at a constant speed with a form of resistance. The speed and resistance are preprogrammed and controlled with a machine. An example is a stationary bicycle, such as those in therapeutic settings or fitness centers. Isokinetic exercises are often used for the purpose of rehabilitation after an athlete experiences an injury or to strengthen weakened muscles when a person is recovering from a stroke or accident.
3. The figure shows a continuous passive motion machine.
4. A continuous passive motion machine is an electrical device used as a supplement or substitute for manual ROM exercise. Machine-assisted ROM is sometimes preferred during the rehabilitation of clients who have experienced burns or who have had knee or hip replacement surgery because the machine precisely controls the degree of joint movement and can increase it in specific increments throughout recovery.

Activity C

1. b   2. e   3. d   4. a   5. c

Activity D

1. Factors such as sedentary lifestyle, health problems, compromised muscle and skeletal function,

obesity, advanced age, smoking, and high blood pressure can impair a client's fitness and stamina.

2. Fitness tests provide an objective measure of a person's current fitness level and potential for safe exercise. They also help to establish safe parameters for the level and duration of exercise.

3. Recovery index is the guide for determining a person's fitness level. Examiners calculate the client's recovery index by taking a 30-second pulse rate 1, 2, and 3 minutes after the test. It is calculated as

recovery index = (100 × test duration in seconds)/2 × total of three 30-second pulse assessments

4. The walk-a-mile test measures the time it takes a person to walk 1 mile. The person is instructed to walk 1 mile on a flat surface as fast as possible. The examiner calculates the time from start to finish and interprets the results.

5. Maximum heart rate is calculated by subtracting a person's age from 220. Thus, a 20-year-old has a maximum heart rate of 200 bpm, whereas a 50-year-old has a maximum heart rate of 170 bpm.

SECTION II: APPLYING YOUR KNOWLEDGE

Activity E

1. The initial requirements for a client before starting on a safe exercise program include a preexercise fitness evaluation from a health care provider or a certified sports trainer. The target heart rate should be determined per the fitness level. An appropriate level of metabolic energy equivalent should be determined because fitness levels vary from client to client.

2. The nurse should prescribe activities such as water skiing and moving heavy furniture for a client with 6 to 7 METs.

SECTION III: PRACTICING FOR NCLEX

Activity F

1. **Answers: a, c, e**
   RATIONALE: When performing ROM exercises for an immobile client, the nurse should raise the level of the bed, avoid forceful joint movements, and move the client closer to the edge of the bed. Raising the level of the bed and moving the client closer to the edge of the bed protects the nurse from injuries resulting from unnecessary stretching and bending. The nurse should not repeat each exercise five times or begin with feet exercises and work upward. The nurse should repeat each exercise only three times and stop if the client complains of pain or discomfort. The nurse should begin exercises at the client's neck and work downward.

2. **Answer: a**
   RATIONALE: Isometric exercises help to preserve and increase muscle mass, strength, and tone and

to define muscle groups. Isometric exercises are not useful in preventing joint deformities, stiffness of joints, or skin breakdown. Skin breakdown can be prevented by frequent repositioning of the client. Regular ROM exercises help to prevent joint deformities and stiffness of joints by preventing muscular contractures.

3. **Answer: d**
   RATIONALE: Aerobic exercise is an isotonic exercise that involves rhythmically moving all parts of the body at a moderate to slow speed without hindering the ability to breathe. Bodybuilding, weight lifting, and holding a yoga position are isometric exercises that improve blood circulation, but do not promote cardiorespiratory function.

4. **Answers: a, b, d**
   RATIONALE: The nurse should recommend squeezing a softball, combing the hair, and finger climbing on the vertical surface of a wall to exercise the arm on the surgical side. The nurse need not ask the client to swim or rotate the arm because the client initially needs to use small groups of muscles that are in a weakened state.

5. **Answer: c**
   RATIONALE: An ECG is an assessment that provides reliable results for fitness levels. The walk-a-mile test, step test, and aerobic fitness tests are submaximal fitness tests that are less demanding and do not stress a person to exhaustion. Therefore, the results of submaximal fitness tests are less reliable than the results obtained through ECG testing.

6. **Answer: a**
   RATIONALE: Walking is the most ideal exercise for this client, considering their age and diabetic condition. Cycling, running, and jogging are vigorous and strenuous, causing strain on the knee joints, which the client should avoid.

7. **Answer: c**
   RATIONALE: The nurse should ask the client to balance periods of physical activity with periods of rest. Older adults should drink plenty of water and eliminate their intake of caffeinated and alcoholic beverages before and during physical activity to avoid depleting fluid volume. The nurse should ask the client to take precautions, such as wearing safe shoes with nonskid soles (not smooth soles) to prevent falls.

8. **Answer: a**
   RATIONALE: When the client constantly ignores objects placed on their right side, the nurse confirms unilateral neglect in the client. Ability of the client to differentiate warm and cold on both sides, combing the hair on both sides, and observing objects placed on either side are not signs of unilateral neglect.

9. **Answers: b, c, d**
   RATIONALE: When caring for a client who has been ordered a continuous passive motion machine, the nurse should instruct the client on techniques for relaxation, which will empower the client with

techniques for controlling pain. The nurse should compare assessment findings with the unaffected extremity to provide comparative data. The nurse should assess vital signs and mobility of the affected extremity to provide a baseline of data for future comparisons. The nurse should provide pain medication before, not after, exercise is completed to control pain before it intensifies with exercise. The nurse should adjust the machine to a lower-than-prescribed rate and degree of flexion to provide gradual progression to prescribed parameters.

10. Answer: d
RATIONALE: The nurse should always approach the client from the left side because the client's perception and attention are limited to the unaffected side. The nurse should suggest the client turn their head from side to side for a panoramic view of the environment, rather than view the environment from one side. The nurse should not place the signal cord on the right-hand side of the client; items of safety should always be placed on the left-hand side of the client. The nurse should have the client locate and touch the right arm and other body structures on the right side to retrain the client's brain to recognize and integrate parts of themselves.

11. Answer: c
RATIONALE: The nurse is assisting the client in performing circumduction. If the nurse places the arm at the client's side and bends the forearm toward the shoulder and then straightens it again, it is called flexion, extension, and hyperextension of the elbow.

12. Answer: d
RATIONALE: The nurse should ask the client to avoid the use of electric blankets, which could interfere with an accurate interpretation of the test results. The client is required to wear the Holter monitor for 24 hours, not 12 hours. Clients use a treadmill, which measures peripheral oxygen, when recording a stress ECG, not an ambulatory ECG.

13. Answer: d
RATIONALE: The step test involves about 76 steps per minute. The prescribed platform height for men is 20 inches, and for women it is 16 inches. A step up (or a step down) is considered one step.

14. Answer: b
RATIONALE: A client with a fitness level of 60 is said to have a below-average fitness classification. A value of less than or equal to 55 indicates poor, between 64 and 56 indicates below average, between 65 and 79 is average, and between 80 and 89 is good.

15. Answer: c
RATIONALE: The nurse should support the joint being exercised because supporting reduces discomfort. All pillows and positioning devices should be removed because they interfere with the exercises. The nurse should move each joint only until there is resistance but no pain; this method

exercises each joint to its point of limitation. A systematic, repetitive pattern should be followed because following a routine prevents overlooking a joint.

SECTION IV: REVIEWING WHAT YOU HAVE LEARNED

Activity G
1. Isometric
2. Fitness
3. Abduction

Activity H
1. False. The ability of the muscles to respond to stimulation is referred to as tone. Strength means the power of the muscles to perform.
2. True

Activity I

	Active Exercise	Passive Exercise
Definition	Therapeutic activity performed independently by the client after proper instruction	Therapeutic activity in which the client is assisted with movement
Uses	Focused on a part of the body in a weakened condition	Provided when the client cannot move one or more parts of the body
Examples	• Squeezing a soft ball • Finger-climbing the vertical surface of a wall • Swinging a rope attached to a doorknob	• Range-of-motion exercises • Use of a continuous passive motion machine

Activity J
Seven factors that can compromise a client's fitness and stamina are (1) sedentary lifestyle, (2) health problems, (3) compromised muscle and skeletal function, (4) obesity, (5) advanced age, (6) smoking, and (7) high blood pressure.

Activity K
The machine controls the degree of joint movement, which can be increased in specific increments throughout the recovery. Pain may interfere with a client's independent effort to exercise the artificial joint.

Activity L
1.
   a. The nurse should determine the client's body composition, evaluate trends in vital signs, and assist with fitness tests. Determining factors for body composition include anthropometric measurements such as height, weight, body mass

index, skinfold thickness, and midarm muscle circumference. After a period of modified exercise, vital signs may decrease, thus reducing the potential for heart-related complications. Two methods of fitness testing are a stress electrocardiogram and an ambulatory electrocardiogram.

b. First, the person's maximum heart rate, which is the highest limit for heart rate during exercise, must be established. Maximum heart rate is calculated by subtracting a person's age from 220. The target heart rate is 60% to 90% of the maximum heart rate. Metabolic energy equivalent, which is the measure of energy and oxygen consumption during exercise, varies with fitness levels.

2.

a. Older adults need to eliminate their intake of caffeinated and alcoholic beverages before and during physical activity to avoid depleting fluid volume. The nurse should ensure that clients drink sufficient water to ensure fluid replacement.

b. The nurse can help the clients in the following ways:
- Encourage older adults to socialize by participating in group activities.
- Assist clients with cognitive impairment to participate in physical activities.
- Assist senior clients in performing passive range-of-motion (ROM) exercises daily to prevent muscle atrophy and disuse syndrome.
- Encourage clients to swim or exercise in water, which minimizes stress on joints.
- Ask clients to take precautions such as wearing safe shoes with nonskid soles to prevent falls.

Activity M

There are no definite answers to this activity. Students may choose to discuss their thoughts with peers or instructors.

CHAPTER 25

SECTION I: ASSESSING YOUR UNDERSTANDING

Activity A

1. Spica
2. Sling
3. Braces
4. Cylinder
5. Traction
6. Fixator
7. Hip
8. Manual
9. Counterpull
10. Fiberglass

Activity B

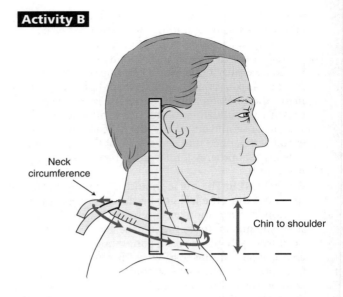

Neck circumference

Chin to shoulder

1. The figure shows vertical and circumferential measurements for cervical collar size.
2. The procedure is used to determine the proper collar size of the client. The nurse measures the neck circumference and the distance between the shoulder and the chin. The nurse then compares measurements with the size guide suggested by the collar manufacturer.
3. The figure shows an external fixator.
4. An external fixator is a metal device inserted into and through one or more broken bones to stabilize fragments during healing. Although the external fixator immobilizes the area of injury, the client is encouraged to be active and mobile.

Activity C

1. a **2.** d **3.** b **4.** c

Activity D

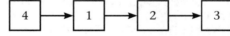

$$4 \rightarrow 1 \rightarrow 2 \rightarrow 3$$

Activity E

1. Plaster of Paris is inexpensive and easy to apply, but it has several disadvantages. It takes 24 to 48 hours to dry and is prone to drying and cracking at the edges. It softens when wet and is heavy.
2. Most clients who require mechanical immobilization have suffered trauma to the musculoskeletal system. Such injuries are painful and heal less rapidly than injuries to the skin or soft tissue. They require a period of inactivity to allow new cells to restore integrity to the damaged structures. Purposes of mechanical immobilization include relieving pain and muscle spasm, supporting and aligning skeletal injuries, restricting movement while injuries heal, maintaining a functional position until healing is complete, allowing activity while

restricting movement of an injured area, and preventing further structural damage and deformity.
3. A splint is a device that immobilizes and protects an injured body part. Splints are used before or instead of casts or traction. Splints often are applied as a first-aid measure for suspected sprains or fractures.
4. Because of diminished tactile sensation, older adults may be unaware of skin pressure from a splint, cast, traction, or other mechanical device. The skin of an older person should be assessed daily for redness or other signs of pressure. If the older person cannot change positions, the caregiver is responsible for ensuring that pressure is relieved at least every 2 hours.
5. Nurses provide care for the pin site to prevent infection. Pin sites are locations where pins, wires, or tongs enter or exit the skin. In conjunction with an external fixator and skeletal traction, pin site care is essential to prevent infection. Insertion of pins impairs skin integrity and provides a port of entry for pathogens. (Refer to Skill 25-5.)
6. When the cast is removed, the skin usually appears pale and waxy and may contain scales or patches of dead skin. The skin is washed as usual with soapy, warm water, but the semi-attached areas of skin are left in place; they are not forcibly removed. Applying lotion to the skin adds moisture and tends to prevent the rough skin edges from catching on clothing. Eventually, the dead skin fragments will shed.

SECTION II: APPLYING YOUR KNOWLEDGE
Activity F
1. The nurse should wash their hands thoroughly or perform an alcohol-based hand rub and then wear clean gloves to reduce the transmission of pathogens. The nurse should then pour a cleaning agent on a cotton tip applicator and clean the skin at the pin site, moving outward in a circular manner so that it prevents microorganisms from moving toward the area of open skin.
2. To assess the client, the nurse should review the medical records for trends in the client's temperature, white blood cell count, reports of pain, and the frequency for treating pain so that the data can be used in case of infection. The nurse should also inspect the area around the pin insertion site for redness, swelling, increased tenderness, and drainage to provide data for current and future comparisons. The nurse should also examine the pin for signs of bending or shifting to identify potential problems with maintaining traction and the desired position.

SECTION III: PRACTICING FOR NCLEX
Activity G
1. **Answer: a**
   RATIONALE: To reduce pain and swelling, the nurse should elevate the cast on pillows or other supports. The nurse cannot administer pain-relieving medication without the physician's prescription. Providing written instructions on cast care will not reduce the pain or swelling, and placing the bed at a comfortable height to prevent backache is an intervention for a client with pin site insertion.
2. **Answers: a, c, e**
   RATIONALE: Inflatable and traction splints such as pneumatic splints, Thomas splints, and Russell traction are intended for short-term use. They are usually applied just after the injury and are removed shortly after a more thorough assessment of the injury is made. Immobilizers and molded splints are used for longer periods.
3. **Answer: b**
   RATIONALE: The nurse should look for trends in the client's temperature, white blood cell count, and reports of pain and frequency of treating pain to determine whether there is any infection. Checking for dry skin or the client's pulse rate is a part of obtaining vital signs. Checking if the pin is bent or shifted identifies problems with maintaining traction and the desired position.
4. **Answers: b, c**
   RATIONALE: Molded splints provide prolonged support and limit movement to prevent further injury and pain. They maintain the body part in a functional position to prevent contractures and muscle atrophy during immobility. A cervical collar, not a molded splint, reduces load-bearing force on the cervical spine. A cast immobilizes the injured structure. It is placed around an injured body part after it has been restored to the correct anatomic alignment.
5. **Answer: b**
   RATIONALE: When a spica cast is applied to a lower extremity, the cast is trimmed in the anal and genital areas to allow for the elimination of urine and stool. A bivalved cast facilitates bathing and skin care, whereas a body cast is a larger form of a cylinder cast that encircles the trunk of the body instead of an extremity. A cylinder cast encircles an arm or leg and leaves the toes or fingers exposed.
6. **Answer: a**
   RATIONALE: To promote healing of a musculoskeletal injury, the nurse should encourage senior clients to consume a diet rich in protein, calcium, and zinc. Teach clients who are lactose intolerant to use milk or calcium substitutes. The nurse need not ask the client to avoid vitamin D supplements. Encourage sun exposure for 10 to 30 minutes daily for vitamin D absorption and weight-bearing exercises if the older person can tolerate these activities.
7. **Answer: b**
   RATIONALE: When the cast is removed, the skin usually appears pale and waxy and may contain scales or patches of dead skin. The unexercised

muscle is usually smaller and weaker. The joints may have a limited ROM and the flexibility will be less for the first few days. There may be minor, not major, swelling on the affected area after cast removal, which is normal.

8. **Answer: b**
    RATIONALE: Buck traction and Russell traction are forms of skin traction in which the pulling effect on the skeletal system is applied by devices, such as a pelvic belt and a cervical halter, to the skin. Manual traction involves the use of hands and muscular strength. Skeletal traction is the pull exerted directly on the skeletal system by attaching wires, pins, or tongs into or through a bone, and an external fixator is used to insert into and through one or more broken bones to stabilize fragments during healing.

9. **Answer: a**
    RATIONALE: Hip fractures are common in senior persons, especially postmenopausal women, who are not treated for osteoporosis. The fracture may result from weakness of the bone and may lead to a fall, or a fall may cause the fracture of a weakened bone. With aging, bones become brittle and weak, resulting in a longer healing time for fractures. Joints become stiffer, not more flexible because of decreased synovial fluid.

10. **Answers: a, b, c**
    RATIONALE: An improperly applied or ill-fitting brace can cause discomfort, deformity, and skin ulcerations from friction or prolonged pressure. Ill-fitting braces do not cause muscle contractures. Molded splints maintain the body part in a functional position to prevent contractures and muscle atrophy during immobility. Permanent stiffness is the result of prolonged dependence on cervical collars, not ill-fitting braces.

11. **Answer: a**
    RATIONALE: The nurse should not provide a pillow if the client's head or neck is in traction because it could disturb the pull and counterpull. Reducing the amount of weights or changing the client's position could interfere with the pulling effect and cause more damage. A pressure-relieving device is used to prevent skin breakdown if the client is confined to bed for a long duration.

12. **Answer: b**
    RATIONALE: To facilitate circulation, the nurse should avoid more than 90 degrees of flexion, especially when there is an elbow injury. Slipping the flexed arm in the canvas sling will only enclose the forearm, but it will not facilitate circulation. Positioning the apex of the triangular sling under the elbow will facilitate in making a hammock of the arm, whereas positioning the knot at the side of the neck of a triangular sling will reduce pressure and friction.

13. **Answer: a**
    RATIONALE: A cast is removed prematurely if complications develop. In most cases, casts are removed when they need to be changed and

reapplied or when the injury has healed sufficiently and the cast is no longer necessary. Cast edges are kept soft to minimize skin irritation, and a bivalved cast is removed when there is a need to provide hygiene to the client.

14. **Answer: d**
    RATIONALE: Clients with a hip spica cannot sit during elimination, so the nurse protects the cast from soiling using a plastic wrap and positions the client on a small bedpan known as a fracture pan. Tucking in an adult diaper is not possible in a hip spica cast because the cast is trimmed only near the genital and anal areas. Inserting an indwelling catheter is not a good idea because it can lead to urinary tract infection. Providing a bedpan to the client will not be useful because the client will not be able to position him or herself on the bedpan.

15. **Answer: c**
    RATIONALE: The nurse can assess by seeing that the splint is filled with air to the point at which it can be indented one-half inch (1.3 cm) with the fingertips. The injury should be examined and treated within 30 to 45 minutes after application of the splint; otherwise, circulation may be affected. Asking the client if the splint feels heavy and touching the splint to determine whether it is cold are secondary measures. Pushing a fingertip between the cast and injured part is not appropriate because the client will experience pressure and pain.

16. **Answers: c, d, e**
    RATIONALE: Although narcotic analgesics are effective in relieving musculoskeletal pain, senior clients are more susceptible to developing adverse effects such as constipation, mental changes, and depressed respirations. Dilated pupils and a pale skin are not effects that are seen in senior clients after the consumption of narcotic analgesics.

17. **Answer: a**
    RATIONALE: Nurses should tell the clients not to write anything on the cast because nurses and physicians write important notes on the cast and, in addition, fiberglass casts are porous. Elevating the cast on a pillow or support helps to reduce swelling and pain. The nurse should apply an ice pack, not a hot pack, to the cast near the injured area to reduce swelling and control bleeding. The nurse should, in fact, encourage clients to ambulate as soon as possible or exercise in bed because movement prevents complications from immobility.

18. **Answer: c**
    RATIONALE: To facilitate skin care and personal hygiene, the nurse should bathe the backs of clients who are in a supine position for a prolonged time. Covering metal pins with cork prevents accidental injury; cleaning the skin around the insertion site with an antimicrobial agent reduces the risk of infection. The nurse should insert padding within the sling if it tends to wrinkle because padding helps cushion, prevents interference with circulation, and reduces the risk of dry skin.

SECTION IV: REVIEWING WHAT YOU HAVE LEARNED

Activity H

1. Molded
2. Spica

Activity I

1. True
2. True
3. False. A trapeze is a triangular piece of metal hung by a chain over the head of the bed.

Activity J

1. External fixator
2. Body cast
3. Skeletal traction

Activity K

1. c
2. a
3. d
4. b

Activity L

	Plaster of Paris	Fiberglass
Application	Takes 24 to 48 hours to dry, depending on the size of the cast	Dries in 5 to 15 minutes
Cost	Inexpensive	Expensive
Durability	Prone to cracking or crumbling at the edges	Durable
Weight	Heavy	Light
Weight Bearing	Delayed until thoroughly dried	Immediate
Effect of Water	Softens when wet	Unaffected by water

Activity M

a. The figure shows the skin traction devices of (A) a pelvic belt and (B) a cervical halter.
b. These devices are used to reduce muscle spasms, re-align bones, relieve pain, and prevent deformities.

Activity N

1. Mechanical immobilization relieves pain and muscle spasm, supports and aligns skeletal injuries, restricts movement while injuries heal, maintains a functional position until healing is complete, allows activity while restricting movement of an injured area, and prevents further structural damage and deformity.
2. A cast is a rigid mold placed around an injured body part to immobilize it after it has been re-stored to correct anatomic alignment.
3. Clients with immobilizing devices may have one or more of the following nursing diagnoses:

- Acute pain
- Impaired physical mobility
- Risk for disuse syndrome
- Risk for peripheral neurovascular dysfunction
- Impaired bed mobility
- Risk for impaired skin integrity
- Risk for ineffective tissue perfusion
- Self-care deficit: bathing/hygiene

SECTION V: APPLYING YOUR KNOWLEDGE

Activity O

1. Older adults often have diminished tactile sensation that interferes with their ability to feel the consequences of pressure on their skin, such as a pressure ulcer that may be forming.
2. Insertion of a pin impairs skin integrity and provides a port of entry for pathogens, which could lead to infections.

Activity P

1.
   a. The nurse should measure the client's neck circumference and the distance between the shoulder and the chin. They should then compare the measurements with the guide suggested by the collar manufacturer to determine the proper collar size.
   b. The nurse should perform neuromuscular assessments by seeing if the client can elevate both shoulders, flex and extend the elbows and wrists, generate a strong hand grip, spread the fingers, and touch the thumb to the little finger on each hand.

Activity Q

There are no definite answers to this activity. Students may choose to discuss their thoughts with peers or instructors.

SECTION VI: GETTING READY FOR NCLEX

Activity R

1. **Answers: a, c, d**
   RATIONALE: The nurse should cover open wounds with a clean material to absorb blood and prevent dirt and additional pathogens from entering. They should select rigid materials such as a flat board or rolled-up newspaper to use as a splint to provide support while restricting movement. The nurse should use wide tape or fabric strip to confine the injured part to the splint so as to prevent displacement and reduce the risk of compromising circulation. The skin is swabbed with acetone and alcohol to remove fiberglass resins. A client whose arm or leg is in a cast is encouraged to exercise fingers and toes respectively.
2. **Answers: a, b**
   RATIONALE: To gather data about the client's neuromuscular function, the nurse needs to monitor the mobility of the client's fingers. Sensations in the exposed fingers indicate intact neurologic

function. Elevating the cast on pillows or other support helps reduce swelling and pain. Applying an ice pack at the level of injury helps reduce swelling and controls any bleeding. Depressing the nailbeds and observing the time taken for color to return is a vascular assessment.

CHAPTER 26

SECTION I: ASSESSING YOUR UNDERSTANDING

Activity A

1. Isometric
2. Dangling
3. Cane
4. Forearm
5. Platform
6. Sum
7. Prosthetic
8. Platform
9. Flexion
10. Axillary

Activity B

1. A walking belt is used to help the client ambulate.
2. A walking belt is applied around the client's waist. If the client loses their balance, the nurse can support them and prevent injuries. When helping a client ambulate, the nurse walks slightly behind the client, holding the walking belt or the client's own belt and supporting the client's arm.

Activity C

1. c   2. a   3. d   4. b

Activity D

Activity E

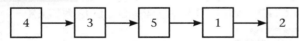

1. Some of the techniques that a nurse can teach a client to increase muscular strength and the ability to bear weight include the following:
   - Isometric exercises with the lower limbs
   - Isotonic exercises with the upper arms
   - Dangling at the bedside
   - Using a device called a tilt table
2. The quadriceps muscles include the rectus femoris, vastus intermedius, vastus medialis, and vastus lateralis, which cover the front and side of the thigh. Together, they aid in extending the leg. Exercising the quadriceps muscles, therefore, enables clients to stand and support their body weight.
3. Clients who will use a walker, cane, or crutches need upper arm strength. An exercise regimen to strengthen the upper arms typically includes the following:
   - Flexion and extension of the arms and wrists
   - Raising and lowering weights with the hands
   - Squeezing a ball or spring grip
   - Performing modified hand push-ups in bed
4. A tilt table is a device that raises the client from a supine to a standing position. It helps clients adjust to being upright and bearing weight on their feet. Just before using a tilt table, the nurse applies elastic stockings. These stockings help to compress vein walls, thus preventing pooling of blood in the extremities that may trigger fainting. After being transferred from the bed or stretcher to the horizontal tilt table, the client is strapped securely to prevent a fall. The feet are positioned against the footrest. The entire table is then tilted in increments of 15 to 30 degrees until the client is in a vertical position.
5. A cane must be the right height for the client. The cane's handle should be parallel with the client's hip, providing elbow flexion of approximately 30 degrees. Removing a portion of the lower end can shorten wooden canes. Depressing metal buttons in the telescoping shaft can shorten or lengthen aluminum canes.
6. Clients may return from surgery with an immediate postoperative prosthesis, which is a temporary artificial limb. It consists of a walking pylon, a lightweight tube attached to a shell made of plaster or plastic on the stump, and a rigid foot. A belt with garters keeps the temporary prosthesis in place. The belt is loosened while the client is in bed and is tightened during ambulation.

SECTION II: APPLYING YOUR KNOWLEDGE

Activity F

1. The nurse should perform the following procedure when applying the prosthetic leg to a client:
   - Cover the prosthetic foot with the stocking and shoe of choice.
   - Apply the nylon sheath, if used, and the appropriate number or ply of stump socks.
   - Place a nylon stocking over the stump socks, allowing a long portion of the toe to extend from the base of the stump.
   - Stand and position the prosthetic limb next to the residual limb.
   - Pull the toe of the nylon stocking through the valve at the base of the socket.
   - Pump the stump up and down as the nylon stocking is completely removed.
   - Replace the plug within the valve opening.
   - Fasten all slings if something other than a suction socket type of prosthesis is used.
2. The nurse is responsible for ensuring that the incision heals and that no complications, such as joint contractures or infection, develop. Complications delay rehabilitation. Contractures interfere with limb and prosthetic alignment, which ultimately affects the client's ability to walk.

SECTION III: PRACTICING FOR NCLEX

Activity G

1. **Answer: c**
    RATIONALE: To prepare the client for ambulation, the nurse can use a tilt table to help the client stand. Debilitated clients require physical conditioning before they can ambulate again. Other techniques for increasing muscular strength and the ability to bear weight include performing isometric exercises with the lower limbs, performing isotonic exercises with the upper arms, and using a device called a tilt table. A walking belt applied to the waist of the client helps the nurse to provide support when the client is ambulating.

2. **Answer: b**
    RATIONALE: The nurse should teach the client to perform isometric exercises to reestablish their ability to walk. Isometric exercises are used to promote muscle tone and strength, which are inherent in maintaining mobility. Inactive clients and those who have been immobilized in casts or traction may require focused periods of exercise to reestablish their previous ability to walk. Walking belts help the nurse support the client during ambulation if the client were to lose balance. Dangling helps to normalize blood pressure, which may drop when the client rises from a reclining position. A tilt table is a device that helps a client to adjust to being upright and bearing weight on their feet.

3. **Answer: c**
    RATIONALE: The nurse assists the client to dangle to normalize the client's blood pressure, which may drop when the client rises from a reclining position. The client would be required to perform isometric exercises to improve muscle tone and strength; isotonic exercise would help the client to improve upper arm strength. The nurse would use a tilt table to help the client to bear weight on their feet.

4. **Answer: a**
    RATIONALE: The quadriceps muscles aid in supporting body weight. The quadriceps muscles include the rectus femoris, vastus intermedius, vastus medialis, and vastus lateralis, which cover the front and sides of the thigh. Together they aid in extending the leg. Exercising the quadriceps muscles, therefore, enables clients to stand and support their body weight. Gluteal muscles aid in abducting and rotating the leg—functions that are essential for standing. Quadriceps may not necessarily aid the client to walk upright.

5. **Answer: d**
    RATIONALE: The client contracts and relaxes the gluteal muscles in a gluteal setting. A gluteal setting is the contraction and relaxation of the gluteal muscles to strengthen and tone them. To ambulate independently, the client could use the handrails of a parallel bar to practice ambulation. Modified hand push-ups in bed would enable the client to strengthen the upper arm. The client dangles or sits at the edge of the bed to normalize blood pressure.

6. **Answer: c**
    RATIONALE: The nurse should place books under the client's hand in case the bed on which the client is doing their modified push-ups is soft. Removing or replacing the mattress with a firmer one or providing a sturdy armchair may not be an appropriate action for this client.

7. **Answer: b**
    RATIONALE: To prevent circulatory problems, the nurse should instruct the client to avoid crossing the legs or keeping the natural knee flexed for a prolonged period. To promote venous circulation, reduce stump edema, and avoid any joint contractures, the nurse should encourage the client to lie in a supine or prone position periodically during the day. Wearing a nylon sheath beneath the stump sock helps to wick perspiration from the skin toward the sock and reduces friction on the skin; it does not prevent circulatory problems. The nurse should ask the client to dry the socks well before application to prevent any skin breakdown. To prevent overexertion and impaired skin integrity, the nurse should advise the client with a new prosthesis to wear it for short periods initially and then increase the wearing time each day.

8. **Answer: a**
    RATIONALE: The nurse lowers the tilt table and returns it to the horizontal position when symptoms of dizziness and hypotension develop. A tilt table is a device that raises the client from a supine to a standing position. It helps clients adjust to being upright and bearing weight on their feet. After being transferred from the bed or stretcher to the horizontal tilt table, the client is strapped securely to prevent a fall. The feet are positioned against a footrest. The entire table is then tilted in increments of 15 to 30 degrees until the client is in a vertical position. If symptoms such as dizziness and hypotension develop, the table is lowered or returned to the horizontal position. It is not necessary for the table to be used for more than 10 minutes.

9. **Answers: a, b, c**
    RATIONALE: When assisting a client who appears dizzy during ambulation, the nurse should support the client by sliding an arm under the axilla and placing a foot to the side, forming a wide base of support. With the client's weight braced, the nurse should balance the client on a hip until help arrives, or slide the client down the length of the nurse's leg to the floor. The nurse need not place the client on the bed. The nurse should not leave the client alone to go fetch water because the client appears dizzy and could fall.

10. **Answer: a**
    RATIONALE: The nurse should suggest the use of a cane for ambulation for clients who have

weakness in one side of the body. Canes are hand-held ambulatory devices made of wood or aluminum. Clients who require considerable support and assistance with balance use a walker. Clients who need brief, temporary assistance with ambulation are likely to use axillary crutches. Forearm crutches generally are used by experienced clients who need permanent assistance with walking.

11. Answer: b
RATIONALE: The nurse should use an axillary crutch for the client who has a fractured leg in a cast to help the client ambulate at the health care facility. Axillary crutches have a bar that fits beneath the axilla. Clients who need brief, temporary assistance with ambulation are likely to use axillary crutches. A cane is used for clients who have weakness on one side of the body. Clients who require considerable support and assistance with balance use a walker. Platform crutches are used by clients with arthritis who cannot bear weight with their hands and wrists.

12. Answers: a, b, c
RATIONALE: The prosthesis of a client who has been amputated below the knee would include a socket, shank, and ankle/foot system. An above-the-knee prosthesis also includes a knee system. A lightweight tube forms a part of the components of an immediate postoperative prosthesis that is fitted after the amputation.

13. Answers: b, a, d, c
RATIONALE: The client should first position him or herself in front of the chair seat and grip an armrest with one arm while placing the other hand on the walker and using the stronger leg for support. The client then releases the grip on the walker while using the free hand to grasp the opposite armrest and lowering him or herself into the chair.

14. Answers: c, a, b, d
RATIONALE: When a client who uses a walker to ambulate needs to rise from a chair, the client moves to the edge of the chair and repositions the walker. After pushing up on the armrests with both arms until the body weight is centered, the client uses one hand, then the other, to grasp the walker.

15. Answer: a
RATIONALE: A paralyzed client with leg braces who uses crutches to ambulate would use the swing-through gait. The three-point partial-weight-bearing gait would be used by an amputee who is learning to use a prosthesis. A client with a severe ankle sprain would use the three-point non–weight-bearing gait. Clients who have more strength, coordination, and balance would have a two-point gait.

16. Answer: a
RATIONALE: The nurse would observe a four-point gait in the arthritic client who uses crutches to ambulate. A two-point gait is observed in clients who have more strength, coordination,

and balance. A three-point partial-weight-bearing gait is observed in amputees learning to use a prosthesis, in clients with minor injuries to one leg, or in clients with previous injuries showing signs of healing. A three-point non–weight-bearing gait can be observed in clients with one amputated, injured, or disabled extremity.

SECTION IV: REVIEWING WHAT YOU HAVE LEARNED

Activity H
1. Platform
2. Isometric

Activity I
1. True

Activity J
A tilt table, which raises clients from a supine to a standing position, helps them adjust to being upright and bearing weight on their feet.

SECTION V: APPLYING YOUR KNOWLEDGE

Activity K
Lying supine or prone promotes venous circulation, reduces stump edema, and prevents joint contractures.

Activity L
1.
  a. The nurse instructs the client using a walker to
    • Stand within the walker.
    • Hold on to the walker at the padded handgrips.
    • Pick up the walker and advance it 6 to 8 inches.
    • Take a step forward.
    • Support the body weight on the handgrips when moving the weaker leg.
  b. When sitting down, the client should proceed as follows:
    • When the legs are in the front of the chair seat, grip an arm rest with one arm while placing the other hand on the walker and using the stronger leg for support.
    • Release the grip on the walker while using the free hand to grasp the opposite armrest and lower oneself into the chair.
    When getting up from the chair, the client should do the following:
    • Move to the edge of the chair and reposition the walker.
    • Push up on the armrests with both arms until the body weight is centered.
    • Use one hand after the other to grasp the walker.
2.
  a. The nurse should encourage the client to perform exercises that will help strengthen the upper arms. Examples include flexing and extending the arms and wrists, raising and

lowering weights with the hands, squeezing a ball or spring grip, and performing modified hand push-ups in bed.

b. The nurse should assist the client to perform push-ups at least three or four times a day. They can teach the client modified push-ups in several ways depending on the client's age and condition. While sitting in bed, a client may lift the hips off the bed by pushing down on the mattress with the hands. The nurse could place a block or books on the bed under the client's hands. The client should perform push-ups while lying on the abdomen in the following sequence:
- Flex the elbows.
- Place the hands, palms down, at approximately shoulder level.
- Straighten the elbows to lift the head and chest off the bed.

Activity M

There are no definite answers to this activity. Students may choose to discuss their thoughts with peers or instructors.

SECTION VI: GETTING READY FOR NCLEX

Activity N

1. **Answer: c**
   RATIONALE: The client should hold both crutches on the right side, which is the weaker side, and use the left hand to grip the handrail on the left side for additional support. The client should use the arm on the stronger side to grip the handrail. The client should step up by raising the left leg first followed by the right leg, not the right leg followed by the left leg. The stronger muscles should bear the weight, with both legs brought to the same stair.

2. **Answer: d**
   RATIONALE: The nurse should measure from the wrist to the floor to determine the appropriate length of the cane. The nurse should instruct the client to stand erect in shoes that they normally wear when ambulating, not lean forward when standing barefoot with a support. The length of the cane should be adjusted to provide 30-degree elbow flexion with the hand on the grip, not 40-degree.

CHAPTER 27

SECTION I: ASSESSING YOUR UNDERSTANDING

Activity A

1. Inpatient
2. Outpatient
3. Autologous
4. Laser

5. Microabrasions
6. Distended
7. Plume
8. Psychosocial
9. Checklist
10. Reversal

Activity B

1. The figure shows a client performing leg exercises (A) and foot exercises (B).
2. Surgical clients are predisposed to thrombus because they have reduced circulatory volume as a result of preoperative restriction of food and fluids, and blood loss during surgery. Blood tends to pool in the lower extremities of these clients because of their stationary position during surgery and the clients' reluctance to move afterward. With the use of leg exercises, efforts to reduce circulatory complications begin as soon as the client recovers from anesthesia. The effects of strong medication are not related to thrombus. Antiembolism stockings help to prevent thrombi and emboli by compressing superficial veins and capillaries.

Activity C

1. e   2. a   3. d   4. b   5. c

Activity D

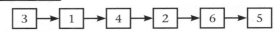

3 → 1 → 4 → 2 → 6 → 5

Activity E

1. The nurse should assess a client's support system before discharge because, if the client cannot manage their postoperative care independently or with the assistance of a supportive family or friends, options relative to extended or skilled nursing care should be explored and discussed. Options for skilled nursing or rehabilitation services may be available for home settings.
2. Nurses should assess the condition of the wound and the characteristics of drainage at least once each shift. They should reinforce or change dressings if they become loose or saturated. Eventually, sutures or staples are removed. Most hospitalized clients are discharged within 3 to 5 days of surgery to continue their recuperation at home.
3. The preoperative period starts when clients, or their families in an emergency, learn that surgery is necessary and ends when clients are transported to the operating room. One major factor affecting the length of the preoperative period is the urgency with which the surgery must be performed.
4. Plume is a substance composed of vaporized tissue, carbon dioxide, and water that may contain intact cells that are released during laser surgery. Plume is accompanied by smoke, an offensive odor, and, for some, burning and itching eyes.
5. If an adult client is under the influence of a mind-altering drug such as a narcotic or is alcohol

intoxicated, obtaining consent must be delayed until the drug has been metabolized. However, in a life-threatening emergency, a court may waive the need to obtain written or verbal consent from a client who requires immediate surgery based on substituted judgment—that is, if the court believes that if the client had the capacity to consent, they would have done so.

6. The nurse should instruct the client preoperatively to leave valuables at home. If the client forgets or does not follow this instruction, they must entrust valuables to a family member. Otherwise, health care agency personnel itemize the valuables, place them in an envelope, and lock them in a designated area. The client signs a receipt and the nurse notes the items' whereabouts in the client's medical record.

SECTION II: APPLYING YOUR KNOWLEDGE

Activity F

1. The nurse can ensure that the client has a clean bowel before the surgery by administering a prescribed enema or a laxative to the client the evening before the surgery. This procedure may be repeated in the morning. If bowel surgery is scheduled, antibiotics may be prescribed to destroy intestinal microorganisms.

2. A clean bowel is important during pelvic surgery because it allows for improved visualization of the surgical site and prevents trauma to the intestine or accidental contamination of the abdominal cavity with feces.

SECTION III: PRACTICING FOR NCLEX

Activity G

1. **Answer: b**
   RATIONALE: Surgery for the removal of a superficial cyst is classified as elective surgery because the surgery is planned at the client's convenience. Failure to remove the cyst will not lead to a catastrophe. It is not classified as optional surgery because this type of surgery is performed at the client's request. Urgent surgery is necessary and done within 1 or 2 days. Emergency surgery is required immediately for survival.

2. **Answer: d**
   RATIONALE: A breast biopsy comes under "diagnostic surgery" because the surgeon removes and studies the tissue to make a diagnosis. Exploratory surgery is performed for more extensive means to diagnose a problem, such as the exploration of unexplained pain in the abdomen. A curative surgery is performed to remove defective tissue to restore function. Cosmetic surgery is performed to correct defects or improve the appearance of a person. Palliative surgery, not a biopsy, is done for the enhancement of function without cure.

3. **Answers: a, c, e**
   RATIONALE: The client remains in the outpatient surgical suite for a brief time and is discharged by mid-afternoon or early evening when the client is awake and alert, vital signs are stable, pain and nausea are controlled, oral fluids are retained, the client voids a sufficient quantity of urine, and the client has received discharge instructions. The client is not discharged when they are just out of anesthesia, and being able to walk independently is not a criterion for discharge.

4. **Answer: d**
   RATIONALE: When applying antiembolism stockings to a client, the nurse should turn the stockings inside out before applying because it facilitates threading the stocking over the foot and leg. The nurse should avoid massaging the legs to prevent dislodging a thrombus if one is present. The client's legs should be elevated, not lowered, for at least 15 minutes before applying the stockings to promote venous circulation. Removing the stockings twice a day and then reapplying them allows for assessment and hygiene.

5. **Answer: a**
   RATIONALE: To be a directed donor, the person must be at least 17 years of age. Having a hematocrit level within safe range is a criterion for autologous donation, not directed donation. The person must donate blood 3 to 20 days before the anticipated date of use, and the donor should not have received a blood transfusion within the past 6 months.

6. **Answers: a, b, d**
   RATIONALE: The nurse can suggest forced coughing for clients with moist lung sounds, thick sputum, and abdominal or chest incisions. Clients with chronic pain and severe muscle spasms may not always be suitable for forced coughing because it can be very painful for them.

7. **Answer: a**
   RATIONALE: A preoperative checklist is a form that identifies the status of essential presurgical activities and is completed before surgery. It does not identify the type of surgery required to be performed on the client, nor does it prepare the client spiritually, emotionally, and physically before the surgery. The preoperative checklist does not allow the nurse to monitor for complications. Frequent assessment after the operation allows the nurse to monitor the client for complications.

8. **Answer: a**
   RATIONALE: The intraoperative period involves transporting the client to a receiving room and then onto the operating room. Assessing whether the client has developed any allergies is done when the nurse is completing the preoperative checklist. Psychosocial preparation of the client is done before surgery, but it is not part of the intraoperative period. The nurse checks for completion of the client's skin preparation during the preoperative period, not during the intraoperative period.

9. **Answer: b**
   RATIONALE: Improper documentation of a client's history and physical examination is the main factor responsible for an incomplete preoperative checklist. Unavailability of surgical equipment, agency policy, and the availability of an anesthesiologist are not factors a nurse checks using the preoperative checklist. The nurse does need to check whether the client has removed their dentures during this process.

10. **Answers: a, b, d**
    RATIONALE: Laser surgery is used as an alternative to many previously conventional surgical techniques such as reattaching the retina, removing skin tattoos, and revascularizing ischemic heart muscle. However, it is not used to replace decayed teeth or adjust dislocated bones. Decayed teeth are usually replaced with artificial teeth or dentures, whereas dislocated bones are fixed through mechanical immobilization.

11. **Answer: d**
    RATIONALE: The major advantage of regional anesthesia is the decreased risk of respiratory, cardiac, and gastrointestinal complications. Regional anesthesia does not increase but decreases mobility to the specific anesthetized area, and the client does not lose consciousness. Team members must monitor the client for signs of allergic reactions, changes in vital signs, and toxic reactions. In addition, they must protect the anesthetized area while sensation is absent because the client is at risk of injury.

12. **Answer: c**
    RATIONALE: The nurse should immediately tilt the client's head and lift the chin or insert an artificial airway for a client who has developed a complication of airway occlusion. A client is placed in the Trendelenburg position when in shock. A nasogastric tube is inserted inside the client and then connected to suction if there is lack of motility, not if there is airway occlusion. A client is administered prescribed intravenous fluid if they have developed complications of hemorrhage.

13. **Answer: b**
    RATIONALE: The nurse should palpate the pedal pulses to validate if arterial blood flow to the foot is present and strong. The nurse should help the client to a position of comfort (such as supine or low Fowler's) to foster rest and relaxation instead of a lateral position, which could affect the client's breathing. The air pump should be secured at the bottom of the bed to ensure protection from damage and to prevent injury to the client. The nurse should check that the air tubes are untwisted and not compressed under the client or the wheels of the bed to ensure the unobstructed delivery of air.

14. **Answer: c**
    RATIONALE: The nurse should provide discharge instruction to the client as to how they should take care of the incision site. Identification of purulent

drainage and their characteristics, level of pain, need for analgesia, as well as ensuring client airways are initial postoperative assessments checked by the nurse systematically, not by the client.

15. **Answers: a, d, e**
    RATIONALE: Before administering preoperative medications, the nurse should check the client's ID bracelet, ask about drug allergies, obtain vital signs, ask the client to void, and ensure that the surgical consent form has been signed. Allaying the client's fears and explaining the process of the surgery are interventions related to preparing the client emotionally and spiritually for the surgery.

16. **Answer: c**
    RATIONALE: Many older adults may be on anticoagulation therapy, including self-therapy with low-dose aspirin, which has to be addressed as an important preoperative consideration. Senior clients are susceptible to urinary tract infection and allergies, but these are not part of preoperative considerations. Wound healing in senior clients may occur more slowly because of age-related skin changes and impaired circulation and oxygenation.

17. **Answers: b, c, d**
    RATIONALE: Laser technology requires unique safety precautions. In some cases, prescription glasses with side shields are allowed, but not contact lenses. Because lasers produce heat, fire and electrical safety are paramount. Volatile substances such as alcohol and acetone are not used around lasers because of their flammability. Surgical instruments are coated black to avoid absorbing scattered light that causes them to heat. Sometimes the client's teeth are covered with plastic or a rubber mouth guard to shield metal fillings. For the same reason, no jewelry is allowed.

18. **Answer: b**
    RATIONALE: As part of presurgical skin preparation, the nurse should use electric hair clippers to remove hair from the designated area to prevent microabrasions caused by razor blades. Depilatory agents are used around bony prominences like the knuckles or ankles, where razors are ineffective. The nurse should apply a moisturizer to the skin but dry it thoroughly so that moisture is eliminated. Because the nurse is performing presurgical skin preparation, the skin needs to be assessed for lesions, not the hair.

SECTION IV: REVIEWING WHAT YOU HAVE LEARNED

Activity H
1. Thrombus
2. Curative

Activity I
1. True
2. True

Activity J

1. Anesthesiologist
2. Directed donors

Activity K

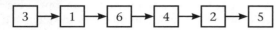

3 → 1 → 6 → 4 → 2 → 5

Activity L

1. A pneumatic compression device promotes circulation of venous blood and relocation of excess fluid into the lymphatic vessels. The device consists of an extremity sleeve with tubes that connect to an electrical air pump. The sleeved extremity can be compressed either intermittently or sequentially from distal to proximal areas. The pumps may cycle one to four times per minute.
2. Three methods of preparing the skin for surgery are to (1) cleanse the particular area with soap for several days before surgery; (2) shave the area before surgery if hair is likely to interfere with the incision; and (3) use electric clippers for hair removal, which is generally preferable to shaving.

SECTION V: APPLYING YOUR KNOWLEDGE

Activity M

1. Volatile substances are highly flammable, and lasers produce heat. The combination could result in a fire.
2. Reduced circulatory volume results from preoperative restrictions of food and fluids and blood loss during surgery.

Activity N

1.
   a. Risk factors that increase the likelihood of perioperative complications are dehydration, malnutrition, obesity, smoking, diabetes, cardiopulmonary disease, drug and alcohol abuse, bleeding tendencies, low hemoglobin and red cells, and pregnancy.
2.
   a. General preoperative information includes preoperative medications—when they are given and their effects; postoperative pain control; explanation and description of the postanesthesia recovery room or postsurgical area; discussion of the frequency of assessing vital signs and use of monitoring equipment; and explanation and demonstration of deep breathing, coughing, and leg exercises.
   b. Depending on the time of admission, physical preparations may include skin preparation, attention to elimination, restriction of food and fluids, care of valuables, donning of surgical attire, and disposition of prostheses.

Activity O

There are no definite answers to this activity. Students may choose to discuss their thoughts with peers or instructors.

SECTION VI: GETTING READY FOR NCLEX

Activity P

1. **Answer: a**
   RATIONALE: Deep breathing reduces the postoperative risk for respiratory complications such as atelectasis (airless, collapsed lung areas) and pneumonia (lung infection), both of which can lead to hypoxemia. Coughing, not deep breathing, is a natural method for clearing secretions from the airways. Deep breathing does not ease postoperative pain and discomfort or decrease the risk for circulatory complications. Leg exercises reduce the risk for circulatory complications.
2. **Answers: b, d, e**
   RATIONALE: The period of fluid restriction before surgery may be shortened for older adults to reduce their risk for dehydration and hypotension. The nurse should assess the client's vital signs, weight, and skin turgor before fluid restriction to establish a baseline for comparison.

CHAPTER 28

SECTION I: ASSESSING YOUR UNDERSTANDING

Activity A

1. Wound
2. Inflammation
3. Phagocytosis
4. Proliferation
5. Remodeling
6. Enzymatic
7. Transparent
8. Drains
9. Sutures
10. Binder

Activity B

1. The image is that of a transparent dressing.
2. The chief advantage of a transparent dressing is that it allows the nurse to assess a wound without removing the dressing. In addition, it is less bulky than gauze dressings and does not require tape because it consists of a single sheet of adhesive material. It commonly is used to cover peripheral and central intravenous insertion sites.

Activity C

1. c   **2.** a   **3.** d   **4.** e   **5.** b

Activity D

3 → 1 → 4 → 2

Activity E

1. Inflammation is the physiologic defense, immediately after tissue injury, which lasts for

approximately 2 to 5 days. The purpose of inflammation is to:
- Limit the local damage
- Remove injured cells and debris
- Prepare the wound for healing

2. Generally, the integrity of skin and damaged tissue is restored by:
- Resolution, a process by which damaged cells recover and reestablish their normal function.
- Regeneration or cell duplication
- Scar formation, which is the replacement of damaged cells with fibrous scar tissue. Fibrous scar tissue acts as a nonfunctioning patch. The extent of scar tissue that forms depends on the magnitude of tissue damage and the manner of wound healing.

3. Several factors that affect wound healing include
- Type of wound injury
- Expanse or depth of wound
- Quality of circulation
- Amount of wound debris
- Presence of infection
- Status of the client's health

4. The key to wound healing is adequate blood flow to the injured tissue. Factors that may interfere include compromised circulation; infection; and purulent, bloody, or serous fluid accumulation that prevents skin and tissue approximation. In addition, excessive tension and pulling on wound edges contribute to wound disruption and delay in healing. One or several of these factors may be secondary to poor nutrition or impaired inflammatory or immune responses secondary to drugs like corticosteroids and obesity.

5. Two potential surgical wound complications include dehiscence (the separation of wound edges) and evisceration (wound separation with protrusion of organs). These complications are most likely to occur within 7 to 10 days after surgery. They may be caused by an insufficient dietary intake of protein and sources of vitamin C; premature removal of sutures or staples; unusual strain on the incision from severe coughing, sneezing, vomiting, dry heaves, or hiccupping; weak tissue or muscular support secondary to obesity; distension of the abdomen from accumulated intestinal gas; or compromised tissue integrity from previous surgical procedures in the same area.

6. A dressing or a cover over a wound is used to
- Keep the wound clean
- Absorb drainage
- Control bleeding
- Protect the wound from further injury
- Hold medication in place
- Maintain a moist environment

SECTION II: APPLYING YOUR KNOWLEDGE

Activity F

1. The nurse applies the cold compress to reduce the temperature of the client.

2. Before applying the compress, the nurse soaks it in tap water or medicated solution at the appropriate temperature and then wrings out excess moisture. To maintain the moisture and temperature, a piece of plastic or plastic wrap is used to cover the compress, and the area is secured in a towel. As the compress material cools or warms outside the range of the intended temperature, the nurse removes it and reapplies it if necessary.

SECTION III: PRACTICING FOR NCLEX

Activity G

1. **Answer: a**
RATIONALE: The nurse should document the wound as an incision wound because it is a clean separation of skin and tissue with smooth, even edges. An abrasion is a wound in which the surface layers of the skin are scraped away. A laceration is a separation of skin and tissue in which the edges are torn and irregular. An ulceration is a shallow crater in which skin or mucous membrane is missing.

2. **Answer: d**
RATIONALE: An ulceration is a shallow crater in which skin or mucous membrane is missing. An incision wound can be described as a clean separation of skin and tissue with smooth, even edges. A laceration is described as a separation of skin and tissue in which the edges are torn and irregular. An abrasion is a wound in which the surface layers of the skin are scraped away.

3. **Answer: a**
RATIONALE: When caring for a client with an open wound, the nurse can describe the inflammation stage of the wound repair process as the physiologic defense immediately after tissue injury. Proliferation is a period during which new cells fill and seal the wound. Proliferation follows the inflammation phase. Resolution is the process by which damaged cells recover and reestablish their normal function; it is part of the proliferation phase. Remodeling, which follows the proliferation phase, is the period during which the wound undergoes changes and maturation. This phase follows the proliferation phase.

4. **Answer: d**
RATIONALE: During the first stage of inflammation, local changes occur. The blood vessels constrict to control blood loss and confine damage. This is followed by the migration of leukocytes and macrophages to the site of injury, after which the body produces more and more white blood cells to take their place. Increased white blood cells, particularly neutrophils and monocytes, suggest an inflammatory and, in some cases, infectious process.

5. **Answer: b**
RATIONALE: In second-intention healing, the wound edges are widely separated, leading to a more time-consuming and complex reparative process. First-intention healing, also called healing

by primary intention, is a reparative process during which the wound edges are directly next to each other. With third-intention healing, the wound edges are widely separated and are later brought together with some type of closure material. However, edges that are close to each other do not require closure material.

6. **Answer: b**
RATIONALE: The nurse should understand that the client is in stage II of pressure ulcer development. A stage II pressure ulcer is red and is accompanied by blistering or a skin tear. Stage I is characterized by intact but reddened skin that remains red and fails to resume its normal color when pressure is relieved. A stage III pressure ulcer has a shallow skin crater that extends to the subcutaneous tissue. It may be accompanied by serous or purulent drainage caused by a wound infection. Stage IV of a pressure ulcer is characterized by deeply ulcerated tissue exposing the muscles and bones.

7. **Answer: a**
RATIONALE: The nurse should understand that factors such as depression, poor appetite, cognitive impairment, and physical or economic barriers that interfere with adequate nutrition in older adults may impair wound healing. Age-related changes like diminished collagen and blood supply affect wound healing. Decreased subcutaneous tissue could result in increased susceptibility to pressure ulcers and shear-type injuries in older adults.

8. **Answer: a**
RATIONALE: The nurse should use gauze to care for the scraped knee. Gauze dressings are made of woven cloth fibers that are highly absorbent, making them ideal for covering fresh wounds that are likely to bleed or wounds that exude drainage. A transparent dressing allows the nurse to assess a wound without removing the dressing. Hydrocolloid dressings such as DuoDERM are self-adhesive, opaque, air- and water-occlusive wound coverings. Hydrocolloid dressings help keep the wounds moist. A bandage is a strip or roll of cloth wrapped around a body part to help support the area around the wound.

9. **Answer: b**
RATIONALE: A transparent dressing allows the nurse to assess the wound (in this case, the intravenous catheter site) without removing the dressing. In addition, it is less bulky than gauze dressings and does not require tape because it consists of a single sheet of adhesive material. A hydrocolloid dressing is an opaque, air- and water-occlusive wound covering that keeps the wound moist, which promotes wound healing. Gauze is ideal for treating fresh wounds that are likely to bleed.

10. **Answer: a**
RATIONALE: When caring for a wound with a closed drain, the nurse cleans the insertion site in a circular manner. After cleaning, the nurse places a precut drain sponge or gauze, which is open to its

center, around the base of the drain. In case of an open drain, a safety pin or a long clip is attached to the drain as it extends from the wound; this prevents the drain from slipping in the tissue. To shorten an open drain, the nurse pulls it from the wound for the specified length. The nurse then repositions the safety pin or clip near the wound to prevent the drain from sliding back internally within the wound.

11. **Answer: c**
RATIONALE: The nurse should use a Steri-Strip to close the superficial laceration. Adhesive Steri-Strips, also known as butterflies because of their winged appearance, can hold a weak incision together temporarily. Sometimes Steri-Strips are used instead of sutures or staples to close superficial lacerations. A hydrocolloid dressing is an opaque, air- and water-occlusive wound covering that keeps the wound moist, which promotes wound healing. Gauze is ideal for treating fresh wounds that are likely to bleed. A bandage is a strip or roll of cloth wrapped around a body part.

12. **Answer: a**
RATIONALE: The nurse should use a spiral turn to wrap the sprained arm of the client. A spiral turn partly overlaps a previous turn. The amount of overlapping varies from one-half to three-fourths of the width of the bandage. Spiral turns are used when wrapping cylindrical parts of the body, such as the arms and legs. A figure-of-eight turn is best when bandaging a joint such as the elbow or knee. A spica turn is a variation of the figure-of-eight pattern. It differs in that the wrap includes a portion of the trunk or chest. A recurrent turn is especially beneficial when wrapping the head or the stump of an amputated limb.

13. **Answer: c**
RATIONALE: The nurse could use the spica turn technique to bandage a client's chest. A spica turn is a variation of the figure-of-eight pattern. It differs in that the wrap includes a portion of the trunk or chest. A figure-of-eight turn is best when bandaging a joint such as the elbow or knee. Spiral turns are used when wrapping cylindrical parts of the body such as the arms and legs.

14. **Answer: a**
RATIONALE: The nurse uses the sharp debridement technique to promote healing in clients with extensive necrotic tissue from the healthy area of the wound with sterile scissors, forceps, or other instruments. This method is preferred if the wound is infected because it helps quick and proper healing. The procedure is done at the bedside or in the operating room if the wound is extensive. Enzymatic debridement is appropriate for uninfected wounds or for clients who cannot tolerate sharp debridement. Autolytic debridement, or self-dissolution, is a painless, natural physiologic process that allows the body's enzymes to soften, liquefy, and release devitalized tissue.

15. Answer: a

RATIONALE: Before performing ear irrigation on the client with a foreign body lodged in their ear, the nurse should conduct a gross inspection of the client's ear because the foreign body may be a bean, pea, or other dehydrated substance that may swell when irrigated, causing it to become even more tightly fixed. Ear irrigation removes debris from the ear. Ear irrigation is contraindicated if the tympanic membrane is perforated. When performing ear irrigation, the nurse should avoid occluding the ear canal with the tip of the syringe because the pressure of the trapped solution could rupture the eardrum. After the irrigation, the nurse places a cotton ball loosely within the ear to absorb drainage but not to obstruct its flow.

16. Answer: d

RATIONALE: Diminished immune response from reduced T-lymphocyte cells predisposes older adults to wound infection. Age-related changes like the thinning dermal layer of skin and decreased subcutaneous tissue result in increased susceptibility to pressure ulcers and shear-type injuries in older adults. Diabetes or other conditions that may interfere with circulation increase the older adult's susceptibility to delayed wound healing and wound infections.

SECTION IV: REVIEWING WHAT YOU HAVE LEARNED

Activity H

1. Leukocytosis
2. Hydrocolloid

Activity I

1. True
2. False. Inflammation, the physiologic defense occurring immediately after tissue injury, lasts approximately 2 to 5 days.

Activity J

1. Proliferation
2. Resolution
3. Douching

Activity K

1. b
2. e
3. d
4. a
5. c

Activity L

In *first-intention healing* (healing by *primary intention*), the wound edges are directly next to each other. In *second-intention healing*, the wound edges are widely separated, leading to a more time-consuming and complex reparative process. In *third-intention healing*, the wound edges are widely separated and must be brought together with some type of closure material. This reparative process results in a broad, deep scar.

SECTION V: APPLYING YOUR KNOWLEDGE

Activity M

1. Transparent dressings do not require layers of gauze or tape; they consist of a single sheet of adhesive material.
2. Moist wounds heal more quickly because new cells grow more rapidly in a wet environment.

Activity N

1.
   a. The nurse performs ear irrigation as under:
   - Performing a gross inspection of the ear if a foreign body is suspected because a bean, pea, or other dehydrated substance can swell if the ear is irrigated, causing it to become even more tightly fixed
   - Removing solid objects with an instrument if they are not deep within the ear
   - Directing the solution toward the roof of the auditory canal
   - Not occluding the ear canal with the tip of the syringe because the pressure of the trapped solution could rupture the eardrum
   b. Placing a cotton ball loosely within the ear after the irrigation—the nurse should place a cotton ball loosely within the ear to absorb drainage without obstructing its flow

2.
   - Use a circular turn to anchor and secure the bandage where it starts and ends. This step simply involves holding the free end of the rolled material in one hand and wrapping it around the area, bringing it back to the starting point.
   - A spiral turn partially overlaps a previous turn. The amount of overlapping varies from one-half to three-fourths of the width of the bandage. Use spiral turns when wrapping cylindrical parts of the body such as the arms and legs.
   - A spiral-reverse turn is a modification of a spiral turn. The roll is reversed or turned downward halfway through the turn.
   - A figure-of-eight turn is best when bandaging a joint such as the elbow or knee and consists of making oblique turns that alternately ascend and descend, simulating the number eight.
   - A spica turn is a variation of the figure-of-eight pattern. It differs in that the wrap includes a portion of the trunk or chest.
   - A recurrent turn is made by passing the roll back and forth over the tip of a body part. Once several recurrent turns are made, the bandage is anchored by completing the application with another basic turn such as the figure-of-eight. A recurrent turn is especially beneficial when wrapping the stump of an amputated limb or the head.

SECTION VI: GETTING READY FOR NCLEX

Activity O

1. Answer: d
   RATIONALE: Cold application numbs the sensation of pain and prevents swelling. Hot applications, not cold applications, speed healing, relieve muscle spasm, and promote circulation.

CHAPTER 29

SECTION I: ASSESSING YOUR UNDERSTANDING

Activity A

1. Gastrostomy
2. Sump
3. Esophagus
4. Nasointestinal
5. Tungsten
6. Orogastric
7. Lumen
8. Endoscope
9. Bolus
10. Intubation

Activity B

1. The figure shows the method of obtaining the NEX measurement.
2. Before inserting a tube, a nurse should obtain the client's NEX measurement (the length from the nose-to-the-earlobe-to-the-xiphoid process) and mark the tube appropriately. The first mark on the tube is made at the measured distance from the nose to the earlobe. It indicates the distance to the nasal pharynx, a location that places the tip at the back of the throat but above where the gag reflex is stimulated. A second mark is made at the point where the tube reaches the xiphoid process, indicating the depth required to reach the stomach.

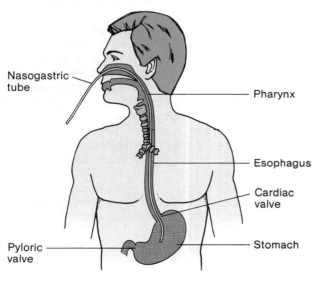

Nasogastric tube
Pharynx
Esophagus
Cardiac valve
Pyloric valve
Stomach

3. The figure shows the nasogastric intubation pathway.
4. Because nasogastric tubes remain in place for several days, clients complain of discomfort in the nose and throat. If the tube's diameter is too large or pressure from the tube is prolonged, tissue irritation or breakdown may occur. Furthermore, gastric tubes tend to dilate the esophageal sphincter, a circular muscle between the esophagus and the stomach. The stretched opening may contribute to gastric reflux, especially when the tube is used to administer liquid formula. If gastric reflux occurs, the liquid could enter the airway and interfere with respiratory function.

Activity C

1. b   **2.** c   **3.** d   **4.** a   **5.** e

Activity D

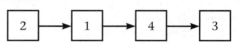

2 → 1 → 4 → 3

Activity E

1. Intubation basically means the placement of a tube into a body structure. Intubation is performed on a client to remove gas or fluids, or to administer liquid nourishment.
2. Narrow tubes tend to curl during insertion because they are very flexible. Therefore, some are supplied with a stylet that helps to straighten and support it during insertion. Almost all have a weighted tip that helps the tube to descend past the stomach. Checking the placement of the distal end is more difficult; these tubes also become obstructed more easily.
3. Usually, nurses insert nasogastric tubes. Additional nursing responsibilities include keeping the tube patent or unobstructed, implementing the prescribed use, and removing the tube when it has accomplished its therapeutic purpose.
4. Tube feedings are used when clients have an intact stomach or intestinal function but are unconscious, have undergone extensive mouth surgery, have difficulty swallowing, or have esophageal or gastric disorders.
5. A bolus feeding is the least desirable because it distends the stomach rapidly, causing gastric discomfort and increased risk of reflux. Some clients experience discomfort from the rapid delivery of this quantity of fluid. Clients who are unconscious or who have delayed gastric emptying are at a greater risk of regurgitation, vomiting, and aspiration with this method of administration.
6. In home and long-term care settings, registered dietitians may be helpful in the ongoing assessment of tube feedings. For older adults living on a fixed income, dietitians can suggest ways to prepare less costly, home-blended formulas that meet the client's nutritional needs.

SECTION II: APPLYING YOUR KNOWLEDGE

Activity F

1. If a senior client has developed hyperglycemia, the nurse should instill diluted formula and gradually increase the concentration. Most tube-feeding formulas are highly concentrated; therefore, the hydration status of the older client must be closely monitored. If a senior client is receiving tube feedings with full-strength formula concentrations, it is important to check capillary blood glucose at intervals until the client's results are within normal range.

2. Tube-feeding formulas may vary based on the older client's condition. Several lactose-free tube-feeding formulas on the market today may be beneficial to senior clients who experience malabsorption syndromes. Clients at risk for pressure sores benefit from formulas fortified with zinc, protein, and other nutrients.

SECTION III: PRACTICING FOR NCLEX

Activity G

1. **Answer: a**
   RATIONALE: Intermittent feeding involves the gradual instillation of liquid nourishment four to six times a day, whereas a bolus feeding involves the instillation of liquid nourishment four to six times a day in less than 30 minutes. A cyclic feeding is the continuous instillation of liquid nourishment for 8 to 12 hours, and a continuous feeding schedule is the instillation of liquid nutrition without interruption.

2. **Answer: d**
   RATIONALE: The nurse should ask the client to exhale when each nostril, in turn, is occluded. The nurse should ask the client to clear nasal debris by blowing into a paper tissue. Presurgical skin preparation is not done to the nose before the insertion of a nasointestinal tube. Asking the client to perform nebulization is not correct because that is done when the client is having respiratory problems. The nurse inspects each nostril for size, shape, and patency only after the client has finished clearing nasal debris by blowing into a paper tissue.

3. **Answer: c**
   RATIONALE: Ambulation helps the tube move through the pyloric valve into the small intestine. Moving the client into the Fowler position for 2 hours on both sides promotes movement through intestinal curves. Observing the graduated marks on the tube enables monitoring of the tube's progression and approximate anatomic location. A radiograph is obtained when the tube has reached the prescribed distance.

4. **Answer: b**
   RATIONALE: The first step that a nurse should do when removing an intestinal decompression tube is to disconnect the tube from the suction source. Next, the tape that secures the tube to the face is removed, and the tube is withdrawn 6 to 10 inches at 10-minute intervals. When the last 18 inches remains, the tube is pulled gently from the nose. A radiograph is obtained to verify the correct placement when it is being inserted in the client, not when it is being removed.

5. **Answer: c**
   RATIONALE: The main goal of preintubation assessment is to determine which nostril is most suitable for inserting the tube. Determining whether there is any nausea and vomiting; the ability to swallow, cough, and gag; or even checking the level of consciousness are different contributing factors of preintubation assessment, not the main goal.

6. **Answer: a**
   RATIONALE: Gastric sump tubes are used exclusively for removing fluid and gas from the stomach. Nasointestinal tubes, not gastric sump tubes, are used to provide nourishment and to remove gas and liquid contents from the small intestine. Intestinal decompression tubes, not the gastric sump tube, reduce trauma to intestinal tissue.

7. **Answer: c**
   RATIONALE: In cyclic feeding, tube feeding is given to clients during the late evening because, during the day, clients eat some food orally. As oral intake increases, the volume and duration of the tube feeding gradually are decreased. Hence, tube feeding the client in the afternoon, early morning, or just after lunch is not a good idea. Cyclic feeding is used to wean clients from tube feedings yet continuing to maintain adequate nutrition.

8. **Answer: d**
   RATIONALE: As a rule of thumb, the gastric residual should be no more than 100 mL or no more than 20% of the previous hour's tube-feeding volume. If the gastric residual is more than 100 mL, overfilling the stomach can cause gastric reflux, regurgitation, vomiting, aspiration, and pneumonia.

9. **Answers: a, b, c**
   RATIONALE: Enteral nutrition is provided via the stomach or small intestine rather than by the oral route by a liquid tube-feeding formula. Although a nasogastric tube can be used, it is more likely that liquid formula will be administered through a nasointestinal or a transabdominal tube, which is longer in length and smaller in diameter.

10. **Answer: b**
    RATIONALE: Before demonstrating the procedure, the nurse should provide detailed written instructions that include the names of the medicine and formula, and names and contact numbers in case of an emergency, among other things. In addition, depending on the client's self-confidence and competence in self-administering tube feedings, health care providers often make a referral to a home health agency for postdischarge nursing support.

11. Answer: a
  RATIONALE: To monitor the tube's progression and approximate anatomic location, the nurse should observe the graduated marks on the tube. Following the markings on the tube before inserting manually will not provide the tube's anatomic location. Never reinsert the stylet when the tube is in the client because reinsertion might cause trauma to the client and damage to the tube. Ambulation helps the tube to move through the pyloric valve into the small intestine.

12. Answer: c
  RATIONALE: To maintain patency, it is best to flush feeding tubes with 30 to 60 mL water immediately before and after administering a feeding or medications, every 4 hours if the client is being continuously fed, and after refeeding the gastric residual. Giving ice chips or occasional sips of water to a client who is otherwise not taking food orally promotes tube patency. However, it must be given sparingly because water is hypotonic and draws electrolytes into the gastric fluid. Cranberry juice and carbonated beverages are used as flushing solutions, although water is best. Formula tends to curdle when it comes in contact with cranberry juice, which detracts from the efficacy of this approach.

13. Answer: b
  RATIONALE: A bolus feeding schedule is the least desirable because it distends the stomach rapidly, causing gastric discomfort and the increased risk of reflux. Intermittent feedings fill the stomach gradually, at a slower rate, thereby reducing the bloated feeling. A cyclic feeding is used to wean the client from tube feedings. A continuous feeding is administered at a rate of approximately 1.5 mL/minute. Continuous feeding creates some inconvenience because the pump must go wherever the client goes.

14. Answers: a, c, e
  RATIONALE: The main causes of gastrostomy leaks are a clamped gastrointestinal tube when the feed is infusing, disconnection between the feeding tube and the gastrointestinal tube, and underinflation of the balloon beneath the skin. When a client is administered with tube-feeding formula, the pressure on the abdomen is increased, not reduced, which could lead to gastrostomy leaks. Instillation of highly concentrated nutritional formula does not cause gastrostomy leaks, but leads to hydration.

15. Answer: d
  RATIONALE: Because the client is complaining of a vomiting feeling, and the nurse has confirmed that the client's bowel sounds are less than five per minute, the nurse should identify it as risk for aspiration. The client is not discharged or eating independently, so self-care deficit is not applicable. The client does not have any problem with the

prescribed nutrition formula or swallowing it, so a nursing diagnosis for imbalanced nutrition and impaired swallowing would be incorrect.

16. Answer: c
  RATIONALE: To prevent air from entering the tube, the nurse pinches the feeding tube just as the last volume of water is administered. To prevent leaking, the nurse should clamp or unplug the feeding tube. To provide access to formula, the nurse should connect the tubing to a nasogastric or nasoenteral tube. The gradual opening of the clamp on the tubing helps to purge air from the tube.

17. Answer: a
  RATIONALE: To reduce middle ear inflammation, the nurse should insert a small-diameter feeding tube. Middle ear inflammation is caused by the narrowing or obstruction of the eustachian tube from the presence of a tube in the pharynx. The nurse provides nasal and oral hygiene when the client's oral and nasal mucous membranes are dry. The client's neck is maintained in a neutral position when there is a plugged feeding tube resulting from a kinked tube. Tubing is filled with water when there is air in the stomach, and the client complains of nausea and vomiting.

SECTION IV: REVIEWING WHAT YOU HAVE LEARNED

Activity H
1. Gavage
2. Nasointestinal

Activity I
1. True.
2. False. Enteral nutrition is nourishment provided via the stomach or small intestine.

Activity J
1. NEX measurement

Activity K
1. c
2. a
3. b

Activity L
1. The figure shows the nasogastric intubation pathway from the nose into the stomach. See Figure 29-1 in your textbook.
2. There may be trauma to the nose during insertion. The tube may enter the airway instead of the stomach and cause respiratory distress. The client may vomit during the insertion and aspirate the vomitus into the airway. Clients may complain of nose and throat discomfort. Tissue irritation or breakdown may occur. Gastric tubes tend to dilate the lower esophageal (cardiac) sphincter, contributing to gastric reflux. If gastric reflux occurs, the

liquid could irritate the esophageal tissue; it also could enter the airway and interfere with respiratory function.

Activity M

1. Causes of gastrostomy leaks are as follows:
   - Disconnection between the feeding delivery tube and the G-tube
   - Clamped G-tube while tube feeding is infusing
   - Mismatch between the size of the G-tube and the stoma
   - Increased abdominal pressure from formula accumulation, retching, sneezing, or coughing
   - Underinflation of the balloon beneath the skin
   - Less-than-optimal stoma and stomal location
2. Gastric or intestinal tubes are used to provide nutrition; administer oral medications that the client cannot swallow; obtain a sample of secretions for diagnostic testing; remove substances, typically poisons, from the stomach; remove gas and liquid contents from the stomach or intestine; and control gastric bleeding.

SECTION V: APPLYING YOUR KNOWLEDGE

Activity N

Water is hypotonic and draws electrolytes into the gastric fluid, depleting serum electrolytes.

Activity O

1.
   a. The nurse provides a written instruction sheet that includes the following:
      - Places to obtain equipment and formula
      - The amount and schedule for each feeding and flush, using household measurements
      - Guidelines for delaying a feeding
      - Special instructions for skin, nose, or stomal care including frequency and types of products to use
      - Problems to report such as weight loss, reduced urination, weakness, diarrhea, nausea and vomiting, and breathing difficulties
      - Names and phone numbers of people to call if questions arise
      - Date, time, and place for continued medical follow-up
   b. Depending on the data collected during client care, the nurse may identify one or more of the following nursing diagnoses:
      - Imbalanced nutrition: less than body requirements
      - Self-care deficit: feeding
      - Impaired swallowing
      - Risk for aspiration
      - Impaired oral mucous membranes
      - Diarrhea
      - Constipation

2.
   - Assemble all necessary equipment.
   - Insert the tube nasally into the stomach.
   - Thread excess tubing through a sling of folded gauze taped to the forehead after confirming gastric placement.
   - Ambulate the client, if possible.
   - When the radiograph indicates that the intestinal tube has advanced beyond the stomach, change the client's position.
   - Observe the graduated marks on the tube.
   - Request X-ray confirmation that the tube has reached the prescribed distance.
   - Secure the tube to the nose after confirming its distal location.
   - Coil the excess tubing and attach it to the client's pajamas or gown.
   - Connect the proximal end to a wall or portable section source.

Activity P

There are no definite answers to this activity. Students may choose to discuss their thoughts with peers or instructors.

SECTION VI: GETTING READY FOR NCLEX

Activity Q

1. **Answers: a, b, d, e**
   RATIONALE: Aspiration clears the path above the obstructing debris. Instillation allows direct contact between the irrigating solution and the debris. Clamping the tube duration gives the substance in solution time to physically affect the obstructing debris. Measurement and documentation provide data for accurate intake and output. Reinstilling the aspirated fluid returns partially digested nutrients and electrolytes to the client, which is useful in checking gastric residual, which may reobstruct the tubing if it is reinstilled.
2. **Answers: a, b, c**
   RATIONALE: Highly concentrated formula, rapid administration, and bacterial contamination are the common causes of diarrhea in the client. Incorrect tube placement creates the potential for aspiration. Inadequate calorie intake contributes to unhealthy weight loss.
3. **Answer: b**
   RATIONALE: Older adults are at an increased risk for fluid and electrolyte disturbances; as a result, they may develop hyperglycemia when receiving tube feedings. Most tube-feeding formulas are highly concentrated; therefore, the client's hydration status must be closely monitored. Malabsorption syndromes, change in skin turgor, and elevation of body temperature are not signs of hyperglycemia in older adults receiving tube feedings.

CHAPTER 30

SECTION I: ASSESSING YOUR UNDERSTANDING
ACTIVITY A

1. Voided
2. Anuria
3. Oliguria
4. Dysuria
5. Catheterization
6. Straight
7. Continuous
8. Incontinence
9. External
10. Bedpan

Activity B

1. The figure shows major structures of the urinary system.
2. The urinary system consists of the kidneys, ureter, bladder, and urethra. These major components, along with some accessory structures such as the ring-shaped muscles called the internal and external sphincters, work together to produce urine, collect it, and excrete it from the body.

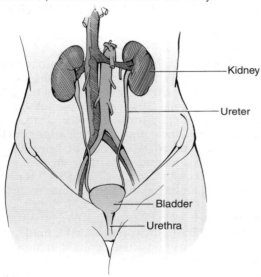

Kidney

Ureter

Bladder

Urethra

Activity C

1. d   **2.** a   **3.** e   **4.** b   **5.** c

Activity D

$$5 \rightarrow 3 \rightarrow 1 \rightarrow 4 \rightarrow 2$$

Activity E

1. The common disorders associated with polyuria include the following:
   - Diabetes mellitus—an endocrine disorder caused by insufficient insulin
   - Diabetes insipidus—an endocrine disease caused by insufficient antidiuretic hormone

2. A urinary catheter is used for various reasons:
   - To keep incontinent clients dry (catheterization is a last resort that is used only when all other continence measures have been exhausted)
   - To relieve bladder distention when clients cannot void
   - To assess fluid balance accurately
   - To keep the bladder from becoming distended during procedures such as surgery
   - To measure residual urine
   - To obtain sterile urine specimens
   - To instill medication within the bladder
3. Application of the catheter correctly and managing care appropriately can prevent potential problems that may accompany the use of a condom catheter, such as the following:
   - Restriction of blood flow to the skin and tissues of the penis, resulting from a tight sheath
   - Skin breakdown resulting from the accumulation of moisture beneath the sheath
   - Leakage
4. Older adults are likely to experience urinary urgency and frequency because of normal physiologic changes such as diminished bladder capacity and degenerative changes in the cerebral cortex.
5. Many resources are available to assist older adults in evaluating and treating incontinence, such as the following:
   - Health care facilities offer special incontinence clinics and physical therapy departments to teach pelvic muscle exercises.
   - The National Association for Continence (http://www.nafc.org) is an excellent source of information for products, resources, and continence programs.
   - Clients should be taught to compile a log of urinary elimination patterns.
   - Suggest that paralyzed clients with reflex incontinence use cutaneous triggering (lightly massaging or tapping the skin above the pubic area).
6. Oliguria indicates the inadequate elimination of urine. Sometimes oliguria is a sign that the bladder is being only partially emptied during voiding. Residual urine, or more than 50 mL urine that remains in the bladder after voiding, can support the growth of microorganisms, leading to infection. In addition, urinary stasis or lack of movement can cause dissolved substances such as calcium to precipitate, leading to urinary calculi (stones).

SECTION II: APPLYING YOUR KNOWLEDGE
Activity F

1. When a closed drainage system is used to collect urine from the catheter, the nurse should do the following:
   - Coil excess tubing on the bed, and keep the section from the bed to the collection bag vertical because dependent loops in the tubing interfere with gravity flow.

- Ensure that the tubing is not compressed and the drainage is not obstructed. The tubing may be placed over the client's thigh.
- Position the drainage system lower than the bladder to avoid a backflow of urine.
- Suspend the drainage bag from the wheelchair below the level of the bladder.
- Secure the drainage bag to the lower part of an intravenous pole, or allow the client to carry the bag by hand when ambulating.

2. To reduce the potential for the drainage system to become a reservoir of pathogens, the entire drainage system is replaced whenever the catheter is changed and is replaced at least every 2 weeks in clients with a urinary tract infection.

SECTION III: PRACTICING FOR NCLEX

Activity G

1. **Answers: c, a, d, b**
   RATIONALE: Urination takes place several times each day. The need to urinate becomes apparent when the bladder distends with approximately 150 to 300 mL of urine. The distention with urine causes increased fluid pressure, stimulating stretch receptors in the bladder wall and creating a desire to empty it of urine.

2. **Answer: b**
   RATIONALE: To avoid the clean-catch specimen from being contaminated by microorganisms or substances other than those in the urine, the external structure through which the urine passes must be cleaned. Collecting the sample in a clean container over a period of 24 hours or using a catheter to collect the sample may not prevent the contamination of the urine. A void specimen is collected in a clean container, a 24-hour specimen is collected over a period of 24 hours, and a catheter is used to collect a catheter specimen.

3. **Answer: c**
   RATIONALE: Diuretic medication could have led to the increase in urinary volume of the client. The other common causes that could have led to an increase in urine volume are high fluid intake and endocrine diseases. Gallbladder disease would affect the color of the urine, making it appear brown in color; infection would cause the urine to appear cloudy. Kidney dysfunction would lead to a decrease in the volume of urine, not an increase.

4. **Answer: a**
   RATIONALE: Stasis could cause the client's urine to appear cloudy. The presence of blood would cause the urine to appear reddish brown in color, whereas water-soluble dyes would cause the urine to appear orange, green, or blue. Dehydration would cause the client's urine to appear dark amber in color.

5. **Answer: c**
   RATIONALE: The nurse could use the term "proteinuria" to document urine containing plasma proteins. Hematuria is the term used for urine containing blood. The presence of pus in the urine can be termed as pyuria. Albuminuria is the term used for urine containing albumin, a plasma protein.

6. **Answer: d**
   RATIONALE: Dysuria is difficult or uncomfortable voiding and is a common symptom of trauma to the urethra or a bladder infection. Anuria means the absence of urine, whereas oliguria indicates the inadequate elimination of urine. Polyuria means greater-than-normal urinary volume.

7. **Answer: a**
   RATIONALE: The presence of urinary stones is a common problem faced by clients with oliguria. Oliguria indicates an inadequate elimination of urine. Residual urine in the bladder after voiding can support the growth of microorganisms, leading to infection. Urinary stasis can lead to precipitation of dissolved substances such as calcium, leading to urinary stones. Common disorders associated with polyuria include diabetes mellitus and diabetes insipidus. In aging men, an enlarging prostate gland, which encircles the urethra, interferes with complete bladder emptying.

8. **Answer: d**
   RATIONALE: The nurse should use a urinal, which is a cylindrical container for collecting urine, for a client who is confined to the bed. Clients who can ambulate should be assisted to the bathroom to use the toilet. Clients who are weak or who cannot walk to the bathroom may use a commode. Clients confined to bed use a urinal or bedpan.

9. **Answers: b, c, d**
   RATIONALE: A urinary catheter is used for a client with urinary incontinence to keep the client dry, to measure residual urine, and to instill medication into the bladder. The other reasons for the use of a urinary catheter are to relieve bladder distention when clients cannot void, to keep the bladder from becoming distended during procedures such as surgery, and to obtain sterile urine specimens. Continence training to restore control of urination involves teaching the client to refrain from urinating until an appropriate time and place. Inserting a retention catheter is the least desirable approach to managing incontinence because it is the leading cause of urinary tract infections.

10. **Answer: c**
    RATIONALE: A urine bag is a bag attached by adhesive backing to the skin surrounding the genitals. It is more often used to collect urine specimens from infants. A straight catheter is a urine drainage tube inserted but not left in place, whereas a retention catheter is a urine drainage tube that is left in place over a period of time. A condom catheter is a flexible sheath that is rolled around the penis.

11. Answer: b
RATIONALE: The nurse should suggest that weight reduction is a possible nursing intervention for the client who complains of loss of small urination when laughing or sneezing. The client's incontinence can be classified as stress incontinence. The nurse should suggest a clothing modification for clients who are unable to control urination because of inaccessibility of a toilet or a compromised ability to use one. The nurse should suggest absorbent undergarments as an intervention for a client with loss of urine without any identifiable pattern or warning. Cutaneous triggering is suggested for a client with spontaneous loss of urine when the bladder is stretched with urine but without prior perception of a need to void.

12. Answer: d
RATIONALE: Bladder irritation secondary to infection is the possible cause for the client's condition. Loss of perineal and sphincter tone is the possible cause for the loss of small amount of urine when intra-abdominal pressure increases. Damage to motor and sensory tracts in the lower spinal cord is the cause for spontaneous loss of urine when the bladder is stretched with urine, but without prior perception of a need to void. Loss of urine without any identifiable pattern or warning could be caused by altered consciousness secondary to head injury.

13. Answer: a
RATIONALE: When providing catheter care, the nurse washes the meatus and a nearby section of the catheter to reduce microorganism colonization. The nurse should don clean gloves and wash the meatus, the catheter where it meets the meatus, the genitalia, and the perineum with warm, soapy water to remove gross secretions and transient microorganisms. The nurse places a pad under the hips of a female client and beneath the penis of a male client to protect the bed linen from becoming wet or soiled. The nurse should wash their hands or perform an alcohol-based hand rub because it reduces the potential for transmitting microorganisms.

14. Answers: b, d, a, c, e
RATIONALE: A closed system is irrigated without separating the catheter from the drainage tubing. To do so, the catheter or drainage tubing must have a self-sealing port. After cleaning the port with an alcohol swab, the nurse pierces the port with an 18- or 19-gauge 1.5-inch needle. The nurse then attaches the needle to a 30- to 60-mL syringe containing sterile irrigation solution. The nurse pinches or clamps the tubing beneath the port and instills the solution; they release the tubing for drainage. The nurse records the volume of irrigant as fluid intake or subtracts it from the urine output to maintain an accurate intake and output record.

15. Answers: a, c, e, b, d
RATIONALE: The steps involved in providing continuous irrigation are as follows. The nurse hangs the sterile solution on the intravenous pole and then purges the air from the tubing. The nurse then connects the tubing to the catheter port for irrigation and regulates the rate of infusion according to the medical records. The nurse then monitors the appearance of the urine and the volume of the drainage system.

16. Answer: c
RATIONALE: Chronic residual urine is likely to increase the risk of urinary tract infection in senior clients. Diminished bladder capacity and relaxation of pelvic floor muscle tone is likely to cause the client to experience urinary urgency. Enlargement of the prostate, a common problem among older men, can totally obstruct urinary outflow and make catheterization difficult or impossible.

17. Answer: a
RATIONALE: Double voiding means a client voids, then waits for a few more minutes to allow any residual urine to be voided. Clients who have been prescribed diuretic therapy should access the toilet within 30 to 120 minutes after the administration of the medication. Teaching older adults to structure activities with planned toilet breaks every 60 to 90 minutes results in less urine in the bladder and, thus, diminishes urge incontinence. Routine toilet schedules every 90 to 120 minutes must be offered to clients who become incontinent from a lack of assistance.

18. Answer: d
RATIONALE: Before providing a bedpan to a client who has been confined to the bed, the nurse palpates the lower abdomen for signs of bladder distention because it indicates bladder fullness. Before placing the bedpan, the nurse warms it by running warm water over it to demonstrate concern for the client's comfort. When placing the bedpan, the nurse should raise the top linen enough to determine the location of the client's hips and buttocks because this prevents unnecessary exposure. Placing the adjustable bed in the high position promotes the use of good body mechanics.

19. Answer: a
RATIONALE: Dehydration causes the client's urine to appear dark amber in color. Liver disease would cause the urine to appear brown, whereas blood would make the urine appear reddish brown. Water-soluble dyes cause the urine to appear orange, green, or blue.

SECTION IV: REVIEWING WHAT YOU HAVE LEARNED

Activity H
1. Polyuria
2. Bedpan

Activity I

1. True.
2. True.
3. False. A retention catheter is an indwelling catheter left in place for a period of time.

Activity J

1. Hematuria

Activity K

1. The figure shows suspension of a drainage system.
2. The drainage system is always placed lower than the bladder to avoid backflow of urine. When transporting the client in a wheelchair, the nurse should suspend the drainage bag from the chair below the level of the bladder. The drainage bag can be secured to the lower part of an IV pole for an ambulating client. If the client can ambulate without support, the nurse can allow the client to carry the bag below the bladder level.

Activity L

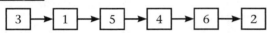

$$3 \rightarrow 1 \rightarrow 5 \rightarrow 4 \rightarrow 6 \rightarrow 2$$

Activity M

1. The four physical characteristics of urine include volume, color, clarity, and odor.
2. A urinary catheter may be used to keep incontinent clients dry; relieve bladder distention when clients cannot void; assess fluid balance accurately; keep the bladder from becoming distended during procedures such as surgery; measure the residual urine; obtain sterile urine specimens; and instill medication within the bladder.
3. The potential problems of using condom catheters are restriction of blood flow to the skin and tissues of the penis, if the sheath is applied tightly; skin breakdown from accumulation of moisture beneath the sheath; and frequent leakage.

Activity N

1. The first-voided specimen is most likely to contain substantial urinary components that have accumulated during the night.
2. The rate of urine production is normally reduced at night.

Activity O

1. Possible nursing diagnoses include the following:
   - Self-care deficit: toileting
   - Impaired urinary elimination
   - Risk for infection
   - Situational low self-esteem
   - Risk for impaired skin integrity
2. The nurse should
   - Plan to clean the meatus and surrounding areas at least once a day.
   - Gather clean gloves, soap, water, washcloth, towel, and a disposable pad.
   - Wash hands or perform an alcohol-based hand rub.
   - Place disposable pads beneath the hips of a female client or the penis of a male client.
   - Don clean gloves and wash the meatus, the catheter where it meets the meatus, the genitalia, and the perineum with warm soapy water.
   - Remove soiled materials and gloves; repeat hand hygiene measures.

Activity P

There are no definite answers to this activity. Students may choose to discuss their thoughts with peers or instructors.

SECTION V: GETTING READY FOR NCLEX

Activity Q

1. **Answer: a**
   RATIONALE: The nurse should document spontaneous loss of urine without an urge to void as reflex incontinence caused by damage to sensory tracts in the lower spinal cord. Stress incontinence is the loss of small amounts of urine when sneezing, coughing, or laughing. Functional incontinence is the lack of control over urination because of inaccessibility to a toilet or a compromised ability to use one. Urge incontinence is the need to void frequently with short-lived ability to sustain control of the flow.
2. **Answer: b**
   RATIONALE: The client should bend forward and apply hand pressure over the bladder to increase abdominal pressure, which helps overcome the resistance of the internal sphincter muscle. Massaging or tapping the skin lightly above the pubic area is called cutaneous triggering. Relaxing the urinary sphincter in response to physical stimulation is called voiding reflex. Contracting and relaxing the muscles alternatively for 10 seconds is one of the techniques of a Kegel exercise.
3. **Answers: b, c, d, e**
   RATIONALE: Soiled tissue should be left in the fracture pan until the time of disposal. Slipping the fracture pan just beneath the buttocks ensures proper placement, while raising the head of the client's bed simulates the natural position for elimination. Palpating the client's lower abdomen is an assessment to check for bladder fullness. Warming a metallic bedpan with running water before placing it beneath the client's buttocks demonstrates concern for the client's comfort.

CHAPTER 31

SECTION I: ASSESSING YOUR UNDERSTANDING

Activity A

1. Peristalsis
2. Stool
3. Constipation

4. Fiber
5. Iatrogenic
6. Impaction
7. Flatulence
8. Retention
9. Secondary
10. Water

Activity B

1. The figure shows a nurse removing a fecal impaction.
2. This procedure is required when a client has fecal impaction caused by a large, hardened mass of stool that interferes with defecation, making it impossible for the client to pass feces voluntarily.

Activity C

1. b   **2.** c   **3.** d   **4.** e   **5.** a

Activity D

3 → 1 → 4 → 2 → 5

Activity E

1. Clients with musculoskeletal disorders, such as arthritis of the hands, may face the problem of not being able to care for an ostomy appliance or perform colostomy irrigations. In such a situation, an occupational or enterostomal therapist can offer suggestions for promoting self-care.
2. Defecation or bowel elimination is the act of expelling feces from the body with the help of all structures of the gastrointestinal tract, especially the components of the large intestine, which must function in a coordinated manner.
3. A comprehensive assessment of bowel elimination involves collecting data about the client's elimination patterns or bowel habits and the actual characteristics of the feces.
4. Clients often have temporary or chronic problems with bowel elimination and intestinal function such as constipation, fecal impaction, flatulence, diarrhea, and fecal incontinence.
5. Pseudoconstipation (perceived constipation) occurs when clients believe that they are constipated, even though they are not. Pseudoconstipation may occur in people who are extremely concerned about having a daily bowel movement.
6. Diarrhea is the urgent passage of watery stool and is commonly accompanied by abdominal cramping. Simple diarrhea usually begins suddenly and lasts for a short period.

SECTION II: APPLYING YOUR KNOWLEDGE

Activity F

1. The nurse should recommend a diet that is high in fiber, such as raw fruits and vegetables, whole grains, seeds, and nuts. Dietary fiber, which becomes undigested cellulose, is important because it attracts water within the bowel, resulting in bulkier stool that is more quickly and easily eliminated. The incidence of constipation tends to be high among those whose dietary habits lack adequate fiber.
2. Constipation is accompanied by various signs and symptoms, such as complaints of abdominal fullness or bloating, abdominal distension, complaints of rectal fullness or pressure, pain on defecation, decreased frequency of bowel movements, inability to pass stool, and changes in stool characteristics, such as oozing liquid stool or hard small stool.

SECTION III: PRACTICING FOR NCLEX

Activity G

1. **Answer: a b, d**
   RATIONALE: Abnormal stools usually appear black, clay-colored, yellow, and green. Whenever stool appears abnormal, a sample is saved in a covered container for the physician's inspection. All shades of brown are considered normal.
2. **Answer: a**
   RATIONALE: To remove a fecal impaction, the nurse needs to lubricate their finger and then insert it inside the rectum of the client. Placing the client in a Sims position facilitates access to the rectum, but it does not ease the insertion of the finger into the rectum. Lubricating the rectal tube or warming the cleansing solution is not required for digital manipulation of stool. These are steps to follow when inserting a rectal tube and performing an enema, respectively.
3. **Answer: b**
   RATIONALE: Clients with fecal impaction can experience rectal pain as a result of unsuccessful efforts to evacuate the lower bowel. Forceful muscular contractions of peristalsis in higher bowel areas do not lead to rectal pain but do lead to the passing of liquid stool. An insufficient intake of liquids, high fiber, and retained barium from an intestinal radiographic procedure result in constipation.
4. **Answer: c**
   RATIONALE: The nurse should insert a well-lubricated rectal tube inside the client so that the gas can escape through it and provide immediate relief to the client. Administering a cleansing enema and insertion of a rectal suppository is done when the client is constipated as a result of blocked stool. Although prune juice is high in fiber, it will not help in this case because it will only make the client feel more bloated and uncomfortable.
5. **Answer: b**
   RATIONALE: To get more accurate findings when testing a client's stool for occult blood, the nurse should cover the entire test space with the stool. Taking the sample from the center of the stool provides more diagnostic value. Placing two drops

of chemical reagent onto the test space promotes a chemical reaction. Applying a thin smear of stool onto the test area ensures thorough contact with the chemical reagent.

6. **Answers: a, b, d**
   RATIONALE: The power pudding recipe consists of one cup wheat bran, one cup applesauce, and one cup prune juice all mixed thoroughly and refrigerated. Senior clients may be taught to incorporate a natural laxative into their diet. Senior clients can begin with one tablespoon per day and increase the amount by small increments daily until ease of bowel movement is achieved. Water and milk are not included in the power pudding recipe.

7. **Answer: c**
   RATIONALE: Fluid intake influences the moisture content of the stool. Bowel motility is altered by a person's emotions, not fluid intake. The type of food consumed by a person influences the color, odor, volume, and consistency of stool and fecal velocity.

8. **Answer: d**
   RATIONALE: To facilitate digital manipulation of the stool, the nurse should insert the lubricated finger to the level of the hardened mass of stool. Moving the finger slowly and carefully facilitates the removal or voluntary passage. Placing the client in Sims position facilitates access to the rectum but does not facilitate digital manipulation of the stool. Lubricating and inserting the finger periodically provides rest and restores patency to the lower bowel.

9. **Answer: a**
   RATIONALE: To purge air from the tubing, the nurse should open the clamp and fill the tubing with the cleansing solution and then reclamp the tubing. Holding the solution container 20 inches above the client's anus does not remove air from the tubing, but does facilitate gravity flow. Lubricating the tip of the tube generously eases insertion. Instilling the solution gradually over 5 to 10 minutes does not purge the air from the tubing, but it does fill the rectum with the solution.

10. **Answers: a, b, c**
    RATIONALE: To promote hydration and avoid dry stool, the nurse should encourage the client to drink at least 8 to 10 glasses of oral fluid per day. Prune juice is high in fiber and promotes bulk in the stool. Apple juice contains pectin, which also adds bulk to the stool. A client is advised to eat bananas and cottage cheese if they have diarrhea.

11. **Answer: b**
    RATIONALE: Nurses must administer them cautiously to clients with intestinal disorders such as colitis because large-volume enemas may rupture the bowel or cause other secondary complications. Large-volume cleansing enemas may create discomfort because they distend the lower bowel. Hypertonic saline enemas draw fluid from body tissues into the bowel. Normal soap-and-water cleansing enemas irritate the local tissue. A large-volume cleansing enema does not increase the fecal velocity of the stool; the type of food consumed by the client affects the fecal velocity.

12. **Answer: d**
    RATIONALE: An oil retention enema should be held within the large intestine for a specified period, usually at least half an hour. Retaining the cleansing enema inside a client for 5 or 10 minutes may result in premature defecation and defeats the purpose of retaining the oil. It is not necessary to retain the enema for an hour.

13. **Answer: c**
    RATIONALE: Older clients can develop healthier bowel elimination habits through the use of bulk-forming products containing psyllium or polycarbophil, which are more effective and less irritating than other types of laxatives. Increasing dosage and overusing laxatives or having a long-standing habit of laxative abuse could actually lead to constipation. Nurses inform senior clients who use mineral oil to prevent or relieve constipation that prolonged use interferes with absorption of fat-soluble vitamins A, D, E, and K.

14. **Answer: a**
    RATIONALE: Some clients with an impaction pass liquid stool, which they may misinterpret as diarrhea. Clients with an impaction need not necessarily have foul breath, weight loss, or poor physical reflexes. Clients with fecal impaction usually report a frequent desire to defecate but an inability to do so. Rectal pain may result from unsuccessful efforts to evacuate the lower bowel.

15. **Answers: b, d, e**
    RATIONALE: Diarrhea may result from emotional stress, dietary indiscretions, laxative abuse, or bowel disorders. Diarrhea is a means of eliminating an irritating substance such as tainted food or intestinal pathogens. Poor or inadequate fluid intake and physical inactivity do not necessarily lead to diarrhea.

16. **Answer: a**
    RATIONALE: When the digital removal of an impaction is required in senior clients, a gentle procedure should be used to prevent bleeding and tissue trauma. Senior clients may have benign lesions such as hemorrhoids or polyps in their lower bowel, which may interfere with the passage of stool. The nurse does not remove the impaction gently to preserve client dignity and self-esteem or to provide privacy and prevent soiling. A healthy bowel elimination habit can be developed in senior clients, not with gentle removal of impaction, but instead with the use of bulk-forming products containing psyllium or polycarbophil.

SECTION IV: REVIEWING WHAT YOU HAVE LEARNED

Activity H

1. 120
2. Iatrogenic

Activity I

1. False. Vegetables such as cabbage and cucumbers are known to produce intestinal gas.

Activity J

1. Peristomal skin
2. Peristalsis
3. Excoriation

Activity K

1. c **2.** d **3.** a **4.** b

Activity L

	Fecal Impaction	Fecal Incontinence
Definition	This large, hardened mass of stool interferes with defecation, making it impossible for the client to pass feces voluntarily.	The client cannot control the elimination of stool.
Causes	• Unrelieved constipation • Retained barium from an intestinal X-ray • Dehydration • Weakness of abdominal muscles	• Neurologic changes that impair muscle activity, sensation, or thought process • Fecal impaction • Intake of a harsh laxative
Symptoms	• Frequent desire but inability to defecate • Rectal pain • Passage of liquid stool	• Loose and watery stool

Activity M

1. The two components of bowel elimination assessment involve collecting data about (1) elimination patterns including frequency, effort required to expel stool, and use of aids and (2) stool characteristics, including color, odor, consistency, shape, and unusual components.
2. Signs and symptoms of constipation include abdominal fullness or bloating; abdominal distension; rectal fullness or pressure; pain during defecation; decreased frequency of bowel movements; inability to pass stool; and changes in stool characteristics such as oozing liquid or hard, small stool.

SECTION V: APPLYING YOUR KNOWLEDGE

Activity N

1. Large-volume enemas may create discomfort from bowel distention or may rupture the bowel in clients with intestinal disorders like colitis, causing secondary complications.
2. Tap water is nonirritating and is an effective cleansing solution.

Activity O

1.
- Place the client in a sitting position in bed, or in a chair beside the toilet.
- Place absorbent pads or towels on the client's lap and hang the container approximately 12 inches above the stoma.
- Wash hands and don gloves.
- Empty and remove the pouch from the faceplate.
- Secure the sleeve over the stoma and fasten it around the client with an elastic belt.
- Place the lower end of the sleeve into the toilet, commode, or a bedpan.
- Lubricate the cone at the end of the irrigation tubing.
- Open the top of the irrigating sleeve and insert the cone into the stoma.
- Hold the cone in place and release the clamp on the tubing.
- Clamp the tubing and remove the cone when the irrigating solution has been instilled.
- Close the top of the irrigating sleeve.
- Remove the belt and sleeve when draining has stopped, clean the stoma, and pat it dry.
- If the client is wearing an appliance, place a clean pouch over the stoma or cover the stoma temporarily with a gauze square.
- Repeat hand hygiene measures after removing gloves.

2.
   a. Two interventions to promote bowel elimination are inserting suppositories and administering enemas.
   b. The nurse should administer a commercially prepared disposable container of hypertonic enema solution by doing the following:
   - Warming the cold container of solution by placing it in a sink of warm water
   - Assisting the client to a Sims position or a knee–chest position
   - Washing hands or using alcohol-based hand rub and donning gloves
   - Removing the cover from the lubricated tip
   - Covering the tip with additional lubricant
   - Inverting the container and compressing the fluid toward the enema tip
   - Inserting the full length of the container's tip through the anus into the rectum
   - Applying gentle, steady pressure on the solution container until the solution has been administered

- Encouraging the client to retain the solution for 5 to 15 minutes
- Discarding the container, removing gloves, and performing hand hygiene measures

Activity P

There are no definite answers to this activity. Students may choose to discuss their thoughts with peers or instructors.

SECTION VI: GETTING READY FOR NCLEX

Activity Q

1. **Answers: c, d, e**
   RATIONALE: The Sims position facilitates access to the rectum. Lubrication eases insertion within the rectum. The nurse instructs the client to breathe slowly and deeply to promote muscle relaxation and to relieve discomfort. Contracting the gluteal muscles tightens the anal sphincters, which is a technique to prevent the premature urge to expel a suppository.
2. **Answer: d**
   RATIONALE: Expect resistance after inserting the tube for 2 inches, which indicates the location of the valve that controls the retention of liquid stool and urine. Lower the external end of the catheter at least 12 inches below the stoma. Cover the stoma with gauze or a large bandage. Remove the catheter and clean it with warm soapy water.

CHAPTER 32

SECTION I: ASSESSING YOUR UNDERSTANDING

Activity A

1. Chemical
2. Scored
3. Verbal
4. Protein
5. Mental
6. Speech
7. Generic
8. Gastrointestinal
9. Stock
10. Password

Activity B

1. The figure shows unit dose medication.
2. A unit dose supply, a self-contained packet that holds one tablet or capsule, is most common in acute care hospitals that stock drugs for individual clients several times in 1 day.

Activity C

1. d   **2.** a   **3.** e   **4.** c   **5.** b

Activity D

1. The frequency of drug administration refers to how often and how regularly the medication is to be given. Frequency of administration is written using standard abbreviations of Latin origin.
2. All medication orders have seven components: the client's name, date and time the order is written, drug name, dose to be administered, route of administration, frequency of administration, and signature of the person ordering the drug. If any one of these components is absent, the nurse must withhold the drug until they have obtained the missing information.
3. Health teaching is especially important before discharge because the client often receives prescriptions for oral medications. Providing health teaching helps to ensure that clients administer their own medications safely and remain compliant. Compliance means that the client follows instructions for medication administration. Even clients who purchase over-the-counter medications may benefit from instruction.
4. Nurses can give medications while a client is receiving tube feedings, but they instill the medications separately—that is, they do not add the medications to the formula. This is done for two reasons. First, some drugs may physically interact with the components in the formula, causing it to curdle or otherwise change its consistency. Also, a slow infusion would alter the drug's dose and rate of absorption.
5. Health agencies are using computerized medication documentation, which involves scanning bar codes on the medication container, the medication administration record (MAR), and the client's ID bracelet, before administering each drug. The computer validates that the nurse is about to give the right dose of the right drug, through the right route, at the right time, and to the right client. The computer also documents the drug's administration based on a password provided by the nurse.
6. As soon as the nurse recognizes a medication error, they check the client's condition and reports the mistake to the prescriber and supervising nurse immediately. Health care agencies have a form for reporting medication errors called an incident sheet or accident sheet. The incident sheet is not a part of the client's permanent record nor does the nurse make any reference in the chart to the fact that they have completed an incident sheet.

SECTION II: APPLYING YOUR KNOWLEDGE

Activity E

1. If an older person has difficulty comprehending information about medication routines, the nurse should include a second responsible person in the discharge instructions to ensure client safety. A referral for skilled nursing visits is appropriate

for homebound older adults who need additional instructions about medication routines after discharge.

2. Education regarding medications must include a visual description of the drug; action, dose, and time of administration; instruction whether food or liquid should accompany administration; a list of potential side effects; and a telephone number for a health care provider to contact should side effects occur.

SECTION III: PRACTICING FOR NCLEX

Activity F

1. **Answer: d**
   RATIONALE: The nurse is permitted to write a medication order if they are legally designated to do so by state statutes. However, the nurse needs to be an advanced practice nurse. A nurse would not be permitted to write a medication order if they are a registered nurse or has a baccalaureate degree. A nurse needs to be legally permitted by the state statute, not the health care facility, to write a medication order.

2. **Answers: a, c, d**
   RATIONALE: A medication order should contain the following seven components: the client's name, date and time the order is written, drug name, dose to be administered, route of administration, frequency of administration, and signature of the person ordering the drug. The age of the client and the name of the nurse are not written on the order.

3. **Answer: c**
   RATIONALE: The chemical name of a drug that is not protected by the company's trademark is known as a generic name, which is written in lowercase letters. Each drug has a trade name that the pharmaceutical company that made the drug uses. A trade name is sometimes called a brand or proprietary name.

4. **Answer: a**
   RATIONALE: The oral route means administration of the drug by swallowing or instillation through an enteral tube. The topical route is the administration of the drug by applying it to the skin or mucous membranes. The inhalant route is the administration of a drug through an aerosol. The parenteral route means the administration of drugs through an injection.

5. **Answer: b**
   RATIONALE: A scored tablet could be used to administer half a tablet to the client per the medication order of the physician. A scored tablet is a solid drug manufactured with a groove in the center. It is convenient when only part of the tablet needs to be administered. Enteric-coated tablets are solid drugs that cannot be broken or crushed; these drugs are coated with a substance that dissolves

beyond the stomach. Some capsules also contain beads or pellets of drugs for sustained release—in other words, drugs that dissolve at timed intervals.

6. **Answer: d**
   RATIONALE: The physician would use the standard abbreviation q.i.d. to indicate that the drug needs to be administered four times a day. The abbreviation q4h indicates that the drug needs to be administered every 4 hours, b.i.d. means twice a day, and t.i.d. indicates that the drug needs to be administered three times a day.

7. **Answer: c**
   RATIONALE: Per the physician's medication order, the drug has to be administered "qh," or on an hourly basis. If the drug needs to be administered immediately, this is indicated by the abbreviation Stat. If it needs to be administered every day, this is represented by the abbreviation qd. Administration of the medication twice a day is indicated by the abbreviation b.i.d.

8. **Answers: a, b, e**
   RATIONALE: To ensure accuracy of the medication order when dictated over the telephone, the nurse should ask the physician to repeat the dosage of the drug, spell out the drug name for confirmation, and have a second nurse listen simultaneously over an extension. The nurse should write "TO," not "VO," at the end of the order to indicate that the order was via the telephone. The order should be written directly on the client's medical record, not a note pad, to avoid errors in memory or repetition.

9. **Answer: a**
   RATIONALE: An individual supply of medication is a container with enough of the prescribed drug for several days or weeks and is common in long-term care facilities such as nursing homes. A unit dose supply is a self-contained packet that holds one tablet or capsule. It is most common in acute care hospitals that stock drugs for individual clients several times in 1 day. A stock supply remains on the nursing unit for use in an emergency so that a nurse can give a drug without delay. Some facilities use automated medication-dispensing systems, which usually contain frequently used medications for that unit, any as-needed medications, controlled drugs, and emergency medications.

10. **Answers: a, c e**
    RATIONALE: When administering controlled substances, the nurse should have an accurate account of their use, record each one used from the stock supply, and count each drug at the change of every shift. Opioids are controlled substances, meaning that federal laws regulate their possession and administration. Nurses count opioids at each change of shift. One nurse counts the number in the supply while another checks the record of their administration or amounts that have been wasted. Both counts must agree, with inconsistencies

accounted for as soon as possible. An individual supply is placed in a container with enough of the prescribed drug for several days or weeks and is common in long-term care facilities such as nursing homes. A stock supply remains on the nursing unit for use in an emergency so that a nurse can give a drug without delay.

11. Answer: a

RATIONALE: The nurse should calculate the drug dosage accurately to avoid medication error before, during, and after administration of the drug. Some of the other precautions include ensuring the five rights of medication administration, preparing medications carefully, and recording their administration. The nurse does need to verify the dosage calculation by a second nurse or ask the physician to mention the dosage in the medication order itself. The nurse also needs to count the number of narcotic drugs in the supply, but these answers do not apply to avoiding a medication error.

12. Answer: b

RATIONALE: Per the physician's medication order, the nurse needs to administer 2.5 mL of the drug to the client at the health care facility. The nurse uses a formula to calculate the amount of drug to administer [desired dose/dose on hand (supplied dose) (quantity)] and applies the formula to the information provided in the medication order: 250 mg. Provided: 500 mg/5 mL. Problem format: 250 mg/500 mg x 5 mL equals 2.5 mL.

13. Answer: d

RATIONALE: Before administering the drug to the client, the nurse compares the MAR with the medical record to prevent any medication errors. Before administration, the nurse reviews the client's drug, allergy, and medical history to avoid potential complications. The nurse should consult a current drug reference concerning the drug's action, side effects, contraindications, and administration information to ensure appropriate administration based on a thorough knowledge base. The nurse should plan to administer the medications within 30 to 60 minutes of their scheduled time because it demonstrates timely administration and compliance with the medical order.

14. Answer: a

RATIONALE: When administering drugs through an enteral tube, the nurse interrupts the tube feeding for 15 to 30 minutes before and after administration of the drug, which should be given on an empty stomach, to facilitate the drug's therapeutic action or absorption. Piercing the end of the sealed gelatin capsule and squeezing out the liquid medication facilitates access to the medication. The nurse opens the shell of a capsule to release the powdered content to facilitate mixing into a liquid form. The nurse adds 15 to 60 mL water to a thick liquid medication to dilute the medication and facilitate instillation.

15. Answers: a, c, d

RATIONALE: The nurse should include the following in the client's education: a visual description of the drug; the action, dose, and time of administration; instructions regarding whether food or liquid should accompany administration; a list of potential side effects; and a telephone number for a health care provider to contact should side effects occur. However, the nurse need not include the name of the health care facility where the client can receive treatment or the client's insurance number should the client require emergency treatment.

SECTION IV: REVIEWING WHAT YOU HAVE LEARNED

Activity G

1. Generic

Activity H

1. True.
2. True.
3. False. The nurse places a drug under the client's tongue for sublingual administration and between the client's cheek and the gum for buccal administration. The drug should remain in place until it dissolves in both cases.

Activity I

1. Medications
2. Enteric coated

Activity J

1. The seven components of a medication order are (1) client's name, (2) date and time the order was written, (3) drug name, (4) dose to be administered, (5) route of administration, (6) frequency of administration, and (7) signature of the person ordering the drug.
2. The medication administration record serves as a source for scheduling and documenting prescribed drugs and the time they are administered.

SECTION V: APPLYING YOUR KNOWLEDGE

Activity K

1. Such actions would impair the integrity of the coating, causing the drug to dissolve prematurely in gastric secretions.
2. Metric measurements are converted to household measurements when giving instructions to clients and family members because nonprofessionals can more easily interpret household measurements.

Activity L

1.
   a. The nurse should withhold the drug until they have obtained the missing information and consult the person who has written the order.

b. The five rights of medication administration are (1) right drug, (2) right dose, (3) right route, (4) right time, and (5) right client.

2. The nurse should
- Have a second nurse listen simultaneously on an extension.
- Record the drug order directly on the client's chart.
- Make sure the order includes all essential components.
- Clarify drug names that sound similar, such as Nicobid or Nitrobid.
- Spell or repeat numbers that could be misinterpreted such as 15 (one, five) and 50 (five, zero).
- Read back the written information to the prescriber.
- Use the abbreviation TO at the end of the order.
- Write the prescriber's name and cosign with name and title.
- Remind the prescriber that the order must be signed as soon as possible according to the agency's policy.

Activity M

There are no definite answers to this activity. Students may choose to discuss their thoughts with peers or instructors.

SECTION VI: GETTING READY FOR NCLEX

Activity N

1. **Answer: a**
   RATIONALE: The Latin abbreviation t.i.d. stands for three times a day. Every 3 hours is written q3h. There is no abbreviation for every third day or for 3 days; that information would be written in full.

2. **Answer: a**
   RATIONALE: Pouring liquids with the drug label toward the palm of the hand prevents liquid from running onto the label. Medications should never be left unattended. If the client is absent, the nurse should return later to administer the medication. The nurse offers a cup of water with solid forms of oral medication. The nurse should encourage the client not to hyperextend the neck when taking the drug, but to keep the head in a neutral position or in slight flexion to protect the airway.

CHAPTER 33

SECTION I: ASSESSING YOUR UNDERSTANDING

Activity A

1. Inunction
2. Transdermal
3. Paste
4. Bronchodilators
5. Otic
6. Sublingual

7. Yeast
8. Inhalant
9. Aerosol
10. Suppositories

Activity B

1. The figure shows an inhaler.
2. Inhalers are hand-held devices for delivering medication into the respiratory passages. They consist of a canister containing the medication and a holder with a mouthpiece through which the aerosol is inhaled.

Activity C

1. e   2. a   3. d   4. b   5. c

Activity D

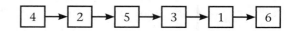

| 4 | → | 2 | → | 5 | → | 3 | → | 1 | → | 6 |

Activity E

1. Skin patches are drugs bonded to an adhesive bandage and applied to the skin. Several drugs are now prepared in patch form, including nitroglycerin, scopolamine, and estrogen. Nicotine withdrawal therapy and contraceptive drugs also are available as skin patches.

2. An otic application is a drug instilled in the outer ear. It usually is administered to moisten impacted cerumen or to instill medications to treat a local bacterial or fungal infection.

3. Nurses warn clients who use over-the-counter decongestant nasal sprays that, if they use the medication too frequently or administer more than the recommended amount, a rebound effect—the swelling of the nasal mucosa—can occur within a short time of drug administration.

4. When giving sublingual or buccal administrations, nurses instruct clients not to chew or swallow the medication. Eating and smoking also are contraindicated during the brief time needed for the medication to dissolve.

5. The inhalant method of medication administration is effective because the lungs provide an extensive area from which the circulatory system can quickly absorb the drug.

6. There are two types of inhalers: (1) a dry powder inhaler holds a reservoir of pulverized drug and a carrier substance and (2) a metered-dose inhaler that delivers aerosolized medication, which is a liquid drug forced through a narrow channel via a chemical propellant.

SECTION II: APPLYING YOUR KNOWLEDGE

Activity F

1. Ophthalmic medications are supplied either in liquid form and instilled as drops or as ointments applied along the lower lid margin. The nurse should

ask the client to blink (rather than rub) the eyes to distribute the drug over the surface of the eye. The eye is a delicate structure susceptible to infection and injury, just like any other tissue. Therefore, nurses take care to keep the applicator tip of the medication container sterile.

SECTION III: PRACTICING FOR NCLEX

Activity G

1. **Answer: a**
   RATIONALE: When caring for a client who has been prescribed hydrocortisone, the nurse should clean the area with soap and water before applying the inunction to promote absorption. The inunction should be applied with the fingertips, a cotton ball, or a gauze square, not with the palm. The inunction should be warmed, not cooled, if it is applied to a sensitive area by holding it in the hand or placing the sealed container in warm water. The inunction should be rubbed into the skin rather than applying it lightly.

2. **Answer: c**
   RATIONALE: The nurse should ask the client to lubricate the applicator tip with water-soluble jelly before application. The nurse should ask the client to administer the application preferably before going to bed to retain the medication for a prolonged period. The client should be asked to empty their bladder just before application. The client should remain recumbent for at least 10 to 30 minutes, not just 5 minutes.

3. **Answer: a**
   RATIONALE: The nurse uses the cutaneous route to administer nitroglycerin to dilate the coronary arteries in a client. Cutaneous applications are drugs rubbed into or placed in contact with the skin. Drugs to be administered sublingually are placed under the tongue and are left to dissolve slowly and become absorbed by the rich blood supply in the area. An otic application is instilled in the outer ear. A drug that has to be administered through a buccal application is placed against the mucous membranes of the inner cheek. These routes, however, are not used to administer nitroglycerin to the client.

4. **Answer: c**
   RATIONALE: A paste is a drug in a thick base that is applied but not rubbed into the skin. Transdermal applications are drugs that are bonded to an adhesive and applied to the skin. Sublingual applications are drugs that are placed under the tongue and left to dissolve slowly. Buccal applications are drugs placed against the mucous membrane of the inner cheek.

5. **Answer: a**
   RATIONALE: When using a patch, the nurse should be aware that patches are mostly used in the upper part of the body such as the chest, shoulders, and upper arms. Small patches can be applied behind the ear. Each time a new patch is applied, it is placed in a slightly different location. After application of the patch, it may take approximately 30 minutes for the drug to reach a therapeutic level. Thereafter, the patch provides a continuous supply of medication. In fact, the drug may still be active for up to 30 minutes after removal of the patch.

6. **Answer: d**
   RATIONALE: To avoid skin irritation, the nurse should rotate the site of the application of the medication. The nurse should avoid applying the paste with bare fingers to prevent self-absorption. The nurse should tape the edges of the application paper to seal the drug between the paper and the skin. The nurse can prevent the intake of excess drug by ensuring that one application is removed before applying another. Any residue on the skin should also be removed.

7. **Answer: a**
   RATIONALE: When administering eye medication to a client who has developed a sty, the nurse positions the client supine or sitting with their head tilted back and slightly to the side the medication is to be instilled to prevent the drug from passing into the nasolacrimal duct or being blinked onto the cheek. Instructing the client to look toward the ceiling prevents looking directly at the applicator, which usually causes blink reflexes as it comes close to the eye. To provide a natural reservoir for liquid medication, the nurse makes a pouch in the lower lid by pulling the skin downward over the bony orbit. To distribute the instilled medication, the nurse should instruct the client to close the eyelids gently and then blink several times.

8. **Answer: b**
   RATIONALE: The nurse should be aware that bronchodilators cause hypertension and tachycardia. Either or both of these effects increase the risks for complications, especially in older adults with underlying cardiovascular disease. Bronchodilators may not cause bronchitis or asthma in a client.

9. **Answers: a, c, e**
   RATIONALE: An otic application is a drug instilled in the outer ear. It usually is administered to moisten impacted cerumen or instill medications to treat a local bacterial or fungal infection. However, the medication should preferably not be used to remove foreign bodies because it may cause the object to swell and become more tightly fixed. Otic application by itself may not help in clearing the auditory canal.

10. **Answer: a**
    RATIONALE: To avoid swelling of the nasal mucosa, the nurse should suggest using a nasal spray containing only normal saline solution. Swelling of the nasal mucosa occurs when administering

medication frequently or administering more than the recommended dosage. The nurse could also suggest that the client follow the label directions. Using a spray that contains a reduced dosage of the prescribed medication, antiinflammatory medication, or antiallergy medication would not improve the client's condition.

11. Answer: d

RATIONALE: The nurse should instruct the client to breathe through the mouth as the drops are instilled to prevent the client from inhaling large droplets of medication. To distribute the medication when it is instilled, the nurse should ask the client to breathe as the container is squeezed. To provide support and aid positioning, the nurse could place a rolled towel or a pillow behind the neck if the client cannot sit. The nurse aims the tip of the dropper toward the nasal passage to deposit the drug within the nose rather than into the throat.

12. Answer: c

RATIONALE: The nurse understands that sublingual application is placing the drug underneath the tongue so that it dissolves slowly. Buccal application is placing the drug against the inner cheek. Inunction is medication incorporated into an agent that is administered by rubbing it into the skin. Patches are drugs bonded to an adhesive applied to the skin.

13. Answer: b

RATIONALE: Before administering the nasal medication, the nurse should read and compare the labels on the drug with the MAR at least three times—before, during, and after preparing the drug—to ensure that the right drug is given at the right time by the right route. Administering the medication within 30 to 60 minutes of the scheduled time demonstrates timely administration and compliance with the medical order. The nurse should compare the MAR with the written medical record to prevent medication error. To avoid potential complications, the nurse should review the client's drug, allergy, and medical history.

14. Answer: a

RATIONALE: The nurse should be aware that a suppository cream can be used to treat a client with a vaginal yeast infection. Scopolamine is used to treat motion sickness. Nitroglycerin cream is used to dilate the coronary arteries. Estrogen is used to treat the symptoms of menopause.

15. Answer: d

RATIONALE: A dry powder inhaler holds a reservoir of pulverized drug and a carrier substance. Dry powder inhalers depend on the client's inspiratory effort to deliver the medication into the lungs. A metered-dose inhaler delivers aerosolized medication, which is a liquid drug forced through a narrow channel via a chemical propellant.

SECTION IV: REVIEWING WHAT YOU HAVE LEARNED

Activity H

1. Topical
2. Transdermal
3. Nitroglycerin

Activity I

1. False. The nurse places a drug under the client's tongue for sublingual administration and between the client's cheek and the gum for buccal administration. The drug should remain in place until it dissolves in both cases.

Activity J

1. Rebound effect
2. Spacer

Activity K

	Dry Powder Inhaler	**Metered-Dose Inhaler**
Description	Holds a reservoir of pulverized drug and a carrier substance	Delivers aerosolized medication, which is a liquid drug forced through a narrow channel via a chemical propellant
Method of Medication Delivery	Depends on the client's inspiratory effort to deliver the medication into the lungs	Compression of the container releases a metered dose of aerosolized drug.
Ease of Use	Simple	Complicated

Activity L

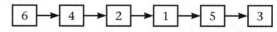

6 → 4 → 2 → 1 → 5 → 3

Activity M

Ophthalmic applications are drugs placed onto the mucous membrane of one or both eyes. Ophthalmic applications are available in liquid form instilled as drops and as ointments applied along the lower lid margins.

SECTION V: APPLYING YOUR KNOWLEDGE

Activity N

1. Application to the skin enables the drug to migrate through the skin and eventually be absorbed into the bloodstream.
2. Removal of hair before application of a skin patch may promote adhesion of the device.

Activity O

1.
- Apply the skin patch to any skin area on the upper body (e.g., chest, shoulders, upper arms) with adequate circulation.
- Apply each new patch in a different skin location than the previous one.
- Remove old patches when applying new ones.
- Date and initial each patch.

2.
  a. When instilling ear medication, the nurse
  - Manipulates the ear depending on the client's age to straighten the auditory canal
  - Tilts the client's head away from the ear into which the medication will be instilled
  - Compresses the container and instills the prescribed number of drops on the side of the ear canal rather than directly onto the tympanic membrane
  - Presses and releases the tragus, the projection of skin-covered cartilage at the opening of the external ear, to facilitate moving the medication toward the eardrum
  - Places a small cotton ball loosely in the ear to absorb excess medication
  - If a bilateral administration is prescribed, waits at least 5 minutes before instilling medication in the opposite ear

  b.
  - For a young child, the nurse pulls the ear down and back.
  - For an adult, the nurse pulls the ear up and back.

Activity P

There are no definite answers to this activity. Students may choose to discuss their thoughts with peers or instructors.

SECTION VI: GETTING READY FOR NCLEX

Activity Q

1. **Answers: a, c, d**
   RATIONALE: The client should shake the canister properly to distribute the drug in the pressurized chamber. Floating the canister in a water bowl shows the amount of medication in the canister; the higher the canister floats, the less medication it contains. The client is instructed to breathe in when the canister is depressed. The client should exhale slowly through pursed lips, not open lips. They should hold the breath for only 10 seconds to allow the medication to reach the lungs.
2. **Answer: a**
   RATIONALE: Placing a rolled towel or pillow beneath the neck facilitates support and aids with positioning. The tip of the container should be placed just inside, not outside, the nostril to confine the spray within the nasal passage. When spraying into one nostril, the person administering the spray should occlude the other nostril. The client should remain in position for approximately 5 minutes, not just 1 minute, to promote local absorption.

CHAPTER 34

SECTION I: ASSESSING YOUR UNDERSTANDING

Activity A

1. Axilla
2. Tuberculin
3. Intramuscular
4. Bunching
5. Radial
6. Needlestick
7. Reconstitution
8. Filter
9. Insulin

Activity B

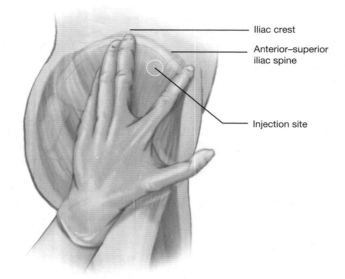

- Iliac crest
- Anterior–superior iliac spine
- Injection site

1. The figure shows the ventrogluteal site for administering intramuscular injections.
2. The muscles in this injection site are the gluteus medius and the gluteus minimus, which are large and, therefore, can hold a fair amount of injected medication with minimal postinjection discomfort.
3. The palm of the hand is placed on the greater trochanter with the index finger on the anterior superior iliac spine. The middle finger is moved as far as possible away from the index finger along the iliac crest. The injection is done into the center of the triangle formed by the index finger, the middle finger, and the iliac crest.

Activity C

1. d   2. c   3. b   4. a

Activity D

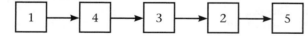

| 1 | → | 4 | → | 3 | → | 2 | → | 5 |

Activity E

1. The parenteral route is a route of drug administration other than oral or through the gastrointestinal tract. This term is commonly used when referring to medications given by injection.
2. All syringes contain a barrel that holds the medication, a plunger located within the barrel that moves back and forth to withdraw and instill the medication, and a tip or hub.
3. A lower dose of parenteral medications may be indicated for senior clients to prevent adverse effects. Age-related changes and possible chronic diseases may impair the older person's ability to absorb and metabolize medications.

4. Pinching the muscular tissue together may be needed to avoid striking bone when administering an intramuscular injection if the older person has decreased subcutaneous fat.
5. Conventional syringes and needles are being redesigned to avoid needlestick injuries, thus reducing the risk for acquiring a blood-borne viral disease such as hepatitis or AIDS.
6. It is important to rotate insulin injection sites because, over time, the injection sites tend to undergo changes that interfere with insulin absorption. To avoid lipoatrophy and lipohypertrophy, the sites are rotated each time an injection is administered.

SECTION II: APPLYING YOUR KNOWLEDGE

Activity F

1. Typically, low-dose insulin syringes are used to deliver insulin in 30 to 50 units or less. A standard insulin syringe can administer up to 100 units of insulin.
2. The nurse should combine the different insulins just before administration. When injected within 15 minutes of being combined, they act as if they had been injected separately. Otherwise, when mixed together, insulins tend to bind and become equilibrated. This means that the unique characteristics of each are offset by those of the other.

SECTION III: PRACTICING FOR NCLEX

Activity G

1. **Answer: b**
   RATIONALE: If the medication will be used for more than one administration, the preparer writes the date and time on the vial label and initials it. In some cases, when the directions provide several

options in diluent volumes, the preparer also writes the amount on the vial. However, the nurse does not write the client's name, illness, or syringe details on the vial label.

2. **Answers: b, c, d**
   RATIONALE: The nurse places an injection in this site in the middle third of the thigh, with the client sitting or in a supine position. The rectus femoris site is in the anterior aspect of the thigh. The nurse places one hand on the client's knee and the other below the trochanter when trying to locate the vastus lateralis site, not the rectus femoris site. The nurse palpates the posterior iliac spine and the greater trochanter to locate the appropriate landmarks of the dorsogluteal site.

3. **Answer: a**
   RATIONALE: A 25-gauge needle is used most often because medications administered subcutaneously usually are not viscous. For intradermal injections, nurses usually use a 25- to 27-gauge needle, whereas a 22-gauge needle that is 1.5- to 2-inch long is usually adequate for depositing medication in most intramuscular sites.

4. **Answer: b**
   RATIONALE: To reduce injection discomfort, the nurse should ask the client to take a deep breath prior to the injection to help bring focus to breathing techniques and not on the injection itself. Although local anesthetics like EMLA are used to reduce discomfort, nurses do not ask the clients to massage the injection site themselves. In addition, EMLA can take 60-120 minutes after application to create the desired effect, making it impractical. The nurse should not ask the client to avoid ambulating for 10 minutes after receiving the injection; the client should be asked to ambulate or move the are of injection as much as possible to reduce pain.

5. **Answer: d**
   RATIONALE: To prevent injecting glass particles into the client, the nurse should remove the filter needle and attach a sterile needle for administering the injection. Inserting the filter needle into the ampule ensures sterility of the needle. Tapping the barrel of the syringe near the hub distributes all the medication to the lower portion of the ampule. Using a needle with a very small gauge is not a good idea because finer glass particles will either clog the needle shaft or enter the barrel.

6. **Answer: c**
   RATIONALE: Before mixing any drugs, the nurse should consult a drug reference or compatibility chart because some drugs interact chemically when combined. Needle gauge, which refers to the diameter of the needle, and the tissue where the needle needs to be inserted do not make any difference when combining two drugs. Nurses should remember to withdraw exact amounts of the prescribed drugs, not equal amounts of drugs, from the

different containers before mixing. A filter needle is used to act as a barrier against glass particles. It does not stop or promote the chemical reaction between two drugs.

7. **Answer: c**
   RATIONALE: The nurse should aspirate and dispose of the entire contents of the excess medication from the vial container in the presence of a witness to comply with federal laws to prevent illegal drug use. Nurses do not dilute excess medication with saline solution to prevent illegal drug use, nor do they label the vial container containing the excess medication.

8. **Answer: b**
   RATIONALE: The nurse should numb the skin of the client with an ice pack before the injection is administered. The nurse should apply pressure to the injection site when removing the needle to reduce discomfort. Likewise, the nurse should instill the medication slowly and steadily to the client and change the needle before administering a drug that is irritating to the tissue.

9. **Answer: d**
   RATIONALE: Adding 0.1 to 0.2 mL air to the syringe flushes all the medication from the syringe at the time of injection. A nurse can flush all the medication from a syringe regardless of the gauge of the needle or the shaft length of the needle. Attaching a long- or short-shaft needle with a small or big gauge to the syringe does not affect the flushing action. Filter needles do not promote flushing, but act as a barrier for glass particles when withdrawing medication from glass ampules.

10. **Answers: a, d, e**
    RATIONALE: Currently, there are three different safety injection devices with plastic shields that cover the needle after use, injections with needles that retract into the syringe, and gas-pressured devices that inject medications without needles. Injections with reusable needles that are immersed in an alcohol solution or boiling water, or injections with disposable needles that are cleaned with spirit-based cotton swabs are conventional syringes and needles.

11. **Answer: b**
    RATIONALE: For the vastus lateralis site, the nurse places one hand above the knee and the other below the greater trochanter. The nurse places the palm of the hand on the greater trochanter and the index finger on the anterior superior iliac spine to locate the ventrogluteal site. For a deltoid site, the nurse has the client lie down, sit, or stand with the shoulder well exposed. The rectus femoris site is located by placing the injection in the middle third of the thigh with the client sitting or supine.

12. **Answer: a**
    RATIONALE: Heparin dosages are very small in volume, and they may require a tuberculin syringe to ensure accuracy. The nurse removes the needle

after withdrawal of the drug from a multidose vial and replaces it with another before administration. The nurse should rotate the sites with each injection to avoid a previous area where there has been local bleeding. Massaging the site is contraindicated because this can increase the tendency for local bleeding.

13. **Answers: b, c, d**
    RATIONALE: Bunching is preferred for infants, most children, and thin adults. Depending on the client's size, regardless of whether they are diabetic or obese, the nurse either bunches the tissue or stretches it taut before administering the injection.

14. **Answer: d**
    RATIONALE: Irritating medications are commonly given intramuscularly because deep muscles have fewer nerve endings. Intradermal injections, such as tuberculin, are commonly used for diagnostic purposes. Subcutaneous injections are given when the medication, such as insulin or heparin, is to be instilled between the skin and muscle and absorbed fairly rapidly. Intravenous injections, such as intravenous fluids or antineoplastic drugs, are administered via peripheral and central veins.

15. **Answer: b**
    RATIONALE: The ventrogluteal site has no large nerves or blood vessels, and it is usually less fatty and cleaner because fecal contamination is rare at this site compared with the dorsogluteal site. The gluteus maximus muscle in the dorsogluteal site can hold large amounts of injected medication. Massaging any intramuscular injection site immediately after administration is not recommended because it can lead to further complications.

16. **Answer: c**
    RATIONALE: Rolling the vial of insulin containing an additive between the palms mixes the insulin without damaging the protein molecules. The nurse should not insert the needle in the insulin itself to avoid coating the needle. Administering within 15 minutes of mixing avoids equilibration. Withdrawing specific units of insulin from the vial containing the insulin with the additive helps in preparing the prescribed dose.

SECTION IV: REVIEWING WHAT YOU HAVE LEARNED

Activity H
1. Barrel
2. Intradermal

Activity I
1. False. Needle length varies from 0.5 to 2.5 inches.
2. False. Lipoatrophy is the breakdown of subcutaneous fat at the site of repeated insulin injections.

Activity J
1. d   2. a   3. c   4. b

Activity K
1. A caregiver is injecting medication into the middle third of the thigh (vastus lateralis site).
2. The nurse injects into the anterior aspect of the thigh with the client sitting or supine. The rectus femoris injection site may also be used for infants.

Activity L
1. Five factors to consider when selecting a syringe and needle are the (1) type of medication, (2) depth of tissue, (3) volume of prescribed drug, (4) viscosity of the drug, and (5) size of the client.
2. Prefilled cartridges, which contain parenteral medication, are sealed glass cylinders made to fit in a specially designed syringe. The cylinders have an attached needle.

SECTION V: APPLYING YOUR KNOWLEDGE

Activity M
1. The smaller the number of the needle's gauge, the larger its diameter will be.
2. Conventional syringes and needles are being redesigned to reduce the risk for transmission of blood-borne viral diseases.

Activity N
1. While mixing insulins, the nurse should
   - Roll the vial of the insulin containing an additive between the palms.
   - Clean the rubber stopper of both vials of insulin.
   - Instill an amount of air equal to the volume that will be withdrawn from the vial containing the insulin with the additive.
   - Withdraw the needle and use the same syringe to instill air and withdraw the prescribed number of additive-free insulin units.
   - Invert the vial with additive-free insulin immediately after having instilled air and withdraw the prescribed number of additive-free insulin units.
   - Insert the needle into the vial with additive-containing insulin and withdraw the second amount.
   - Ask another nurse to check the label on the insulin and the number of units in the syringe.
   - Swab the rubber stopper of the vial containing the insulin with additive and pierce it with the needle of the partially filled syringe.
   - Withdraw the specified number of units from the vial containing the insulin with the additive.
   - Ask another nurse to check the label on the insulin and the number of units in the syringe.
   - Administer within 15 minutes of mixing.
2. If an accidental needlestick injury occurs, the nurse should
   - Report the injury to a supervisor.
   - Document the injury in writing.
   - Identify the client if possible.

- Obtain HIV and hepatitis B virus client status results.
- Obtain counseling on the potential for infection.
- Receive the most appropriate postexposure prophylaxis.
- Be tested for the presence of antibodies at appropriate intervals.
- Monitor for potential symptoms and obtain medical follow-up.

SECTION VI: GETTING READY FOR NCLEX

Activity O

1. **Answers: c, d, e**
   RATIONALE: The nurse should insert the needle, aspirate, and then inject the medication to ensure proper administration. A large muscle provides a location with the capacity for depositing and absorbing the drug. Withdrawing the needle and immediately releasing the skin create a diagonal path that prevents leaking into the subcutaneous and dermal layers of tissue. The Z-track method is administered into large muscles; therefore, the deltoid muscle would not be used. When using the Z-track method, the nurse should not massage the injection site so that the medication remains sealed.

2. **Answer: d**
   RATIONALE: The nurse should snap off the ampule's neck away from the body to protect the hands and face from any small glass particles. The nurse should invert the ampule, not hold it at an angle because inversion facilitates withdrawing the medication. Tapping an ampule correctly distributes all the medication to the lower portion of the bottle. The rim of the ampule should be avoided as an insertion point because this area may be contaminated.

CHAPTER 35

SECTION I: ASSESSING YOUR UNDERSTANDING

Activity A

1. Intravenous
2. Dementia
3. Percutaneous
4. Bolus
5. Pharmacist
6. Xiphoid
7. Medication
8. Antineoplastic
9. Implanted

Activity B

1. The figure shows the piggyback arrangement done during secondary infusion.
2. The piggyback arrangement or secondary infusion is advantageous because it is administered in tandem with a currently infusing primary intravenous solution.
3. The figure shows the placement of an implanted catheter.
4. The main advantage of an implanted catheter is that it provides the greatest protection against infection. Moreover, it can sustain approximately 2,000 punctures without leaking and can remain in place for several years barring complications.

Activity C

1. c   **2.** a   **3.** d   **4.** b

Activity D

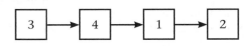

Activity E

1. To avoid the hazards of infiltrating tissue with medications delivered intravenously, it is appropriate to collaborate with the prescribing practitioner on the possibility of administering the same drug by another route.
2. Bolus administrations are given either through a port in an existing intravenous line or through a medication lock.
3. A medication lock is a plug that, when inserted into the end of an intravenous catheter, allows instant access to the venous system.
4. Antineoplastic drugs are medications used to destroy or slow the growth of malignant cells and are commonly referred to as chemotherapy or just chemo.
5. A central venous catheter is a venous access device that extends to the superior vena cava and provides a means of administering parenteral medication in a large volume of blood.
6. Health care personnel should explain the purpose and potential side effects for each drug administered, especially by the intravenous route.

SECTION II: APPLYING YOUR KNOWLEDGE

Activity F

1. Older adults who are discharged with medical devices for medications or treatments are likely to qualify for skilled nursing for follow-up in home or other independent settings, such as assisted living facilities.
2. Increasing emphasis on early discharge may require the nurse to teach older adult clients, family caregivers, or both how to flush venous access equipment.

SECTION III: PRACTICING FOR NCLEX

Activity G

1. **Answer: b**
   RATIONALE: The nurse removes a refrigerated secondary solution at least 30 minutes before administration so that the solution becomes slightly warm and promotes comfort during instillation. Removing the solution 30 minutes before administration does not ensure medication accuracy but having a second nurse double-check does. To prevent medication errors and ensure client safety, nurses should check the client's identity and documented drug allergies.

2. **Answers: a, b, c**
   RATIONALE: Nurses and caregivers can absorb antineoplastic drugs through skin contact, inhalation of tiny fluid droplets or dust particles on which the droplets fall, or oral absorption of drug residue during hand-to-mouth contact. Antineoplastic drugs cannot be absorbed through radiation of heat or chemical vapors.

3. **Answer: a**
   RATIONALE: One of its best features of a medication lock is that it eliminates the need for a continuous, and sometimes unnecessary, administration of intravenous fluid. It can be flushed with saline and heparin to maintain patency, but this is a secondary feature. An implanted catheter, not a medication lock, can sustain approximately 2,000 punctures. To verify patency of a medication lock, nurses need to obtain a blood return.

4. **Answer: c**
   RATIONALE: Older adult clients tend to metabolize and excrete drugs at a slower rate. This factor may predispose them to toxic effects from the accumulation of medications. They have decreased visual acuity and manual dexterity, but nurses can give additional instructions with time allowed for repeated practice. Older adult clients with dementia face confusion and disorientation with an acute illness, but this factor does not lead to toxic effects. Diminished protein components in the blood of older adult clients may lead to more "free drug."

5. **Answer: b**
   RATIONALE: The nurse should reclamp the catheter of the central venous catheter to prevent complications such as air embolism. To administer medication according to a prescribed rate, the nurse releases the clamp of the catheter tubing and regulates the rate of infusion. Removing the needle from the port when the medicated solution has instilled terminates current use of the catheter. Instilling 5 mL normal saline in the tubing maintains patency.

6. **Answers: a, b, d**
   RATIONALE: Nurses should observe older adult clients who are receiving intravenous medications such as anticoagulants, sulfonamides, opiates, and antimicrobials for adverse effects. Normal saline and insulin usually do not lead to adverse effects when administered per the physician's prescribed orders.

7. **Answer: b**
   RATIONALE: To reduce skin discomfort, the nurse should apply a local anesthetic topically. The administration of intravenous solution is stopped if there are complications and when the physician orders it. Replacing the special needle or changing the self-sealing port is not a good idea. Implanted catheters have a self-sealing port pierced through the skin with a special needle when administering intravenous medications or solutions.

8. **Answer: d**
   RATIONALE: A secondary infusion is the administration of a parenteral drug that has been diluted in a small volume of intravenous solution, usually 50 to 100 mL, over 30 to 60 minutes. All the other intravenous volume solutions and rate of flow are incorrect.

9. **Answer: b**
   RATIONALE: If the client's condition changes for any reason, the first thing that a nurse should do is cease the administration immediately. The nurse should then call for the lead physician and take emergency measures to protect the client's safety. The nurse does not reduce the prescribed rate of intravenous medication on their own without the lead physician's permission.

10. **Answer: d**
    RATIONALE: Covering the drug preparation area with a disposable paper pad is done to absorb small drug spills. Nurses should wear one or two pairs of surgical latex, nonpowdered gloves to reduce the potential of skin contact, and they should avoid inhalation of the drug spill.

11. **Answer: b**
    RATIONALE: The nurse should use sterile normal saline to fill the intravenous tubing before administration to maintain patency. Nurses do not use sterile bacteriostatic water for flushing, but for injection. Sterile isopropyl alcohol is used for cleaning the skin. Sterile hydrogen peroxide is usually used to disinfect and clean medical equipment.

12. **Answer: c**
    RATIONALE: The nurse should identify excess fluid volume as the nursing diagnosis because the client complains about a bloated abdomen and frequent urination. The client does not have risk for injury or infection because the intravenous equipment is sterilized and placed appropriately by the nurse per the physician's orders. The client is bound to experience a little bit of discomfort, but not acute pain, from the intravenous administration.

13. Answers: a, d, e

RATIONALE: Hanging the secondary solution higher than the primary solution instills the solution under greater hydrostatic pressure. Releasing the roller clamp on the secondary solution initiates infusion. Regulating the rate of flow by counting the drip rate and adjusting the roller clamp establishes the maintenance rate of flow to instill the solution. The nurse should clamp the tubing when the solution has instilled to prevent backfilling with the primary solution. Inserting the modified adapter within the port provides access to the venous system.

SECTION IV: REVIEWING WHAT YOU HAVE LEARNED

Activity H

1. Bolus
2. Percutaneous

Activity I

1. False. Volume-control sets are a substitute for a separate secondary infusion. They eliminate the need for additional fluid.
2. False. Hickman and Broviac catheters are examples of tunneled catheters.

Activity J

1. Antineoplastic drugs

Activity K

1. c
2. d
3. a
4. b

Activity L

	Tunneled Catheters	Percutaneous Catheters
Method of Insertion	Inserted into a central vein with the distal end exiting the skin around the xiphoid process. The catheter is secured in subcutaneous tissue with an external cuff.	Inserted through the skin in a peripheral vein (e.g., the basilic, cephalic, jugular, or subclavian vein) with the distal end terminating in the axillary vein, subclavian vein, or superior vena cava
Uses	Extended therapy	Short-term fluid or medication therapy

Activity M

1. Intravenous administrations are appropriate in the following circumstances:
   - A quick response is needed during an emergency.
   - Clients have disorders that affect their absorption of drugs.
   - Blood levels of drugs need to be maintained at a consistent therapeutic level.
   - It is in the client's interest to avoid the discomfort associated with intramuscular injections.
   - A mechanism is needed to administer drug therapy over a prolonged period.
2. A medication lock allows instant access to the venous system. It thus eliminates the need for continuous and unnecessary administration of intravenous fluids.

SECTION V APPLYING YOUR KNOWLEDGE

Activity N

1. Intravenous drugs cannot be retrieved once they have been delivered.
2. Multiple lumens enable incompatible substances or more than one solution or drug to be given simultaneously.

Activity O

The nurse can use the mnemonic SAS or SASH as a reminder of the steps for administering IV medication into a lock. SAS stands for flush with **S**aline, **A**dminister drug, flush again with **S**aline. SASH refers to flush with **S**aline, **A**dminister drug, flush again with **S**aline, instill **H**eparin. To maintain patency, the nurse usually needs to flush medication locks with saline or heparin every 8 to 12 hours. The nurse should change the medication lock while changing the IV site or at least every 72 hours.

Activity P

There are no definite answers to this activity. Students may choose to discuss their thoughts with peers or instructors.

SECTION VI GETTING READY FOR NCLEX

Activity Q

1. **Answer: a**

   RATIONALE: One or two pairs of nonpowdered surgical gloves can help reduce the potential for skin contact. The nurse should wear a long-sleeved gown with a closed front to avoid any drug contact with the body area. If there is a drug spill, the area requires cleaning with water and detergent at least three times to prevent any adverse effects.
2. **Answer: d**

   RATIONALE: The nurse should wipe the uppermost port of the primary tubing with an alcohol swab to remove colonized microorganisms. The refrigerated secondary solution should be removed at least 30 minutes, not just 10 minutes, before infusion to warm the solution slightly and promote comfort during instillation. The nurse should check the drop factor on the package of the secondary IV tubing and calculate the rate of infusion accordingly, not as per the rate of infusion of the primary solution. The height of the primary solution should be set approximately 10 inches below the height of the secondary solution.

CHAPTER 36

SECTION I: ASSESSING YOUR UNDERSTANDING

Activity A

1. Epiglottis
2. Cilia
3. Viscosity
4. Aerosol
5. Dysphagia
6. Suctioning
7. Oral
8. Nasotracheal
9. Trumpet
10. Pneumonia

Activity B

1. The figure shows a client using aerosol therapy.
2. Aerosol therapy improves breathing, encourages spontaneous coughing, and helps the client to raise sputum for diagnostic purposes.
3. The figure shows the nurse performing percussion.
4. Percussion, rhythmic striking of the chest wall, helps to dislodge respiratory secretions that adhere to the bronchial walls.

Activity C

1. e   **2.** a   **3.** d   **4.** b   **5.** c

Activity D

$$3 \rightarrow 1 \rightarrow 4 \rightarrow 2$$

Activity E

1. There are many factors that can jeopardize airway patency, including the following:
   - Increased volume of mucus
   - Thick mucus
   - Fatigue or weakness
   - Decreased level of consciousness
   - Ineffective cough
   - Impaired airway
2. The structures that protect the airway from a wide variety of inhaled substances include the following:
   - Epiglottis—It is a protrusion of flexible cartilage above the larynx that acts as a lid that closes during swallowing. It helps to direct fluid and food toward the esophagus rather than the respiratory tract.
   - Tracheal cartilage—This ensures that the trachea, the portion of the airway beneath the larynx, remains open.

- Mucous membrane—This is a type of tissue from which mucus is secreted, which lines the respiratory passages.
- Cilia—These are hairlike projections that beat debris upward that collects in the lower airway.

3. The most common methods of maintaining the natural airway are keeping respiratory secretions liquefied, promoting their mobilization and expectoration with chest physiotherapy, and mechanically clearing mucus from the airway by suctioning.
4. Clients at risk for airway obstruction or requiring long-term mechanical ventilation are candidates for an artificial airway. Two common types are:
   - An oral airway
   - A tracheostomy tube
5. An oral airway is a curved device that keeps a relaxed tongue positioned forward within the mouth, preventing the tongue from obstructing the upper airway. It is most commonly used in clients who are unconscious and cannot protect their own airway, such as those recovering from general anesthesia or a seizure.
6. Many older adults with pathologic pulmonary changes have a history of smoking cigarettes since their youth, working in occupations where they inhaled pollutants that affected their lungs, or living for an extended time in industrial areas known for toxic emissions.

SECTION II: APPLYING YOUR KNOWLEDGE

Activity F

Because a tracheostomy tube is below the level of the larynx, clients usually cannot speak. Communication may involve writing or reading the client's lips. Being unable to call for help is frightening; therefore, the nurse should check these clients frequently and respond immediately when they signal.

SECTION III: PRACTICING FOR NCLEX

Activity G

1. **Answers: a, c, d**
   RATIONALE: The nurse should be aware that the lower airway consists of the trachea, bronchi, alveoli, and bronchioles. The upper airway consists of the nose and pharynx, which is subdivided into the nasopharynx, oropharynx, and laryngopharynx.
2. **Answer: b**
   RATIONALE: The tracheal cartilages or rings ensure that the trachea, the portion of the airway below the larynx, remains open. The epiglottis is a protrusion of flexible cartilage above the larynx that acts as a lid that closes during swallowing, helping direct fluid and food toward the esophagus rather than the respiratory tract. Mucous membrane is a type of tissue from which mucus

is secreted. It lines the respiratory passages and traps particulate matter. Hairlike projections called cilia beat debris upward that collects in the lower airway.

3. **Answer: a**
RATIONALE: Aerosol therapy helps in raising sputum for diagnostic purposes. It also improves breathing and encourages spontaneous coughing. Percussion helps to dislodge respiratory secretions that adhere to the bronchial wall. Vibration is using the palms of the hands to shake underlying tissue and loosen retained secretions. Postural drainage is a positioning technique that promotes gravity drainage of secretions from various lobes or segments of the lungs.

4. **Answer: c**
RATIONALE: The nurse should collect a sputum specimen just after the client awakens or after an aerosol treatment because more mucous is available or is in a thin state. It may not be possible to collect enough thin-sputum specimen before the client goes to bed, after physiotherapy, or after percussion is performed.

5. **Answer: a**
RATIONALE: Postural drainage is a positioning technique that promotes gravity drainage of secretions from various lobes or segments of the lungs. Aerosol therapy encourages spontaneous coughing. Vibration uses the palms of the hands to shake underlying tissue and loosen retained secretions. Percussion helps to dislodge respiratory secretions that adhere to the bronchial wall.

6. **Answer: a**
RATIONALE: The nurse should perform percussion for 3 to 5 minutes, not more, in each postural drainage position. Percussion, the rhythmic striking of the chest walls, helps to dislodge respiratory secretions that adhere to the bronchial wall.

7. **Answer: b**
RATIONALE: The nurse should apply a negative pressure from 50 to 95 mm Hg when using a wall suction machine on an infant, whereas 100 to 140 mm Hg of negative pressure is appropriate for adult clients and 95 to 100 mm Hg is appropriate for children, when using a wall suction machine. The nurse does not apply a negative pressure of 45 to 50 mm Hg for infants, children, or adults.

8. **Answer: c**
RATIONALE: The nurse should encourage the client to cough, if coughing does not occur spontaneously, to break up mucus and raise secretions. To maximize the effectiveness of suctioning, the nurse should occlude the air vent and rotate the catheter as it is withdrawn. The nurse should wait until the client takes a breath before advancing the tubing for tracheal suctioning, to ease insertion below the larynx.

9. **Answer: a**
RATIONALE: Nasopharyngeal suctioning involves removing secretions from the throat through a nasally inserted catheter. Nasotracheal suctioning removes secretions from the upper portion of the lower airway through a nasally inserted catheter. Oropharyngeal suctioning removes secretions from the throat through an orally inserted catheter. Oral suctioning is the removal of secretions from the mouth using a Yankauer-tip or tonsil-tip catheter.

10. **Answers: b, d, e**
RATIONALE: Clients who have an upper airway obstruction, require prolonged mechanical ventilation, and are less stable and require oxygenation are likely candidates for tracheostomy. Tracheostomy is a surgically created opening into the trachea. Clients who are recovering from general anesthesia or a seizure are candidates for an oral airway.

11. **Answer: a**
RATIONALE: To prevent aspiration, the nurse should perform suctioning. This also helps to clear saliva from the mouth. Positioning the client supine with the neck hyperextended opens the airway and facilitates insertion of the artificial airway. Holding the airway so that the curved tip points toward the roof of the mouth is done to prevent pushing the tongue into the pharynx during insertion. Rotating the airway over the top of the tongue ensures that the artificial airway follows the natural curve of the upper airway.

12. **Answer: c**
RATIONALE: The nurse should understand that a possible cause of resistance when inserting the catheter is the result of contact between the tip of the catheter and the carina. When suctioning a tracheostomy, the nurse inserts the catheter a shorter distance, approximately 4 to 5 inches, or until resistance is felt because the tube already lies in the trachea. The resistance is caused by contact between the catheter tip and the carina, the ridge at the lower end of the tracheal cartilage where the main bronchi are located.

13. **Answers: a, c, e**
RATIONALE: Tracheostomy care includes cleaning the skin around the stoma, changing the dressing, and cleaning the inner cannula. The nurse need not change the outer cannula or clear the outer airway when performing tracheostomy care.

14. **Answer: b**
RATIONALE: The nurse should be aware that respiratory cilia become less efficient with age, predisposing older adults to a high incidence of pneumonia. Usually the bases of older clients' lungs receive less ventilation, contributing to retention of secretions, decreased air exchange, and compromised ventilation.

15. **Answers: a, b, d**
RATIONALE: Inquiring about a current history of coughing, determining how long the cough has been present, and observing and describing any sputum are important when assessing older clients who have difficulty coughing. Inquiring whether

the physician has been informed and checking the client's medication against the medical order are not appropriate interventions in the given situation. Severity of chronic pulmonary diseases increases with age.

16. Answer: c
RATIONALE: The nurse should be aware that older clients with difficulty swallowing (or dysphagia), often associated with stroke or middle and late stages of dementia, are more vulnerable to aspiration pneumonia. Older adults are at increased risk for cardiac dysrhythmias during suctioning because many have preexisting hypoxemia from illnesses and age-related changes in ventilation.

SECTION IV: REVIEWING WHAT YOU HAVE LEARNED

Activity H

1. Alveoli
2. Nasotracheal

Activity I

1. False. Nurses perform oropharyngeal suctioning with a device called a Yankauer-tip.
2. False. The epiglottis is a protrusion of flexible cartilage above the larynx.

Activity J

1. Airway
2. Tracheostomy

Activity K

1. The figure depicts the lower airway and its related structures. See Figure 36-1 in your textbook.
2. Gases travel through the airway to and from the blood.

Activity L

1. The four natural mechanisms that protect the airway are sneezing or blowing the nose, coughing, expectorating, and swallowing.
2. Two conditions that indicate a need to insert an artificial airway are risk for airway obstruction and long-term mechanical ventilation.

SECTION V: APPLYING YOUR KNOWLEDGE

Activity M

1. The tracheostomy tube is below the level of the larynx, which makes the client unable to speak. The only communication possible is writing or reading the client's lips. Because the client cannot communicate as they are used to, frequent assessments are needed to ensure that the client's needs are being addressed.
2. Hydration helps to keep the mucous membranes moist and the mucus thin, which in turn promotes expectoration.

Activity N

1.
a. To perform the percussion technique, the nurse cups the hands, keeping the fingers and thumb together as if carrying water. The nurse then applies the cupped hands to the client's chest as if trapping air between them and the thoracic wall. The nurse percusses for 3 to 5 minutes, taking care to avoid striking the breasts of female clients and any areas of chest injury or bone disease.
b. To perform the vibration technique, the nurse positions the hands on the client's chest or back during inhalation and then vibrates them as the client exhales to increase the intensity of expiration.

2. The nurse should instruct the client and the family to
   - Plan to perform postural drainage two to four times daily, before and after meals.
   - Administer prescribed inhalant medications before performing postural drainage.
   - Keep paper tissues and a waterproof container nearby for collecting expectorated sputum.
   - Position the client to drain the appropriate lung areas.
   - Cough and expectorate secretions that drain into the upper airway.
   - Remain in each prescribed position for 15 to 30 minutes.
   - Resume a comfortable position after expectorating the usual volume of sputum, or in case of a rapid pulse rate, difficulty in breathing, or chest pain.

SECTION VI: GETTING READY FOR NCLEX

Activity O

1. **Answer: b**
   RATIONALE: The nurse should ask the client to attempt a forceful cough and expectorate into the specimen container to help obtain secretions from the lower airway. The client should rinse the mouth before specimen collection to remove microorganisms and food residue. Collection of the specimen preferably takes place after, not before, an aerosol treatment so that mucus is available or is in a thin state. A specimen of saliva obtained from within the mouth would result in an inconclusive test result; the desired specimen should be from deep within the respiratory passages.

2. **Answer: a**
   RATIONALE: Maintain 2000 to 3000 mL fluid intake for 24 hours to ensure that the client is well hydrated to enable thinning of the mucus. The client should not breathe through the mouth; deep breaths should occur through the nose and out through the mouth; the client should then lean

forward and cough forcefully to enable expansion of the lung surface. The client should be in Fowler position to provide maximum room for lung expansion. The client should avoid milk, which has mucus-producing properties.

3. **Answer: b**
   RATIONALE: The nurse should clean the area around the stoma with diluted peroxide to remove secretions and colonizing microorganisms from the tracheal opening. They should remove the inner cannula and place it in a solution of hydrogen peroxide and saline to loosen protein secretions and reduce colonizing microorganisms. After cleaning the cannula with saline solution, the nurse should wipe it dry with a gauze square to remove large droplets of fluid. When working alone, the nurse should remove the used ties only after the new ones are secure to prevent accidental extubation.

CHAPTER 37

SECTION I: ASSESSING YOUR UNDERSTANDING

Activity A

1. Supine
2. Recovery
3. Esophagus
4. Sternum
5. Bolus
6. Ribs
7. Rescue
8. Hands
9. Consciousness
10. Resuscitation

Activity B

1. The figure shows mouth-to-mouth rescue breathing.
2. During mouth-to-mouth breathing, a rescuer seals the victim's nose, uses their mouth to cover the victim's mouth, and blows air into the victim.

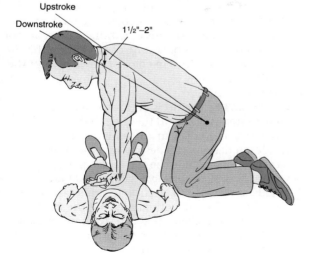

Upstroke

Downstroke   1½"–2"

3. The figure shows correct hand and body position during chest compressions.
4. Health professionals assess whether there is need for chest compressions assessing the client's level of consciousness and responsiveness. Responsiveness is determined initially by shouting and shaking the victim. With the victim in a supine position on a dry, firm surface, a quick assessment taking no more than 10 seconds is performed to determine unresponsiveness and the absence of normal breathing or a pulse.

Activity C

1. c   **2.** a   **3.** d   **4.** b

Activity D

| 4 | → | 2 | → | 3 | → | 1 | → | 5 |

Activity E

1. If the client can speak or cough, or if they are exchanging some air, then these signs indicate that the client has a partial airway obstruction. Infants cannot talk or make the universal choking signs; ability to cry is the best evidence of partial obstruction in this age group.
2. The process of ventilating the lungs through the victim's mouth, nose, or stoma is called rescue breathing.
3. Resuscitation must proceed with CAB (circulation, airway, breathing if the rescuer is a trained health care provider, or hands-only chest compressions if untrained in defibrillation) or cardiopulmonary resuscitation (CPR), a technique used to restore circulation and breathing.
4. Mouth-to-nose breathing is performed when the client is an infant or a small child, or when mouth-to-mouth breathing is impossible or unsuccessful.
5. An AED is a portable, battery-operated device that analyzes heart rhythms and delivers an electrical shock to restore a functional heartbeat.
6. Rescuers and nurses performing rescue breathing should use a one-way valve mask or other protective face shield if available because these devices theoretically reduce the potential for acquiring infectious diseases such as hepatitis and AIDS. However, lack of a barrier device should not interfere with attempting rescue breathing.

SECTION II: APPLYING YOUR KNOWLEDGE

Activity F

1. When performing CPR, older adults are at a greater risk for fractured ribs because of the increased likelihood of osteoporosis. Similarly, those with vascular disease may not receive adequate blood perfusion of the brain during CPR, and they may experience brain damage as a result.
2. Older adult clients who take daily doses of aspirin or other anticoagulant drugs are more apt to bleed internally during chest compressions.

SECTION III: PRACTICING FOR NCLEX

Activity G

1. **Answer: c**
   RATIONALE: When performing the chin lift technique or head tilt technique to open the airway, nurses assist the client to lie in the supine position on a firm surface without twisting the spine. The lateral position, Sims position, and Fowler position are not suitable for performing the chin lift technique or the head tilt technique.

2. **Answer: c**
   RATIONALE: The nurse should observe for signs of partial or complete airway obstruction, such as inability to speak, coughing, audible wheezing, or the client holding the throat. Insufficient chewing, compromised swallowing, and aspiration of vomitus are causes of airway obstruction.

3. **Answer: b**
   RATIONALE: Use of an AED in children from 1 to 8 years of age or in those weighing less than 55 lb is not recommended unless the device can deliver a pediatric "shockable" dose. If a client has an implanted defibrillator or pacemaker, the AED pad is placed 1 inch away from the implanted device. Senior clients are at a greater risk for fractured ribs because of the increased likelihood of osteoporosis when performing CPR. Clients with dementia can also be administered shock with the aid of an AED.

4. **Answer: c**
   RATIONALE: If a person has an implanted defibrillator or pacemaker evidenced by a hard object beneath the skin with an overlying scar, the AED pad must be placed at least 1 inch to the side of the implanted device. Placing the AED pads on the implanted device itself is not recommended. Nurses do not place AED pads between the sternum and vertebrae, but use this site for chest compression in clients and use the brachial artery in the upper arm in infants for promoting circulation.

5. **Answer: a**
   RATIONALE: Periodically, rescuers should perform an assessment after five cycles of compressions and ventilations. They assess the victim to determine whether CPR is effective. Nurses do not assess the client's condition after 10, 15, or 20 cycles of compression and ventilations. When an AED is not available and the arrival of emergency resuscitation personnel is delayed, CPR continues at a rate of 30 compressions to two ventilations.

6. **Answers: a, b, d**
   RATIONALE: After early recognition and providing access of emergency services, the nurse should provide the client with early CPR, arrange for the cardiac defibrillator, and keep the advanced life support services ready for use. The nurse should not waste time checking the pulse or blood circulation of a client with cardiac arrest, but provide emergency care with great speed. Placing the client

in a recovery position is done when the client starts breathing and has a normal pulse rate.

7. **Answer: a**
   RATIONALE: When a person has a complete or partial airway obstruction, the face initially reddens and then becomes pale or blue. Signs of airway obstruction generally occur when the person is eating. They may make a high-pitched sound while inhaling.

8. **Answers: a, b, c**
   RATIONALE: AEDs are located in many public access locations, such as schools, airports, and police stations. However, they are not readily placed at pedestrian subways or amusement parks. Once obtained, the user turns on the AED so that they can observe its monitor screen. Most AEDs have pictorial instructions and the capacity to provide voice instructions.

9. **Answer: d**
   RATIONALE: Nurses give rescue breathing to a client with a laryngectomy by sealing their mouth over the victim's stoma. Because the upper airway is essentially a blind pathway, the nose does not require sealing. A one-way mask is used to reduce the potential for acquiring infectious disease when performing mouth-to-mouth breathing. The nurse covers or closes the client's mouth when performing mouth-to-nose breathing.

10. **Answer: b**
    RATIONALE: Holding the infant prone with the head downward, nurses use the heel of one hand to administer five back slaps between the shoulder blades. The rescuer turns the infant supine and uses two fingers to give five chest thrusts. Nurses alternate between five back blows and chest thrusts, not just turning the client between the supine and prone positions, until the object is dislodged. The rescuer does not use finger sweeps unless they can see the obstructing object.

11. **Answer: a**
    RATIONALE: For assessment of spontaneous breathing, nurses observe for rising and falling of the chest, and listen and feel for air escaping from the client's nose and mouth. Nurses check the client's pulse rate as part of obtaining vital signs, not to assess spontaneous breathing. Nurses do not assess spontaneous breathing of a client on the basis of the change in skin color or movement of the mouth and nose.

12. **Answers: a, b, e**
    RATIONALE: The decision to stop resuscitation efforts often is based on the time that elapsed before resuscitation began and whether the client's condition deteriorates despite resuscitation efforts. Other factors include the age and diagnosis of the victim, as well as objective data, such as arterial blood gas results and electrolyte studies. It is not the wishes of the client's family, but the written evidence of the client, that can stop resuscitation efforts. Resuscitation is not discontinued when rescuers or nurses are exhausted.

13. Answer: d
RATIONALE: The nurse positions their body over the hands to deliver a straight-down motion with each compression. The hands remain in contact with the client's chest when the elbows are locked to avoid rocking back and forth over the client. Nurses either interlock their fingers or extend them after placing the heel of one hand over the other hand on the client's chest for compression. Nurses do not use two fingers when giving chest compression; they use two fingers on an infant's chest when performing the Heimlich maneuver.

14. Answer: b
RATIONALE: If the emergency involves someone within a health care agency, the initial rescuer can alert the resuscitation team by notifying the switchboard operator that assistance is needed and by giving the location of the emergency. When there is a client with cardiac arrest, nurses should not waste time alerting the lead physician or describing the client's age and physical appearance. A nurse can assess the client quickly, but dialing 911 for help when the client is in the health care facility itself would be incorrect.

SECTION IV: REVIEWING WHAT YOU HAVE LEARNED

Activity H

1. Circulation
2. 100

Activity I

1. False. The jaw-thrust maneuver is an alternative method for opening the airway.

Activity J

1. Code
2. Recovery position

Activity K

1. d   **2.** e   **3.** a   **4.** c   **5.** b

Activity L

	Mouth-to-Mouth Breathing	**Mouth-to-Stoma Breathing**
Technique	The nurse uses their mouth or a pocket mask to cover the client's mouth and to blow air into the client	The nurse seals their mouth over the laryngeal stoma of a client with a laryngectomy
Sealing of the Client's Nose	Required	Not required if the tracheostomy tube has an inflated cuff

Activity M

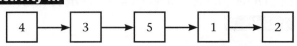

Activity N

1. Signs of an airway obstruction include the following:
   • Coughing and gagging while eating
   • Audibly wheezing
   • Persistently attempting to clear the throat
   • Making hoarse or wet vocal sounds
   • Resisting efforts to be fed
   • Being unable to speak
   • Holding the throat
   • Being unable to breathe
   • Exhibiting cyanosis
2. Basic cardiopulmonary resuscitation cannot be interrupted for more than 7 seconds except when
   • There is a pulse and the client resumes breathing.
   • The rescuer becomes exhausted.
   • The client's condition deteriorates despite resuscitation.
   • Written evidence shows that resuscitation is contrary to the client's wishes.
   • Advanced cardiac life support measures such as defibrillation are administered.

SECTION V: APPLYING YOUR KNOWLEDGE

Activity O

1. This device theoretically reduces the potential for acquiring infectious diseases like hepatitis and AIDS.
2. The monitor would display an error message if the client's skin were diaphoretic or extremely hairy.

Activity P

1. The nurse should give a series of five subdiaphragmatic thrusts to increase intrathoracic pressure equivalent to a cough. They should use the head-tilt and chin-lift maneuver along with continuous administration of upward thrusts to open the client's airway. The nurse should avoid blind finger sweeps unless the object in the airway is visible.
2. If the child is unconscious, the nurse should perform cardiopulmonary resuscitation rather than continue with the Heimlich maneuvers. Chest compression in cardiopulmonary resuscitation creates enough pressure in an unconscious client to eject a foreign body from the airway.

Activity Q

There are no definite answers to this activity. Students may choose to discuss their thoughts with peers or instructors.

SECTION VI: GETTING READY FOR NCLEX

Activity R

1. **Answer: c**
   RATIONALE: When performing CPR on a 6-year-old child, the triage nurse should place the heel of the hand at the center of the chest between the nipples. When performing CPR for infants, the nurse applies compression in the midline one finger width below the nipples and compresses using two thumbs with the hands encircling the chest. When performing CPR for an adult or anyone who has reached puberty, the nurse provides one breath every 5 to 6 seconds at the rate of 10 to 12 per minute.

2. **Answer: d**
   RATIONALE: The nurse should monitor SpO_2 with a pulse oximeter at all times to measure the amount of oxygen bound to hemoglobin. Room air has the equivalent of 21% oxygen, so someone with impaired ventilation would need a device, such as a simple mask or Venturi mask, which delivers more than room air. The client should remain in Fowler position to facilitate chest expansion by lowering abdominal organs away from the diaphragm. The nurse should replace the Venturi mask with a non-rebreather mask if SpO_2 is less than 80% for more than 10 minutes, not equal to 90%.

CHAPTER 38

SECTION I: ASSESSING YOUR UNDERSTANDING

Activity A

1. Terminal
2. Hospice
3. Hydration
4. Death
5. Sucking
6. Autopsy
7. Coroner
8. Mortician
9. Dysfunctional
10. Paranormal

Activity B

1. The figure shows a nurse caring for a client in a home care setup.
2. The nurse caring for a client in a home care setup may help to coordinate community services, secure home equipment, and arrange for nursing visits. The nurse also assesses the toll of client care on

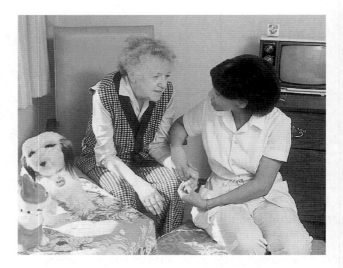

the primary caregiver. The nurse encourages the caregiver to identify relatives or friends who will volunteer relief time with the client.

Activity C

1. d   **2.** c   **3.** e   **4.** a   **5.** b

Activity D

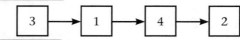

$$3 \rightarrow 1 \rightarrow 4 \rightarrow 2$$

Activity E

1. "Dying with dignity" is the process by which the nurse cares for dying clients with respect, no matter what their emotional, physical, or cognitive state.
2. Brain death is a condition in which there is an irreversible loss of function of the whole brain, including the brain stem.
3. A death certificate is a legal document attesting that the person named on the form has been found dead; it also indicates the presumptive cause of the person's death.
4. Postmortem care or care of the body after death involves cleaning and preparing the body to enhance its appearance during viewing at the funeral home, ensuring proper identification, and releasing the body to mortuary personnel.
5. Multiple organ failure is a condition in which two or more organ systems gradually cease to function. When the supply of oxygen begins to fall below levels required to sustain life, cells (followed by tissues and organs) begin to deteriorate. The cardiovascular, pulmonary, hepatic, and renal systems are most vulnerable to failure.

SECTION II: APPLYING YOUR KNOWLEDGE

Activity F

1. The client refuses to believe that the diagnosis is correct. They assume that the test results are wrong. The client is in the first stage of dying, or denial, where they are using a psychological defense mechanism by refusing to believe the diagnosis.

2. To help the dying person cope, the nurse should
   - Accept the client's behavior to demonstrate respect for the client's individuality.
   - Provide opportunities for the client to express their feelings and help them to meet their individual needs.
   - Try to understand the client's feeling to reinforce their uniqueness.
   - Communicate with the client in a language that encourages them to choose the topic or manner of response.

SECTION III: PRACTICING FOR NCLEX

Activity G

1. **Answer: d**
   RATIONALE: The statement, "Yes, I'm dying ..." indicates that the client is in the depression stage of dying as the client realizes that death will come sooner or later. A client in the denial stage says, "How can it be? No, I'm not dying." A client in the second stage of dying, or anger stage, feels victimized and may say, "What have I done wrong? Why me?" A client in the third stage of dying, or bargaining stage, tries to convince a higher power or God why they need to live and may say, "I have just finished college ...."

2. **Answer: b**
   RATIONALE: Informing the client about preparing an advance directive indicates respect for the rights of the dying client. The nurse should not ask the client to avoid talking about death, avoid any reference to spirituality when talking to the client, or tell the client that the results of the diagnostic test look good. The Bill of Rights for a dying client states that the client has a right to express feelings about death in their own way. It allows the dying client to discuss spiritual experiences and to have their questions answered honestly.

3. **Answer: a**
   RATIONALE: When caring for a dying client, it is often helpful if the nurse offers to secure spiritual counseling, if requested, for the client and family members. Nurses who dedicate their careers to end-of-life care must be compassionate and caring and must understand their own feelings regarding life and death. The client should not be restricted from talking about death with family members; otherwise, it may make the client feel unimportant and unwanted by the family. The nurse must not force or try to convince the client or family members to

agree to organ donation because some people feel very vulnerable and they should not feel pressured into consenting to organ or tissue donation.

4. **Answers: a, b, c**
   RATIONALE: When providing home care for a terminally ill client, the nurse coordinates community services, arranges for home nursing visits, and secures home equipment. Round-the-clock nursing care is provided to clients in a residential care facility. The nurse need not suggest transferring the client to residential care because that is the decision of the client and the client's family.

5. **Answer: a**
   RATIONALE: The nurse should assist the client to a lateral position to prevent choking and aspiration. The client's position should be changed at least every 2 hours to promote comfort and circulation, and to prevent skin breakdown. Asking the client to sleep without a pillow, assisting the client to a semi-Fowler position, and ensuring that the client is supine at all times are not relevant interventions for this client because they do not help to prevent choking or aspiration.

6. **Answer: d**
   RATIONALE: Although the client may designate himself as an organ donor, the nurse should discuss the possibility of organ donation with the client's next of kin. The client's eyes must not be harvested for donation without informing and obtaining permission from the client's surviving spouse or next of kin. A pack of ice is usually placed over the client's eyes to preserve their integrity when harvesting them for donation. It is important to discuss the matter of organ or tissue donation with the client's family members and clarify their doubts regarding organ donation.

7. **Answer: a**
   RATIONALE: Clients who are certified by the physician as having less than 6 months to live are eligible for hospice care. If a client survives beyond 6 months, they continue to receive care as long as the physician certifies that the client continues to meet hospice criteria. Clients with difficult behavior or clients requiring palliative care are not necessarily placed in hospice care. Clients who cannot live independently are referred to residential care.

8. **Answer: d**
   RATIONALE: A client placed under hospice care is provided care by a multidisciplinary team of professionals and volunteers who support the care given by the family. A client in residential care receives subacute or intermediate care in nursing homes or long-term care facilities that provide round-the-clock nursing care for clients who cannot live independently. A client in acute care is provided with sophisticated technology and labor-intensive treatment.

9. **Answer: c**
   RATIONALE: The nurse should provide wrapped ice cubes to be sucked. Sucking is one of the last reflexes to disappear as death approaches. A client with difficulty in swallowing should not be offered water or beverages even in small amounts because it could lead to aspiration followed by pneumonia. Eventually, the client may need intravenous fluids to maintain adequate fluid volume.

10. **Answer: b**
    RATIONALE: Nausea and vomiting may result in inadequate consumption of food. The client may have little interest in eating or may find the effort too exhausting. Poor nutrition leads to weakness, infection, and complications like pressure sores.

11. **Answer: c**
    RATIONALE: The lips of the client may need periodic lubrication as a result of dryness from administration of oxygen. Administration of intravenous fluids and total parenteral nutrition may be required if the client is unable to swallow or suck. Frequent mouth care may be necessary for clients who cannot swallow or expectorate.

12. **Answer: d**
    RATIONALE: The goal of non-narcotic analgesics is to provide relief from pain. Non-narcotic analgesics are not administered to dull consciousness, suppress respirations, or inhibit the client's ability to communicate.

13. **Answers: a, c, d**
    RATIONALE: The nurse should identify him or herself by name, title, and location to provide a more personal communication. The nurse should ask for the family member by name to ensure that the right person is provided with the information. The nurse should speak calmly and explain that the client's condition is deteriorating, rather than tell the family that all answers to queries will be given at the facility because this explains the purpose of the call. The nurse should not ask the family to rush to the facility without explaining the reason because it could lead to confusion or contribute to a traffic accident.

14. **Answers: a, d, e**
    RATIONALE: Irreversible brain death is considered to be present if there is a flat encephalogram for at least 10 minutes, complete absence of central and deep tendon reflexes, and no spontaneous respiration after being disconnected from a ventilator. Unreceptiveness or unresponsiveness to intense (not moderately) painful stimuli confirms brain death. $PaCO_2$ greater than or equal to, not less than, 60 mm Hg after preoxygenation with 100% oxygen indicates brain death.

15. **Answer: a**
    RATIONALE: The nurse should clean secretions and drainage from the skin to ensure delivery of a hygienic body. The dentures need not be removed from the mouth because they maintain the natural contour of the face. The nurse should remove all hairpins or clips to prevent accidental trauma to the client's face. A small rolled towel is placed beneath the chin of the client to close the mouth, not under the head.

SECTION IV: REVIEWING WHAT YOU HAVE LEARNED

Activity H

1. Bargaining
2. Residential
3. Suck

Activity I

1. False. Constipation may be a common consequence of continuous narcotic analgesia.
2. False. Autopsy is the examination of human organs and tissues to determine a cause of death.

Activity J

1. Coroner
2. Death certificate
3. Multiple organ failure

Activity K

1. d   **2.** c   **3.** a   **4.** b

Activity L

	Home Care	**Residential Care**
Role of Nurses	Nurses help to coordinate community services, secure home equipment, arrange for this type of care, and implement interventions in the home.	Nurses perform physical, emotional, spiritual, and social care within the nursing homes or long-term care facilities where they work.
Delivery of Care	Depends on spouse, family members, and nurses who care for the home-bound client	Shared by personnel such as nurses, certified nursing assistants, dietitians, physical and occupational therapists, and activity coordinators who are employed as staff of round-the-clock health care facilities

Activity M

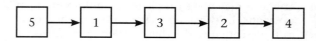

5 → 1 → 3 → 2 → 4

Activity N

1. A terminal illness is a condition from which recovery is beyond reasonable expectation and death is an expected outcome in the near future.
2. Hospice care can be terminated when the client withdraws for any reason to receive treatment not covered in the hospice plan of care or when the client no longer meets the Medicare criteria for hospice care.

SECTION V: APPLYING YOUR KNOWLEDGE

Activity O

1. Urine and stool left in contact with the skin contribute to skin breakdown and may produce foul odors.
2. Mouth breathing and oxygen administration may cause the lips to become excessively dry and uncomfortable.
3. The local health department uses death certificates for information about mortality statistics to identify trends, needs, and problems in the fields of health and medicine.

Activity P

1. Nurses can help clients by providing emotional support and by honoring each client's choices concerning terminal care. Facilitating the client's directives helps to maintain personal dignity and locus of control. If the dying client wants an opportunity to express feelings, a nurse can act as a nonjudgmental listener. Nurses can also provide emotional support to dying clients by acknowledging them as unique and worthwhile. The process in which the nurse cares for a client with respect, regardless of the client's emotional, physical, or cognitive state, is called dying with dignity.
2. Nursing diagnoses for this dying client and their family may include the following:
   - Acute or chronic pain
   - Fear
   - Spiritual distress
   - Social isolation
   - Ineffective role performance
   - Interrupted family processes
   - Ineffective coping
   - Disabled family coping
   - Decisional conflict
   - Hopelessness
   - Powerlessness
   - Dysfunctional grieving
   - Anticipatory grieving
   - Caregiver role strain
   - Death anxiety
   - Chronic sorrow
3.
   a. The nurse should ensure that this client receives appropriate nutrition because poor nutrition could lead to weakness, infection, and other complications such as pressure sores. Client dignity is related largely to personal appearance. A nurse should strive to keep the client clean, well groomed, and free of unpleasant odors. Suctioning helps to remove mucus and saliva that the client cannot swallow or expectorate. A lateral position keeps the mouth and throat free of accumulating secretions.
   b. If the client's swallowing reflexes remain intact, the nurse should offer water and other beverages frequently. As swallowing becomes impaired, the client is at risk for aspiration, followed by pneumonia. Sucking is one of the last reflexes to disappear as death approaches. The nurse should provide a moist cloth or wrapped ice cubes for the client to suck. Eventually, the client may also need intravenous fluids.

Activity Q

There are no definite answers to this activity. Students may choose to discuss their thoughts with peers or instructors.

SECTION VI: GETTING READY FOR NCLEX

Activity R

1. **Answer: a**
   RATIONALE: The client should have full access to information about their health, including positive laboratory findings. The nurse should ask the client to identify goals that could be accomplished in 6 to 12 months, not 24 months because focusing on short-term goals offers an alternative to the defeat the client may feel over not accomplishing unrealistic long-term goals. Encouraging alternative forms of treatment is a form of offering false hope that the client's condition could be improved or that traditional medical care has been incomplete. The nurse could encourage the client to think about memories and previously established goals if this activity helps or inspires the client. Assisting clients with such reminiscence may motivate them toward similar future-related activities.
2. **Answers: a, c, d**
   RATIONALE: Obtaining supplies for cleaning and wrapping the body promotes organization and makes the body presentable before cremation. Contacting individuals involved in organ procurement following death promotes timely harvesting of tissues that do not require oxygenation prior to harvesting, such as skin, corneas, and bones. Asking for the approximate arrival time of the mortuary personnel facilitates efficient time management. The nurse should disconnect all medical equipment attached to the client and apply disposable pads between the legs and under the buttocks to absorb urine and stool.

3. **Answer: a, b, e**

   RATIONALE: Some clients make their wishes to donate organs and tissues known to their family, physician, or nursing personnel prior to dying. Even if the client has a document indicating a desire for organ donation, the next of kin must also provide consent. An organ procurement coordinator is the appropriate resource person to obtain permission, contact an organ procurement agency, and facilitate the removal and preservation of organs by personnel trained for this purpose. Neither a mortician nor a pathologist is involved in organ procurement.

4. **Answer: a**

   RATIONALE: Failure of the client's brain and heart would lead to stupor, cold, and mottled skin. Internal bleeding, jaundice, nausea, vomiting, anuria, oliguria, and itching skin are symptoms of liver and kidney failure. Acute pancreatitis, peptic ulcer, and dyspepsia are symptoms of pancreas and stomach failure. Absent bowel sounds, abdominal distension, blood in the urine, and bowel obstruction are symptoms of intestinal and bladder dysfunction.